Of Diabetic Mothers and Their Babies

Of Diabetic Mothers and Their Babies

An Examination of the Impact of Maternal Diabetes on Offspring Prenatal Development and Survival

Harold Kalter

Professor Emeritus
Department of Pediatrics
College of Medicine
University of Cincinnati
and
Children's Hospital Research Foundation
Children's Hospital Medical Center
Cincinnati, Ohio, USA

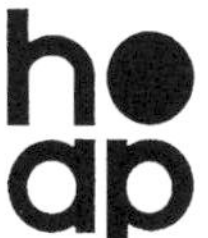

harwood academic publishers

Australia • Canada • France • Germany • India •
Japan • Luxembourg • Malaysia • The Netherlands •
Russia • Singapore • Switzerland

Amsteldijk 166
1st Floor
1079 LH Amsterdam
The Netherlands

Cover design by John F. Kalter.

Kalter, Harold
Of diabetic mother and their babies : an examination of the impact of maternal diabetes on offspring prenatal development and survival
1. Diabetes in pregnancy 2. Abnormalities, Human 3. Fetal death
4. Perinatal death
I. Title
618.3

ISBN 90–5702–617–1

To my wife—

Bella Briansky Kalter

CONTENTS

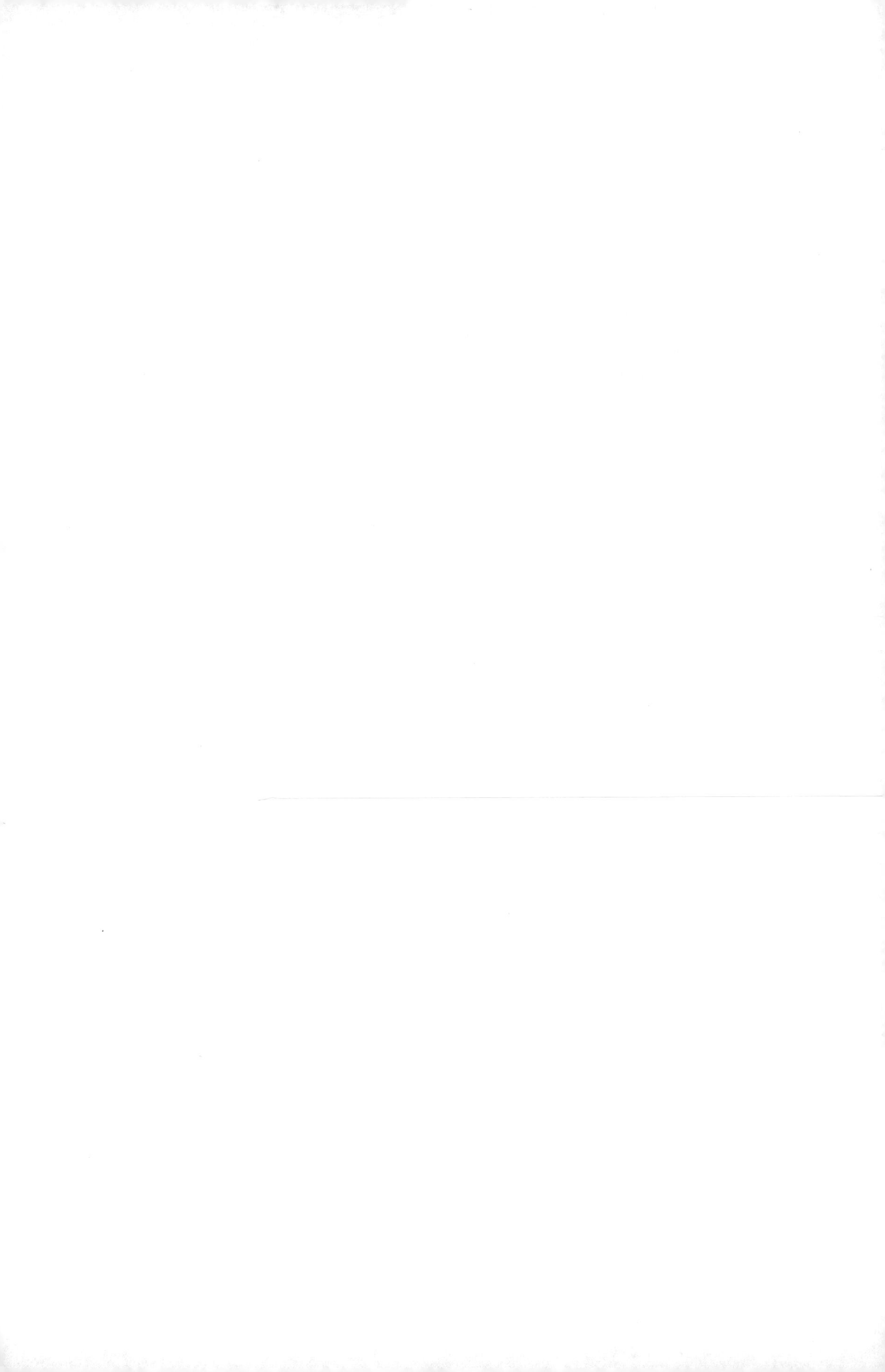

PREFACE

A happy chance led to my interest in the subject of this book. The impetus arose in early 1982 when I received an invitation from an editor of the *New England Journal of Medicine* to write an article reviewing the causes, as then known, of congenital malformations in human beings. Since just about 20 years previously I had been the junior co-author of a review of the same subject in the same journal, I thought it proper, and even more, that it would lead to a far stronger statement, to have Dr. Josef Warkany, the senior partner of that first article, join me in the second. Warkany and *NEJM* agreed to this, and many months later, months of close reading and rereading of medical journals, months of pondering and writing, the manuscript was submitted; and then we were told it was too long! We in turn told the editor it would be impossible to shorten, and finally an unconventional solution (for the journal) was found: it would be published in two parts, on successive weeks (Kalter and Warkany 1983).

The invitation was completely unexpected. The earlier review had mostly been the work of Warkany, a clinician and giant in the world of both clinical and experimental teratology, and so it was obvious why he had been asked to do the writing. He in turn asked me to help him with it because in a previous shared writing I had shown some facility in examining reports of past studies and reflecting on their significance, and perhaps also because we had worked harmoniously on that task (Kalter and Warkany 1959).

As for me, however, by training and long practice I was an experimental teratologist, and following the 1961 review had written nothing more than one or two brief general articles on the subject of human malformations. But my interests were broad, and I had kept myself well informed about new findings and thinking about such matters, partly because of my responsibilities during the years I was editor of the journal *Teratology*, and later as editor of *Issues and Reviews in Teratology,* and also because I did not regard animal teratology entirely as an end in itself, but mainly as a means of illuminating outstanding questions in human teratology. Nevertheless, why I had been chosen for this new review was and remains a mystery. As it turned out, it was a fortunate stroke.

The review that emerged rested on a critical examination and analysis of the vast biomedical literature of the previous several decades that dealt with congenital malformations and their causes. These primary sources—reports of isolated cases, hospital series, epidemiological surveys, vital statistics—contained many suspicions and allegations, as well as, of course, some clear evidence, about the origins of these abnormalities in babies. Our job was to consider this body of evidence in order to come to a balanced assessment of what we considered the understanding of the causes and likelihood of preventing congenital malformations to be at the time.

These causes earlier had been broadly categorized into genic, chromosomal, environmental, and complex or unknown. About the first two generally there was little theoretical that was not settled, and about the last there was little that was clear. Thus, it was the environmental origins of congenital malformations that got most of our attention, especially since that was where the controversies lay. By that year, a considerable number of environmental agents—physical, nutritional, pharmacological, and so on—had been found, under the forced conditions of experimentation, to be teratogenic in animals. But just a mere handful had been unquestionably identified as having caused prenatal damage in human beings. These were ionizing radiation, already identified by the 1920s; the rubella virus, its "story" appearing in 1941; later some other infectious agents; and afterward several therapeutic substances, environmental contaminants, and a small number of others—cytotoxic, anticoagulant, and anticonvulsant drugs, thalidomide, organic mercury, and others.

In addition, some noninfectious maternal illnesses were known sometimes to cause or be associated with fetal maldevelopment, most of them seldom-occurring, however, except for one—insulin-dependent diabetes mellitus. Year after year, studies had added to and made ever more firmly entrenched the belief that women with this condition had children with a severalfold increase in the frequency of serious congenital malformations.

This disease was intriguing for several reasons, which led me to a fuller reading and thinking about it and its harmful effects on prenatal life. First, insulin-dependent diabetes occurs rather commonly in younger women, and their pregnancies being prevalent present a frequent prenatal menace. Next, in distinction to most other human teratogens, which, upon discovery of their harmfulness, had been eliminated or counteracted, this diabetes had all the hallmarks of being a permanent fixture of the human constitution, or at least one that would be around for a long time to come. And last it seemed to me, while writing and after completing the 1983 review, that the basis of the long-held belief in its teratogenicity had not been closely scrutinized, and needed further looking into.

Professional people concerned with pregnancy in diabetic women from the beginning were mainly obstetricians and diabetologists, and their predominant facility was with pregnant and parturient women. Most major congenital malformations are obvious and need no special training to recognize, but nevertheless require judgment to be put into perspective. I am not a physician, but through experience considered myself knowledgeable in the complexities of judging problems regarding fetal maldevelopment.

I thus set out to immerse myself in and become acquainted with what I soon discovered to be the voluminous and wide-flung literature on the subject of pregnancy in diabetic women, beginning with pertinent writings in the decades before the discovery of insulin in 1921. Years of reading and summarizing the frequently opaque and fragmentary reports, of organizing and collating my notes, of making preliminary jottings, led to putting down on "paper," the definitive end-product, here presented.

INTRODUCTION

Long-accepted beliefs are difficult to challenge. They are embedded in everyday thinking and guide everyday behavior. What are accepted as scientific and medical truths may not be quite as fiercely adhered to and as vigorously championed as religious or even political philosophies are. But long-held scientific orthodoxies can be zealously defended, and anyone foolhardy enough to oppose them must be sure of his position and ready to withstand the fire of denunciation.

The "truth" challenged in these pages is the almost universal belief that the babies of women with insulin-dependent diabetes are congenitally malformed more often than babies of nondiabetic women are. Except for a very small number of dissenters speaking out over the years, who were hardly noticed and unfortunately never took great pains to defend their position, an army of clinicians and experimentalists has asserted that there was no question about it, the babies of diabetic women are at increased risk of prenatal madevelopment.

How did this idea get started and what perpetuated it? Before the 1950s, the major question diabetologists and obstetricians caring for pregnant diabetic patients asked was why so many of the babies of such women were born dead or died soon afterward. Malformations did not seem to be part of the answer, so were relegated to the background. Only as the large death rate of these children began to subside, with improving control of the maternal disease, did the malformations in the surviving babies become conspicuous and more of a problem.

It was largely to a survey of births to diabetic women in a Danish hospital, whose account appeared in 1964, that the credit must go for explicitly formulating the idea that diabetes is teratogenic, that is, causes congenital malformations. This was supported by a summarization a few years later of outcomes of pregnancies to diabetic women in hospitals in several countries.

Congenital malformations are not rare. In the overall population, malformations of a serious nature are present in about 3% of newborn children. The usual finding has been that in the births of diabetic women this frequency is about doubled or even trebled. This has been unquestioningly taken for granted, as seen in reports of case studies, diabetes clinic surveys, public health findings, epidemiological inquiries, where it is almost obligatory to begin by stating that diabetes causes malformations, backed by the same often repeated percentages.

From this unquestioned position, a number of extensions implicitly followed. First was the attribution to maternal diabetes of another harmful pregnancy outcome, spontaneous abortion, which it has also been asserted is increased in such instances. Second came programs designed to counteract the increased malformation rate by vigorous management of the disease early in the pregnancies of diabetic women, which, it seemed, achieved their purpose. It can be imagined how many professional reputations had been erected upon these edifices.

Nevertheless, one is permitted to be skeptical. My skepticism arose from a survey I made of the then-known causes of human congenital malformations, which left me feeling that there was more to the story of the teratogenicity of diabetes than the certainty then held about it. How, though, does one verify or refute such impressions about deeply entrenched beliefs? Only by a critical reading of the corpus of the medical literature pertinent to the outcome of pregnancy in diabetic women. The following pages are devoted to outlining and analyzing the facts, as far as they go, in these works. The approach taken has been to examine progress made over the years in the effort to deal with the difficulties besetting the conceptuses of such women regarding viability and development, perinatal death, spontaneous abortion, and congenital malformation.

This "paper trail," has led into many corners, but always to a consistent end. While the record shows a remarkable improvement in newborn mortality, with a constant decrease decade by decade, almost reaching the level in the general population, it has also strengthened the doubt initially felt in the accepted view of diabetes teratogenicity. Exhaustive scrutiny of various sources of information—hospital and clinical surveys, in the aggregate as well as one by one, case histories pertaining to a particular developmental anomaly, studies of indigenous groups, population studies of various individual malformations, reports of the newest spontaneous abortion results, and so on—has led to but one conclusion. Congenital malformations do not occur, and probably have never occurred, more frequently in the children of diabetic women than of nondiabetic women.

How, then, account for the belief that the opposite was the case? Parts are easy to explain. It stems first and most obviously from the loose meaning given to the term malformation by physicians and others caring for diabetic women, even when such a matter was given some thought. It surely needs no words to emphasize how necessary it is for investigators to speak and write the same language always and everywhere. A consensus, such as that taken by workers in clinical teratology and allied fields concerned with abnormal prenatal development, is not only imperative for comparability, it lends intellectual precision to inquiry.

The second error was that the theory was founded on faulty soil. Patients who are cared for in hospital diabetes departments and specialized diabetes clinics are very often unrepresentative of the severity of the disease in all diabetic women in the whole population. And, once founded, its root sank deep. Even so, it might still have led to more judicious perspective had proper control groups been included as a foil against the cases, but controls, of any sort, were rarely employed. Numerous studies of one type or another followed down the years, all with hardly any exception concluding that diabetes was associated with or caused malformations. Many cases of malformed children of diabetic women were published, each fortifying the belief in the prenatal harmfulness of diabetes, with their authors seldom if ever stopping to consider the possibility that these were a biased selection of instances, with no confirmatory value at all. Thus the belief began, grew with each repetition of the belief as fact, until it became dogma.

The task undertaken here was not to overthrow the dogma, but to examine the written record, from as far back as necessary, and to come to an opinion as to its credibility. If it leads to nothing more than a reopening of the question, and an objective reexamination of the facts, it will have been beneficial. It is presented with much trepidation, since its conclusions largely fly in the face of the conventional beliefs about the effects of maternal diabetes on the unborn. But I believe that the case made out will be convincing and will lead to a rethinking about the subject.

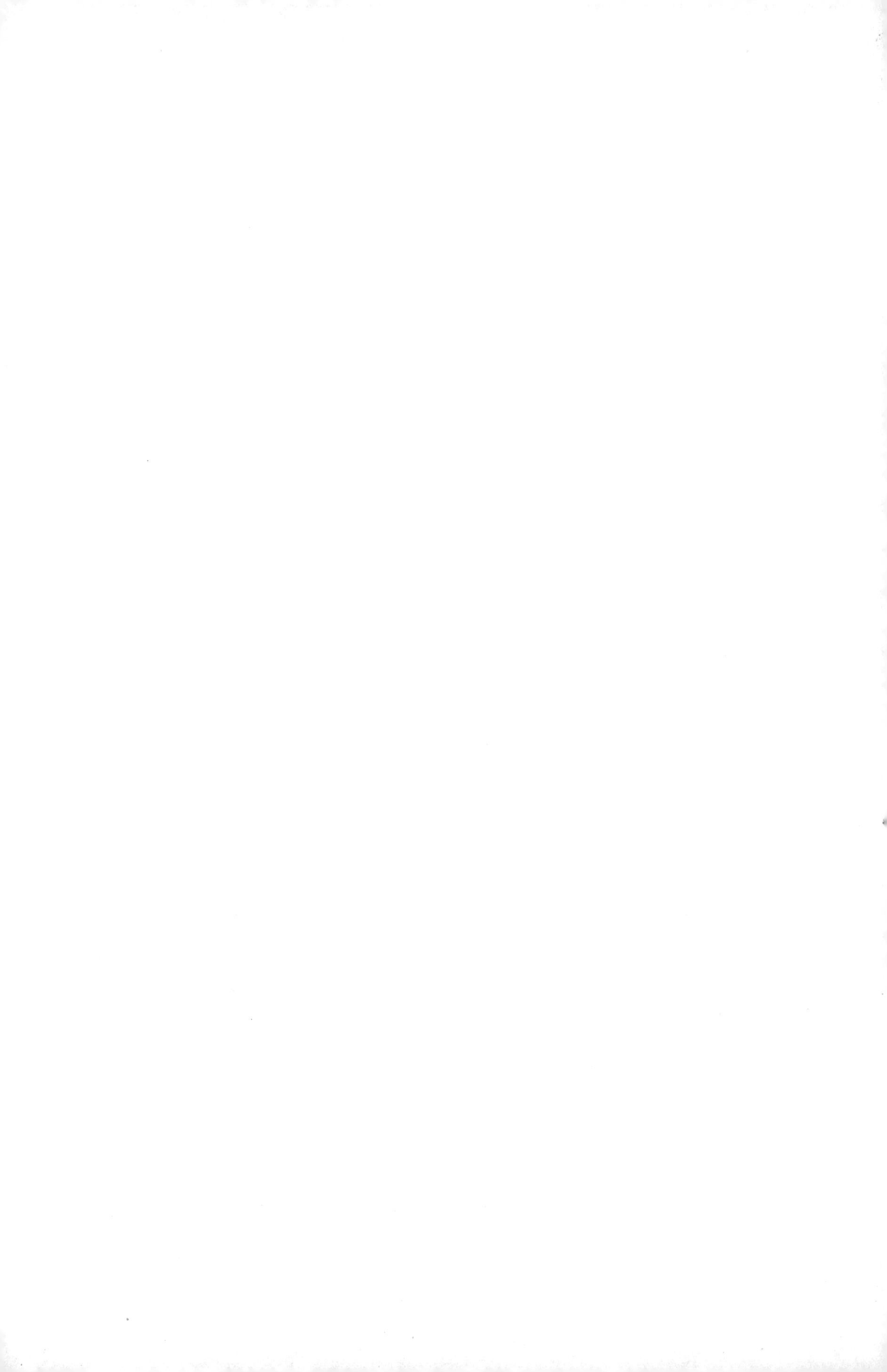

1

THE FRAMEWORK OF DIABETES

The history of medicine, like the chronicle of humankind, is burdened with the unexpected. Major advances, at first offering new-found health, have sometimes been followed by the unanticipated, disclosing new disease. There is no more telling instance of this human endeavor than is seen in the annals of diabetes mellitus, a record of a proud human success in whose train there came disappointment: disappointment that following the apparent conquest of an old lethal disease there soon emerged tough new questions, which upon being addressed in turn gave rise to still others to be overcome.

Diabetes stands at the conjunction of these medical challenges: the unforeseen and unwelcome outcome and the obstinate residuum. Both are glaringly presented by our subjects: the embryos, fetuses, and newborn infants of pregnant diabetic women. The focus, therefore, is on the hazards faced by these subjects. And so, we begin at the end—the death of the newborn.

EARLY CHILDHOOD DEATH

One of the most trumpeted social and medical achievements of many parts of the present-day world is the great reduction during the 20th century in the rate of deaths of children under the age of 1 year, by which, it is customarily acknowledged, the standard of civilization of nations is judged. Years ago it was declared that "infant mortality is the most sensitive index we possess of social welfare..." (Newsholme 1910), and this criterion still reigns (Shapiro et al. 1965, Yankauer 1990). Extraordinary progress thus shines forth from the fact that in the 80 years or so following the end of the First World War the mortality rate of children under 1 year of age in the US underwent a precipitous decline of greater than 90%, from 99.9 to 7.0 per 1000 children born alive (U.S. Bureau of the Census 1960, National Center for Health Statistics 1997). And the same great achievement was realized in many countries in Europe and elsewhere (Chase 1967, Thomson and Barron 1983).

The most perilous time of the first year of life is the first month, especially the first week, since it is in these few days that most of the weak and damaged liveborn babies are eliminated. These earliest deaths, plus those occurring in about the last 2–3 months of pregnancy, are of particular interest here. Together, these are known as "perinatal deaths." Their rate has also greatly declined, falling, for example, in the United States from 32.5 per 1000 total births in 1950 to 10.7 per 1000 in 1985 (Powell-Griner 1986, 1989).

These remarkable reductions were largely brought about by the virtual elimination of many public health problems and pediatric diseases. But advancement has been most uneven. At the same time that many widespread and fearsome causes of neonatal and infant death, disability, and distress—hygienic, nutritional, infectious—were being so impressively ameliorated, barely any headway was made with others.

THE PLACE OF DIABETES IN THIS PICTURE

Diabetes mellitus exemplifies various facets of this uneven progress. The almost insurmountable barrier to reproduction in women that was caused by diabetes was rapidly removed by the discovery of insulin in 1921 and its wide availability soon afterward (Wrenshall et al. 1962, Bliss 1982). However, a new misgiving soon emerged. As the number of pregnancies in diabetic women increased, it became apparent that many offspring did not survive for long. This problem diminished in time, because some of the reasons for the high perinatal mortality were discovered and continually more successfully dealt with.

But this achievement created new puzzles. With the ongoing decline in offspring death a progressive shift took place in the composition of the causes of the deaths that continued to occur; and as some receded in importance the remainder became ever more prominent. What soon became, and what is now, the chief cause of offspring death (in all pregnancies, in fact, not only diabetic ones) were congenital malformations. And with malformations proving to be largely unpreventable they soon demanded and received increasing attention—especially as suspicion arose that maternal diabetes itself may be teratogenic, that is, causes malformations.

At the same time, however, because of a number of methodological and conceptual shortcomings, the teratogenicity of diabetes was sometimes questioned. For example, the definition of congenital malformations that was followed by many diabetologists and obstetricians, and even pediatricians, was not always acceptable, clear, or uniform. The means of diagnosing these malformations was often unstated or variable; ascertainment of pregnant diabetic patients (ie, avenues of their selection for study and treatment) was usually biased; no or poorly matched controls were often obtained for comparison, and so on (Rubin and Murphy 1958, Wilson 1960, Simpson 1978, Mills 1982). These strictures make it necessary to discuss definition and classification of congenital malformations, diabetes in pregnancy, and other things that require clarifying.

Unanswered Questions

Diabetes mellitus, when present in women during pregnancy, profoundly affects the viability, growth, and development of the unborn. This work traces the ideas and practices that have evolved over the years in the attempt to manage these difficulties. It will consider some of the most perplexing of the imperfectly answered or still unanswered of these problems, most prominent among them: whether diabetes causes or is associated with spontaneous abortion, retarded prenatal growth, and congenital malformations, whether such malformations form distinctive patterns, the relation between malformation and perinatal death, whether the form and degree of the maternal disease or presymptomatic stages of the disease are related to these phenomena, and whether control of the disease from before or early in pregnancy can lessen these hazards.

For reasons that will be seen in later text, the decade of the 1950s can be taken as a watershed in the ongoing progress in the treatment and outcome of diabetic pregnancy. Therefore the events and problems encountered in dealing with these pregnancies before insulin was discovered in 1921 and those emerging in the years between this momentous discovery and the 1950s will introduce the subject.

SOURCES OF MATERIAL

The primary sources of information this monograph has depended on are reports of pregnancies of diabetic women by hospital-based physicians in North America (ie, America north of Mexico in conformity with the usage of many geographers (Weber 1992 and thenceforth described as America) and many European countries. The publications were identified by exhaustive search of the medical literature, using the *Quarterly Cumulative Index Medicus* for the older sources, Internet biomedical sources, and, most usefully, the lists of citations in the reports themselves, whose trail led to older and older relevant publications. In addition to these sources, also consulted were publications that reported multicenter, population-based, epidemiologic surveys and public health matters with respect to children born of diabetic women.

The advantages of hospital-based reports compared with vital statistics and other such data are that they are more complete than the commonly underreported data of public records (Greb et al. 1987, Snell et al. 1992). Hospital reports usually provide detailed descriptions of individual pregnancies and offspring and are more informative than public record statistics, especially since they are sometimes supported by autopsy records.

But hospital-based studies also have their drawbacks, requiring cautious interpretation of their observations. An important problem is that the composition of the patients served by different hospitals can vary in many ways, demographically, medically, and so on, and some of these variations are without doubt relevant to this work. For example, some hospitals were primary care facilities, whose patients were drawn from their immediate communities and for the most part were unselected and representative of the disease picture of population of that community. Other reports, on the other hand, emanated from larger hospitals or specialized medical facilities many of whose patients were referred for one reason or another from other hospitals in the area or from outside the area altogether. These patients, being a selected group, were no doubt unrepresentative of the spectrum of the illness present in the entire population. How must the facts from such different sources be handled? The problems of procedure and interpretation that these and other uncertainties presented will be considered in the text that follows.

DEFINITION OF DIABETES IN PREGNANCY

A full discussion of the definition of diabetes in pregnancy is presented later in this text. Here only a few general remarks are necessary. "Diabetes mellitus" is the umbrella term given to what probably covers several etiologically distinct disorders of carbohydrate metabolism. These disorders are characterized by chronic hyperglycemia, in which there is usually an absolute or relative deficiency or reduced secretion or impaired action of insulin. The disease usually occurs in one of two forms: type 1 (insulin-dependent), mostly of juvenile onset, and type 2 (noninsulin-dependent), mostly of adult onset (National Diabetes Data Group 1979, World Health Organization 1985).

In addition to the general classification of diabetes, there are two broad categories of diabetes in pregnancy: diabetes that antedates pregnancy, often called *pregestational diabetes*, and diabetes that occurs during pregnancy, called *gestational diabetes*. Pregestational diabetes is usually insulin-dependent, and gestational diabetes is usually insulin-independent, but either form may vary in insulin dependence. The unfavorable outcomes of diabetic pregnancy that we are mainly concerned with—spontaneous abortion, fetal and neonatal death, and congenital malformation—are associated almost entirely with insulin-dependent pregestational diabetes.

For the sake of developing the historical picture, gestational diabetes and related topics also have much space devoted to them. However, the main focus is on the pregestational variety of diabetes. Hence, when the unqualified term "diabetes" is used, it refers to that variety.

2

THE EARLY YEARS

Diabetes mellitus is an old disease, mentioned in ancient and medieval sources (Barach 1928), although the validity of even that has been disputed (Bottazzo 1993). Nevertheless, the first recorded instance of pregnancy in a woman with diabetes was described only about 175 years ago—barely yesterday (Bennewitz 1824). Even this instance of diabetic pregnancy does not represent the type of diabetes with which we are mainly concerned here. Hadden (1989) and Hadden and Hillebrand (1989) provided many details of this case in translation from the original Latin.

The story of diabetes in pregnancy had its real beginnings even more recently—toward the end of the 19th century. The reason for its much-delayed appearance in human history is simple: before the modern age, diabetes in pregnancy could have happened only rarely, if at all, because diabetic women of reproductive age virtually did not exist. In other words, the form of the disease that occurs at younger ages—the kind this work focuses on—was responsible for a high toll of infertility and early death.

INFERTILITY

Before Insulin

Before the discovery of insulin, the diabetic woman, a rarity in herself, probably never became pregnant for a number of interconnected reasons—physical impairment, profound sterility, reduced life expectancy. Physicians at that time had never or seldom seen pregnancies in the diabetic (Bouchardat 1875, Lecorché 1885, Taylor, 1899).

This dearth, in contrast, for example, with "nephritic and other complications," was commented on by Duncan (1882), who noted in confirming this fact that in a then-current "great work on pregnancy" there was reference to but one such event, Bennewitz's observation, mentioned above. He himself learned of this want when, apparently in response to his inquiries, he heard from colleagues that they had possibly seen only three such occurrences in 157 women with the disease. This revelation apparently led him to collect and publish all such cases he had personal or other knowledge of, which amounted to 22 pregnancies in 15 diabetic women.[1] Sagely commenting on the ways of the world, he prophesied that "attention being called to the subject, the list of cases will soon be augmented."

The sparsity of such pregnancies continued to be (if I may be permitted the oxymoron) amply confirmed. Lecorché (1885) recorded only 7 pregnancies at most in 114 diabetics (a majority of whom, however, developed the disease postmenopausally, that is, were apparently afflicted with a late-appearing form of the disease not at the center of the present discussion). In diabetic women of reproductive age, von Noorden (1910) noted 22 pregnancies in 427 cases; Wiener (1924) in New York City one in 20 women in 6 years; Gray and Feemster (1926) in St. Louis 5 pregnancies in 4 of 205 women; Walker (1928), searching the records of the Middlesex Hospital back for 23 years, found 1 case in 10,000 maternity records; and Skipper (1933) 4 in 190 married diabetics up to age 46 during 1893–1922 in the London Hospital. Various other writers also reported a marked but perhaps not as profound scarcity in the years leading up to the 1920s (cited by Lambie 1926, Eastman 1946).

An early partial explanation of this great infertility was supplied by Graefe (1898), who often found uterine atrophy in diabetic women. Herman (1902) added another element: "When the disease occurs in woman of child-bearing age it usually, when advanced, suppresses menstruation and produces atrophy of the uterus." Parisot (1911) then discovered the basis for the amenorrhea to be lack of ovarian follicles. The structural and functional changes in the reproductive system of diabetic women that possibly underlie infertility were summarized by Lambie (1926). Even 20 years later, not much more was understood of the underlying bases of infertility in diabetic women—no doubt because the problem by then had all but disappeared (Eastman 1946).

After Insulin

Insulin came into widespread use for the general diabetic patient very soon after its discovery in 1921 (Banting and Best 1923, Bliss 1982). But it seems nevertheless that the infertility of women with the disease only slowly abated, since few reports during the earliest years of the insulin era tell of pregnant diabetic women being treated with this new panacea (Reveno 1923, Graham 1924; see Wilder and Parsons 1928). Even in medical centers, they continued to be uncommon; for example, at the Mayo Clinic, only 11 pregnancies were seen in 285 diabetic women of childbearing years (Parsons et al 1926). From these few early cases, just a meager hint of the capability of the new ingredient to promote the fertility of diabetic women could be guessed. But Parsons and colleagues (1926) presciently commented, "The incidence of pregnancy in diabetic women is likely to rise." And in fact, reports had already begun to appear regarding the efficacy of insulin in restoring menstruation and supporting pregnancy (Lambie 1926).

Within a brief period of time, the situation markedly brightened. From 1923 to 1927 worldwide, at least 55 pregnancies of diabetic women had already been recorded in the medical literature (Wilder and Parsons 1928). In the London Hospital

1 A reading of Duncan's paper disclosed a discrepancy with the numbers cited above, given in his summary on p. 283: I counted 29 pregnancies in 16 diabetic women. Duncan apparently omited seven pregnancies of one woman, but gave no reason for this; her symptoms were somewhat erratic from pregnancy to pregnancy, but no more so it seems than was so in the other cases.

alone, 27 of 177 (15%) diabetic women admitted to the hospital from 1923 to 1931 were pregnant (Skipper 1933). Thus, Wilder and Parsons (1928) triumphantly concluded that with insulin administration and an adequate diet, diabetic women achieved regular and normal menstruation, ovulation apparently proceeded normally, and pregnancy was no longer the oddity it had been not long before.

The improved fertility, and its continuation, can be gauged by the records of the prevalence of diabetic pregnancy. Happily, many publications, especially older ones, reported the number of diabetic pregnancies that occurred within a specific period among all the births in given hospitals. These figures are to be interpreted cautiously, however, because records of series collected over various extended and overlapping periods may conceal or distort happenings during the years surveyed. Figures from different hospitals are sometimes discrepant, possibly reflecting widely different sources of patients—referral clinics and centers (although not all were clearly designated as such) or general hospitals serving overall communities. Reporting only viable pregnancies and omitting spontaneous and elective abortions and ectopic pregnancies would account for underestimates. And unspecified inclusion of gestational diabetic pregnancies, that is, diabetes with onset or discovery during pregnancy, would have tended to raise the estimate.

Even these possible misrepresentations could not obscure the signs that the prevalence of diabetic pregnancy greatly and continually increased in these early years (Kramer 1936, Koller 1953) and continued to improve in later ones. From the 1920s through the mid-1990s, it increased in America from a mean of 1.9 to 5.8, and in Europe from 2.0 to 4.3 per 1000 overall population pregnancies. The last figures are close to the rate found in some 55,000 randomly selected pregnancies (Chung and Myrianthopoulos 1975b) in the National Institutes of Health Collaborative Perinatal Study (Berendes and Weiss, 1970; Niswander and Gordon, 1972).

This clearly established that considerable fertility had been restored to diabetic women. It is to be noted, however, that even in the earliest period the prevalence varied greatly from center to center, ranging from 0.5 to 5.2, the latter in a referral center (Randall 1974) Why did the rate continue to rise? Why has a plateau possibly not yet been reached? Is it because the fertility of diabetic women had not, and perhaps has still not achieved its peak? Is it because the prevalence of diabetes is still increasing in women of reproductive age; because ascertainment biases may have given an increasingly erroneous picture? The following may answer some of these questions.

The prevalence of diabetic pregnancy in the US in the earliest period was close to that of diabetes in American women of reproductive age during that era (Spiegelman and Marks, 1946), and the most recent US rate mentioned was approximately equal to that of such women during a later period (Marks et al, 1971). These facts indicate that the fertility of diabetic women was soon virtually restored and has remained so. With restoration accomplished, the prevalence of diabetic pregnancy attained at a given time would therefore depend on the overall prevalence of diabetes in women of reproductive age. It may thus be the widespread increasing prevalence of early-onset diabetes, which it is feared may not yet have culminated, that at least partly accounts for the growth in the rate of diabetic pregnancy (Levy-Marchal and Czernichow 1992).

Other factors perhaps were also at work. The upward trend may have been partly due to the disproportionate number of diabetic pregnancies reported by referral centers, as indicated in some earlier cases (Randall 1947). Countervailing the trend, despite the above-mentioned correlation, is the likelihood that the fertility of diabetic women of reproductive age was still impaired. This is supported by the significantly delayed age of menarche frequently found in diabetic women, especially those with diabetes of juvenile origin (Bergqvist 1954, Post and White 1958, Knorre 1969, Sutherland et al 1981, Kjaer et al 1989a,b) and by recent reports that the total prevalence in the US of known or previously diagnosed diabetes in women ages 20–44 years is much greater than the mean rate of their pregnancies (Drury and Powell 1987, Harris et al 1987).

MATERNAL MORTALITY

Before Insulin

In the years before the discovery of insulin, high maternal death rates were commonplace in the small minority of diabetic women who became pregnant. Of the paltry 16 cases of pregnant diabetic women collected by Duncan (1882), 10 (62%) died soon after or within 1 year of delivery. Nearly the same disastrous percentages were noted in later tallies. Eshner (1907) found 54% maternal mortality in 35 diabetic women (including some mentioned by Duncan), Williams (1909) found 25% in 34 women whose disease predated pregnancy, and Joslin (1915) found 23%, excluding one suicide. Lambie (1926) cited percentages of 25–55% reported in publications from 1894 to 1908.

These records may have referred to less serious instances of the disease; Parsons et al (1926) doubted that the "patients with severe diabetes ever survived pregnancy in the pre-insulin era." Outcomes in the years just preceding the discovery of insulin seem to reflect a possible improvement in this dismal record, but the prospect of any substantial further improvement no doubt remained unimaginable.

After Insulin

In the first years of the insulin era, the diabetic maternal death rate still far exceeded that which was occurring generally. The literature of the period recorded 6 deaths in 73 pregnancies (8.2%) (Bowen and Heilbrun 1932). Great improvements noted later were said to compare favorably with contemporary nondiabetic rates (Kyle 1963). A compilation of reports of diabetic pregnancies surveyed in the 1940s and 1950s shows that maternal diabetic death had declined to about 1.0–1.2% in the US and Europe. This was still about 10 times the overall rate in white women in the US during these years (US Bureau of the Census 1960). Although the decline continued in subsequent years, the gap had not yet closed, since even the low US mortality rate was still about 10 times that in the general population (National Center for Health Statistics 1992).

The diabetic maternal mortality rate has presumably declined even further in recent years, as it has for pregnancies generally (Morbidity and Mortality Weekly Report 1991), if judging only from its infrequent mention in publications of the last several years. However, this may be deceptive, and only if such information is explicitly presented will it be possible to judge the pace of progress.

3

SPONTANEOUS ABORTION

The discovery of insulin brought a rapid, almost miraculous alleviation of the two perils of young diabetic women: infertility and pregnancy-related death. But the newly discovered pancreatic factor had disappointingly little or no impact on another hazard of diabetic pregnancy, perinatal mortality, death of offspring in the late weeks of pregnancy and the first weeks of postnatal life (discussed in Chapter 4). This chapter considers a subject still controversial at this late date, spontaneous abortion.

EARLY STUDIES

Spontaneous abortion (SAB)[2] is a major source of reproductive failure. During the early insulin years, however, with the numerous other problems that caretakers had to contend with, the fact of whether or not SAB was increased in women with diabetic pregnancy was never a major controversy, although there were differences of opinion about it. For example, Skipper (1933) said that SAB was "relatively uncommon," and White (1935) called it "relatively...frequent." Others conceded that at best "the effect is small" (Moss and Mulholland 1951). Perhaps such differences of opinion could be expected of a medical generation that for the most part was not well aware of how prevalent SAB ordinarily is. Today, it is well established that abortions in "recognized pregnancies" (ie, pregnancies that women are aware of because of a missed menstrual period) are extraordinarily common, ranging from 10% to 25% and higher, depending on the type of study and analysis. The lowest estimates (about 10%) were obtained by prospective surveys of already pregnant women in clinical settings (Jansen 1982). Other estimates were 12–15% by retrospective investigations of pregnancy histories (Warburton and

2 Spontaneous abortion (SAB) is defined as death of the conceptus before reaching the age of viability (ie, the time when the conceptus is able to sustain independent life). Until relatively recently, fetal viability was commonly held to be 28 weeks of pregnancy after the first day of the last menstrual period (Hook and Porter 1980). Hence, unelected conceptus death before this time was called "spontaneous abortion." However, over the years medical technology has succeeded in keeping many younger and younger fetuses alive (Anon, 1988b), which has required that the age of viability be redefined. Thus, the widely accepted age of viability has been lowered and at present SAB is generally defined as death of conceptuses before 20 weeks of pregnancy.

Fraser 1964, Naylor 1974, Leridon 1976) and 15–25% by the use of life-table probability procedures (Harlap et al. 1980, Leridon 1977).

Great attention has been given to understanding the etiology and epidemiology of SAB. Although much of the blame has been implicitly directed at the high incidence of chromosomal and morphologic abnormalities that abortuses possess, the connection between these aberrations and embryonic death is very little understood. Nor are the reasons well understood for the many deaths not accompanied by such abnormalities (Boué et al. 1975, Porter and Hook 1980, Carr 1983, Roman and Stevenson 1983, Rushton 1985).

The frequency of SAB reported in the earliest studies of diabetic pregnancies and even in some later ones was at times relatively low, probably at least partly because patients were commonly first seen by physicians at later stages of pregnancy. This limitation and the methodologic inadequacies of many reports, which result in underestimates of abortion, have been pointed out and must be taken seriously (Combs and Kitzmiller 1991).

One such factor was taken into account, in a survey of articles published over a 30-year span that mentioned SAB in diabetic pregnancy, by separately considering pregnancies that were probably observed from a relatively early stage (Kalter 1987). In these the mean SAB frequency was 12.7%, approximating the level usually found in studies of general clinic populations (Warburton and Fraser 1964, Naylor 1974, Leridon 1976). This led to the conclusion that diabetes is probably not associated with an excess occurrence of SAB in recognized pregnancy (though some authors interpreted the facts most bizarrely—Guivarc'h-Levêque et al. 1992).

The survey also revealed that the diabetic SAB rate was substantially the same before and after 1960. This is noteworthy, since it is in marked contrast with the dramatic plunge during the past 30 years or so in the perinatal mortality rate in diabetic pregnancy, a contrast that points to these two entities having different etiologies.

To some investigators, it seemed logical that embryonic death and perinatal death should have common roots, that if diabetes were associated with high levels of death in late pregnancy, it should also be so in early pregnancy. Thus, it was difficult for some authors to relinquish the plausible notion that diabetes was associated with or caused an increased frequency of SAB, as may be judged by their evident reluctance to discard it, despite the contrary or equivocal examples (Eastman 1946).

RECENT STUDIES

Introduction

The evidence provided by the review mentioned previously (Kalter 1987), that SAB is not increased in diabetic pregnancy, has been challenged. Therefore, reexamination is necessary but must be prefaced by recalling that attempts to determine the prevalence of SAB have frequently been hindered by various confusing and intruding factors common to retrospective inquiries, including the following:

faulty maternal recall; biases in the detection of SAB (both of which can result in overestimates as well as underestimates); vagaries of the sampling method; innumerable demographic, social, and biologic confounding variables; and possible environmental influences.

These aspects were fully discussed elsewhere (Harlap et al. 1980, Kalter 1987), but it must be mentioned that they have seldom been given a moment's thought in studies alleging that SAB was increased in diabetic pregnancy.

Reproductive loss also occurs before pregnancy recognition, from the time of conception onward. It is obvious that to discover its full extent, pregnancies must be monitored from soon after conception. The newer evidence that diabetes may be associated with excess abortions came from studies of women enrolled in diabetes programs from early in pregnancy and, when possible, even from before pregnancy had begun. This allowed surveillance over the entire or almost the entire gestation period, including the crucial earliest weeks.

Researchers had probably always realized that the total amount of reproductive loss could only be uncovered if pregnancies were closely monitored from these initial days. But the finding that various harmful reproductive outcomes were associated with high levels of maternal blood glucose early in pregnancy was the stimulus for reexamining the subject from a new perspective (Leslie et al. 1978, Miller et al. 1981, Ylinen et al. 1981a, 1981b). Following this new track would have problematical if it had not been for the discovery of a new blood component, glycosylated hemoglobin, and the newly developed methods of measuring it.

Glycosylated Hemoglobin

The diagnosis and management of diabetes depend on knowledge of the concentration of glucose in blood. Traditionally, measurement was made by a number of nonphysiological means, especially the oral glucose tolerance test. But several difficulties with this procedure—reproducibility, individual variability, confounding factors, and others—made even its periodic use an unreliable measure of previous glycemic state and indicator of effectiveness of metabolic control on pregnancy outcome (O'Sullivan and Mahan 1966, Hadden 1975).

For the first of these purposes especially, a more valid guide is the level of glycosylated hemoglobin, HbA_1. This minor component of hemoglobin A consists of three main fractions, HbA_{1a}, HbA_{1b}, and HbA_{1c}, which compose about 4–5% of the total hemoglobin in normal persons. HbA_{1c} is the largest component, making up about 3% of hemoglobin (Mayer and Freedman 1983). The importance of HbA_1 to the care of diabetics consists in its being the product of a nonenzymatic, nearly irreversible process by which glucose is bound to hemoglobin (Bunn et al. 1976). Considering the protracted life span of red blood cells, HbA_1 represents an average of the plasma glucose concentration during the several weeks preceding its determination.

The relevance of these facts to studies of diabetes became apparent with the discovery that the level of HbA_{1c} may be two to three times greater in diabetic or glucose-intolerant persons than in normal individuals (Rahbar et al. 1968, Rabhar 1969). Moreover, its concentration in diabetics was proportional to the blood glucose level and fell with metabolic management of the disease (Koenig et al. 1976a,b).

Table 3.1 Relation Between Frequency of First-Trimester Spontaneous Abortion (SAB) and Glycosylated Hemoglobin (HbA_1) Levels in Early Stages of Pregnancies of Diabetic Women

Reference	HbA_1/SAB Relation			
	HbA_1 % or SD	SAB/pregs	% SAB	*P*
Wright et al. 1983	≤ 11.5	3/33	9.1	
	> 11.5	7/25	28.0	> .05
	≤ 6 SD	6/45	13.3	
	> 6 SD	4/13	30.8	> .05
	Total	10/58	17.2	
Sheridan-Pereira et al. 1983[a]	≤ 11.0	3/21	14.3	
	> 11.0	2/14	14.3	
	Total	5/35	14.3	
Key et al. 1987	≤ 11.4	3/48	6.2	
	11.5–13.4	8/15	53.3	
	≥ 13.5	11/20	55.0	< .01
	Total	22/83	26.5[b]	
Stubbs et al. 1987[a, c]	4[d]	27/230	11.7	
Mills et al. 1988[a]	≤ 1 SD	10/108	9.2	
	2–5 SD	34/223	15.2	
	> 5 SD	12/42	28.6	> .05
	Total	56/373	15.0	
	Control	69/432	16.0	
Dicker et al. 1988	Group 1	5/59	8.5	
	Group 2	10/35	28.6	
	Total	15/94	16.0	< .01
Lucas et al. 1989	≤ 11.0	14/85	16.5	
	> 11.0	4/20	20.0	> .05
	Total	18/105	17.1[e, f]	
Greene et al. 1989	≤ 9.0 SD	21/198	10.6	
	9.0–12.0 SD	15/61	24.6	
	≥ 12.1 SD	16/44	36.4	> 0.5
	Total	52/303	17.2[g]	
Hanson et al. 1990[h]	≤ 10.1	30/490	6.1	
	> 10.1	11/42	26.2	< .01
	Total	41/532	7.7	
	Control	16/222	7.2	
Gestation and diabetes in France 1991	–	23/249	9.2	
Rosenn et al. 1991[i]	< .8.0 SD	1/12	8.3	
	8.0–11.9 SD	25/144	17.4	
	≥ 12.0 SD	26/59	44.1	< .01
	Total	52/215	24.2	
Diabetes Control Group 1986	Group 1	18/135	13.3	
	Group 2	14/135	10.4	> .05

Table 3.1 ***continued***

Reference	HbA1/SAB Relation			
	HbA_1 % or SD	SAB/pregs	% SAB	*P*
Mello et al. 1997	< .8	3/32	9.4	
	8–10	8/26	30.8	
	> 10	4/12	33.3	> .05
	Total	15/70	21.4	

[a] Multicenter study.
[b] Individual outcomes for insulin-dependent and insulin-requiring women not stated.
[c] Personal communication.
[d] Statistically insignificant difference in mean HbA_1 level between 27 women spontaneously aborting and those not doing so.
[e] Missed or spontaneous abortion.
[f] Diabetes type unspecified.
[g] 51/302 (16.9%) if an electively aborted Turner syndrome were omitted.
[h] Nationwide multihospital study.
[i] Including data from Miodovnik et al. 1985.

The association of diabetic status early in pregnancy, as gauged by this new technique, with frequency of SAB is considered in this chapter and with that of congenital malformations in a later one.

Glycosylated Hemoglobin and SAB

Studies began in the early 1980s regarding the relation of maternal blood glucose level in early diabetic pregnancy, as denoted by HbA_1, to the incidence of SAB. Up to the time of this writing, 13 such studies have been reported. Their primary purpose was to manage the diabetic state from early in pregnancy to mitigate as fully as possible its harmful outcomes. Perhaps because of this, the studies did not all give satisfactory attention to recording data regarding predictors of SAB risk, such as diabetes severity and duration, the proportion of subjects that were primigravid, previous SAB history, and maternal age. But information given in most reports permitted comparisons of one sort or another of the following: between diabetic aborters and nonaborters; between aborters with glycosylated hemoglobin levels above and below the group mean; between intensively and conventionally managed women; between attenders and non-attenders of preconception clinics; between insulin-dependent and non–insulin-dependent pregnancies; and where controls were included, between diabetic and nondiabetic pregnancies. In only 2 of the 13 studies was a statistically significant difference in a risk factor found in one group compared with the other.

The information was obtained by a literature search of the Internet (Ovid) from the time of the first reports in the early 1980s through May 1998, augmented by citations in the identified articles (Table 3.1). The studies varied geographically in the span of years surveyed and in the number of patients sampled, but were similar in almost all other ways: all studies were prospective; patients were seen consecutively and were predominantly pregestational insulin-dependent diabetics;

all were metabolically managed from before or soon after conception; all or almost all patients were white; all pregnancies were confirmed; SAB was defined fairly uniformly; standard methods of measuring glycosylated hemglobin were used.

DETAILED ANALYSES

Birmingham Study

Wright et al. (1983) were among the first to consider this relation. They reported 10 (17.2%) early SAB in 58 consecutive pregnancies of 52 insulin-dependent women, almost all of whom visited the clinic before 14 weeks of gestation. The glycosylated hemoglobin levels at the first visit ranged from 6.1% to 16.9% (mean 11.5%). For comparison, in a group of normal women the range in the early weeks of pregnancy was 4.1–6.9% with a mean of 5.6% (Morris et al. 1985).

The results can be interpreted in several ways. The range was not very different in women who went on to abort than in those who did not abort. The SAB incidence was greater in women with levels above the group mean than in those below the mean, but the increase was far from statistically significant. The same was true whether the comparison was based on the group mean or the standard deviation above the mean for nondiabetic women (see Table 3.1). These findings nevertheless were taken by the authors to indicate that prolonged poor glycemic control in the weeks preceding pregnancy or early in the first trimester contributed to the likelihood of SAB or at least early SAB. This raises the question of whether an overall 17.2% SAB is excessive for women enrolled in a study before week 14 of pregnancy.

Cincinnati Study

A series of studies of the relation between early poor glycemic control and SAB was made by investigators at a center engaged in a long-term study of juvenile diabetics. The initial publication, establishing a baseline, reported 39 (29.5%) SAB in 132 clinically apparent insulin-dependent diabetic pregnancies occurring from June 1978 through January 1983 (Miodovnik et al. 1984). The relevance of the dates will soon become apparent. The abortion frequency at first was associated with diabetes severity, but not confirmed later (Miodovnik et al. 1985).

The first communication in the series considering the association of SAB and glycemic status reported 116 pregnancies in 75 insulin-dependent diabetic women in1978–1984. Of these SAB, 26 (22.4%) occurred before 20 weeks of gestation (Miodovnik et al. 1985). Glycosylated hemoglobin was measured at the first visit to the clinic at about 8–9 weeks of gestation—by one method in patients studied in 1978 to 1980 and by another method in those studied in 1981 to 1984. In both groups, women who aborted had a mean glycosylated hemoglobin level that was significantly greater than those who did not (11.2 versus 9.9% and 12.8 versus 11.3%, respectively). In both groups combined, women with levels of 12% or higher had a significantly increased risk of SAB, although within each group the increase was not statistically significant.

The overall means of the two groups were not presented (and no control group was included), so it is not clear why 12% was chosen as the cutoff for making the comparison. Later, an increased rate was found only in women with glycosylated hemoglobin levels of 13% and higher (Rosenn et al. 1994). Wright et al. (1983) used 11% for comparison because that was approximately the mean in the study group; if 12% had been chosen, no significant difference in incidence of SAB in those above and below that level would have been found.

Methodological imponderables confused the findings. Different methods of measuring glycosylated hemoglobin were used during different periods of the study; how comparable their results were was not discussed. Matters of ascertainment and representativeness of the diabetic women constituting the study groups were also left unclarified, especially with respect to race and ethnicity, factors related to abortion incidence (Porter and Hook 1980) and which were of relevance, since the study emanated from a municipal hospital largely serving an inner-city population.

One further point is appropriate, since it casts doubt even on the reported frequency of abortion. Without explanation, pregnancies that continued beyond 20 weeks and resulted in a congenitally malformed infant were excluded from the study population. The number of these instances was not stated, but obviously their exclusion inflated the calculated incidence of SAB.

A later study noted a slightly lower incidence of SAB (18 of 84, 21.4%) than previously (Miodovnik et al. 1986). It seems the longer this project was carried on, the lower the frequency became. In the next study, reported over a slightly longer period of time, it was 17.7% in 96 pregnancies (Mimouni et al. 1987); not very different from the 12–15% seen in recognized pregnancies (Hertz-Picciotto and Samuels 1988).

The latest study of the series (Rosenn et al. 1994) had the same sort of difficulties as those just mentioned. For example, 16.7% of the patients were nonwhite, whereas census data for 1990 for the city of Cincinnati show that 39.9% of the population were nonwhite (Anon 1990). The study sample thus contained an unrepresentative racial and ethnic distribution, perhaps indicating that many of the patients were self-selected or referred to this municipal, medical school–affiliated hospital because of special problems. These possible biases were not recognized, nor was the fact that blacks, who were not considered separately and comprised 37.8% of the 1990 Cincinnati population (Anon 1990), have an excess of SAB (Harlap et al. 1979).

A Multicenter Study

A painstaking multicenter inquiry had contradictory and puzzling results (Mills et al. 1988a). Insulin-dependent diabetic and control women were enrolled before or within 21 days of conception, with accurate dating of pregnancy ensured by various means. Periodic evaluation thereafter included glycosylated hemoglobin measurement during the first trimester. The SAB rates up to 20 weeks of gestation (excluding ectopic pregnancies and hydatidiform moles) were virtually identical in the diabetic and control women (15.7 and 16.2%, respectively). Despite this, the mean glycosylated hemoglobin level was significantly higher in the diabetic women than in the controls, and the SAB frequency was significantly increased in diabetic women with glycosylated hemoglobin levels greater than their mean, but was not increased in the controls. What these facts may mean is that elevated blood glucose level, by itself, does not pose a risk for miscarriage. Further examples are seen below regarding the inadequacy of elevated maternal blood glucose level to explain apparent deleterious pregnancy outcome.

How is it to be explained that the diabetic women did not have an increased overall SAB rate? Several possibilities were proposed: the fairly well-controlled diabetes produced a lower than normal abortion rate; the diabetic group was a "motivated health-conscious" one; there were other undetected selection biases. However, none of these was believed to be acceptable.

The results left various questions unanswered. Because a large number of subjects was thought necessary to conduct the study, the data were collected at five centers over an unspecified time period. The diabetic subjects were gathered by "public appeals as well as through the medical system," and the control group was collected mostly by solicitations through mailings to various sources (Mills et al. 1983). Matching of the groups was successful, since the control women closely resembled the diabetic women in characteristics indicative of abortion risk. Still, the fact that the study combined information from centers varying in ascertainment, composition, and care of patients must be a caution against uncritical acceptance of even its few positive findings.

It must also be noted that the SAB frequency in the diabetic and control women, though they were monitored from the time of conception or very soon after, was much smaller than has usually been the case in studies of pregnancy loss with such early initiation of monitoring (see eg, Hertz-Picciotto et al. 1988, Wilcox et al. 1988, Steer et al. 1989, Modvig et al. 1990). This was also true of other studies discussed in this section with early initiation of pregnancy monitoring.

Other Studies

Several other studies were carried out and, together with those just discussed, are summarized in Table 3.1. All dealt with pregnancies first seen before 14 to 16 weeks of gestation, at times from as early as conception to about 10 weeks. Some investigators compared the glycosylated hemoglobin level in aborters with nonaborters; others compared the percentage of aborters and nonaborters above and below the mean for the entire group.

Controls were included in only two studies; in both, the incidence of SAB in the diabetic women was no different from that in the controls (Mills et al. 1988a, Hanson et al. 1990). A positive finding in the Mills study—that the glycosylated hemoglobin level was elevated in the diabetic but not the control aborters—was not assessed in the Hanson study.

In two studies the SAB frequency was not different in women with glycemic levels above the mean than in those with levels below it (Sheridan-Pereira et al. 1983, Lucas et al. 1989), whereas in six others it was significantly greater in the former than the latter (Wright et al. 1983, Miodovnik et al. 1985, Key et al. 1987, Greene et al. 1989, Hanson et al. 1990, Mello et al. 1997). But in these six the frequency was similar to that in overall early monitored pregnancies—which seems to mean that low glycemic levels are protective, an explanation already rejected. The results in two studies that monitored women from before conception were contradictory: in one the frequency was lower than in cases not seen that early (Dicker et al. 1988), whereas in the other it was no lower than in the controls (Mills et al. 1988a).

DOSE RESPONSE

The findings can also be considered from the "dose-response" standpoint. The toxicological principle that the magnitude of an adverse effect is proportional to that of the cause is subject to the proviso that there exists a threshold of reaction—an amount of the causal factor below which an effect cannot be demonstrated. If it is postulated that glycohemoglobin levels beyond the normal cause an increase in SAB and if it is assumed that this adverse effect is subject to the toxicological principle enunciated, it follows that beyond the threshold the degree of the response must be proportional to the glycohemoglobin level.

In six instances, it was possible to examine the data in this manner. Two found evidence of a dose-response relation (Rosenn et al. 1984, Key et al. 1987). In the latter, however, heterogeneity of the sample of women monitored confused the outcome (see Table 3.1). In the four others, the evidence was negative, since the frequencies of SAB associated with the two greatest levels were not significantly different from each other (see Table 3.1) (Wright et al. 1983, Mills et al. 1988a, Greene et al. 1989, Mello et al. 1997). This may be explained by some sort of "saturation" principle, but nevertheless the account is again equivocal.

PATHOLOGY OF ABORTUSES

It is surprising that the numerous studies declaring that the SAB frequency is significantly increased in diabetic pregnancy were accompanied, it seems, by only two investigations into the pathology of abortuses from such women. One would have thought it important to look into the basis of the supposed increase, and determine whether it might have been due, for example, to augmentation of the fetal malformation frequency, especially as this was thought to be significantly raised in diabetic pregnancy.

Both pathology studies had negative results. Mills et al.(1988a) reported equal numbers of grossly malformed diabetic and control embryos, and Bendon et al. (1990) found no histological feature different in abortion tissue from diabetic than nondiabetic women. An amniocentesis study determined that chromosome abnormality, not surprisingly, was not increased in fetuses of diabetic women (Henriques et al. 1991). A study, only remotely relevant here, of pregnant rats made diabetic by streptozotocin administration, found a decreased inner cell mass in blastocysts (Pampfer et al. 1990).

CONCLUSION

No consistent evidence was presented by the studies discussed above of an increased SAB frequency in diabetic pregnancy, a conclusion also arrived at, though reluctantly, in a review of the epidemiology of SAB in insulin dependent diabetic women (Smith 1989); nor that SAB frequency is correlated with glycosylated hemoglobin levels in early pregnancy. In most of these studies, however, as in others below, no group of matched nondiabetic pregnant women was included. And only when such a group is as closely and thoroughly monitored and from as early in pregnancy as the index women can a totally convincing answer be forthcoming to these questions. The biases in retrospective as well as even in various forms of prospective studies of the complex phenomenon of SAB have been extensively discussed (eg, Leridon 1977), and ignoring these possible biases can only depreciate the value of a work.

The most vexing difficulty remains explaining the extraordinarily low SAB frequencies in the diabetic women with glycohemoglobin levels below the means for their groups, frequencies far smaller than those generally occurring in pregnancies monitored from soon after their onset. At the same time it must be recognized that SAB frequencies in the women with far greater than normal glycohemoglobin levels fell within the range previously often found in overall early-monitored pregnancies, and thus can hardly be considered unusual.

Essentially, the question is whether the apparently increased rate of SAB found in some studies can be attributed to the maternal disease state or to monitoring the pregnancies from (or almost from) their onset. The danger of neglecting the latter possibility was clearly pointed out by an overall population study that found a total prevalence of spontaneous postimplantation abortion of 31% (Wilcox et al. 1988).

4

PERINATAL MORTALITY

The most tenacious and demanding difficulty presented by the pregnancies of diabetic women has been the excessive rate of fetal and neonatal death. The disastrously high rate that prevailed in the pre-insulin era continued with little improvement for some time after the advent of this miraculous agent. In fact, the situation appeared to worsen because insulin enabled many more diabetic women to become pregnant and an increased number of offspring deaths to occur. Although with the passing years, the rate of these deaths has steadily and appreciably diminished, today, decades later, offspring death is still several times greater in diabetic pregnancies than in the overall population. This chapter examines the general nature and attributes of perinatal mortality and then discusses it in depth.

DEFINITION AND CLASSIFICATION

Offspring death in the last months of pregnancy and the earliest postnatal weeks—stillbirth and neonatal death—is known collectively as "perinatal mortality" (PNM). Its number is considerable and has constituted and continues to constitute a large percentage of offspring mortality from midpregnancy to 1 year of age.

In the 1920s, when such deaths in the general population were beginning to gain increased attention, it was understood that the times that they occurred had to be marked off because only by setting widely agreed-upon limits could comparisons of various sorts be made and progress charted. To assign this specification, it was also necessary to draw another boundary. This followed appreciation that death in the first several months of pregnancy—spontaneous abortion—had to be differentiated from death in the later months because of the cardinal difference between abortuses and stillbirths—the potential of the fetuses surviving to the later months of pregnancy for extrauterine life.

This made it necessary to consider when fetal viability begins. A legal decree regarding this question, based on experience, was promulgated in Great Britain in 1926 with the passage of an act that formally defined stillbirths as intrauterine deaths occurring after 28 weeks of pregnancy (Armstrong 1986). The modifications in this definition that were made over time will be noted elsewhere in the text.

About the same time, it was recognized that stillbirths and the earliest occurring neonatal deaths, which are sometimes difficult to differentiate (Golding 1987), share the prenatal origin of many of their causes and that these causes largely differ from the causes of death of older infants, which are mostly of postnatal origin (Crosse and Mackintosh 1954; Bakketeig et al. 1984). Hence, stillbirth and early neonatal death came to be considered a unit and given a separate term—perinatal mortality (Peller 1923, 1948). This in turn necessitated that early neonatal deaths be kept separate from later ones, with the earlier deaths arbitrarily defined as those occurring in the first week and the later ones as those occurring in the second through fourth weeks after birth. These terms have been useful and enabled clinicians, public health workers, demographers, statisticians, and other investigators, when they accepted these standards, to compare their findings and draw inferences.

Although the definition of early neonatal death has continued to be accepted, that of stillbirth has undergone a change. The original delimitation—28 weeks of gestation—underwent a major shift as over time medical advances made possible the survival of more prematurely born infants, resulting in a reduction of the age of viability and a modification in its definition. Thus, today the widely accepted definition of stillbirth is intrauterine death after 20–22 weeks of pregnancy. This, in turn, led to stillbirth, like neonatal death, becoming subdivided into early and late, the former from 20 through 28 weeks and the latter after 28 weeks of gestation.

These time delineations are based on the method of dating gestational length from the first day of the last menstrual period before pregnancy, the practice of most clinicians and epidemiologists, which is convenient but biologically incorrect. To obtain the more correct figure, 14 days—the usual time between the first day of the last menstrual period and presumed conception—must be subtracted from the conventionally derived age.

Nevertheless, this rule also has its caveats, since whatever starting time is used there is bound to be uncertainty of the gestational length (Berg 1991, Moore 1991, Saunders and Paterson 1991). To attempt to obviate this difficulty and "to eliminate national idiosyncracies," the World Health Organization (1977) recommended that the weight of the conceptus be used as the preferred criterion of stillbirth classification. Thus (at least for international comparison), the minimum of 1000 g or certain fetal measurements (equivalent to 28 weeks of gestation) continues to be taken as indicating the attainment of viability. Details of this topic can be found in a lucid exposition by Hook and Porter (1980).

INFLUENCES ON DIABETIC PERINATAL MORTALITY

The rate of stillbirth and neonatal death in developed countries has steadily decreased ever since statistics for these phenomena were first widely gathered 70 or more years ago (eg, U.S. Bureau of the Census 1961, Chase 1967, Hirst et al. 1968, Powell-Griner 1986, 1989). In addition to strictly medical reasons for this great shift in global demography, a great assortment of situations and conditions exists—biological, demographic, social, cultural, environmental—which directly or indirectly affect the rate of PNM (Woolf 1947, Butler and Alberman 1969, Thomson and Barron 1983, Bakketeig et al. 1984, Golding 1991, Emanuel 1993).

As in the general population, over the years the PNM rate has greatly decreased in diabetic pregnancy, which largely paralleled that in the general population. Similarly, the substratum of factors associated with perinatal death generally is shared by the pregnancies of diabetic women and hence cannot be neglected.

Demographic Factors

The majority of demographic features have been poorly documented in diabetic pregnancy and were seldom mentioned in the many hospital and other records of diabetic pregnancies on which this review is mainly based. For example, in hospitals in many larger US and British cities, where patients were almost certainly of different races, this fact was seldom documented. Even when race was mentioned, the pregnancy outcomes in the different races were almost never listed separately. Similarly, in heterogeneous populations, ethnic facts were rarely noted and socioeconomic variables were ignored, except occasionally indirectly when patients were noted as being private or ward cases. Again, in such instances results for the different groups were hardly ever considered separately. Certain other variables, such as nationality, region, and time, were obviously inherent in the reports themselves.

Sparsity of such details perhaps can be expected of hospital-based phenomena reported from the past by clinicians describing their often comparatively few and incomplete observations, with emphasis on their own particular interests and the interests of their times. Those writing 40 or more years ago could hardly be expected to have known what information the present-day reviewer would need. On the other hand, these lacunae are recompensed by the richness of other details, which are missing or equally inadequate in reports of population-based data.

Thus, of the many factors listed here as influencing PNM, it is possible to consider only the handful that were reported often enough and in useful enough detail to allow their association with the rate and temporal trend of PNM to be judged. An analysis of the roles played by even these few factors can, however, most often only be suggestive.

Gestational and Neonatal Age

Cardinal considerations in a discussion of PNM rate are the demarcations of gestational age and neonatal age. National health statistics reveal that the portion of all perinatal deaths claimed by each of its four components—early and late stillbirths and early and late neonatal deaths—is far from equal. Since 1950, late stillbirths in the United States have comprised about 72% of all stillbirths, and early neonatal deaths comprise about 88% of all neonatal ones. Together, they make up by far the predominant segment of perinatal deaths—about 80% (Powell-Griner 1989).

The number of perinatal deaths reported by individual investigators therefore depended partly on the extent of their observations—greater when both segments of stillbirth and neonatal death were included, less when some were not. With respect to diabetic births, these matters seem not to have caused much difficulty. Regarding stillbirth, most investigators, following the convention in their views about the onset of viability, restricted the reporting of stillbirths to the late variety. This was especially true in Europe, and even more so in Great Britain where this standard was first adopted. Fewer than half of the reports explicitly provided information on gestational age and neonatal age at all, but the customary precept would probably have been adhered to by most physicians. As for neonatal deaths, many articles clearly reported only early deaths. However, even when they not specified, since early neonatal deaths far outweigh later ones, it is likely that the deaths reported composed the majority of all neonatal deaths.

Maternal Age

The most often-mentioned maternal feature relevant to PNM in reports of diabetic pregnancies was the mean or range of maternal age at pregnancy. However, even this was noted in comparatively few instances. Maternal age is important because it is closely associated with overall PNM rate—being slightly increased before about age 20, reaching a low at age 20 to 24, then rising ever more steeply with further advance in age (Sutherland 1949, Thomson and Barron 1983, Bakketeig et al. 1984, Golding 1991).

Maternal age and PNM are no doubt also associated in pregnancies of diabetic women. Therefore, whether in the past, the average age at conception was greater in diabetic women than in the general population, as a result of reduced fertility and increased menarcheal age, must be a consideration. Reduced fertility of women with early-onset diabetes persisted into the early decades of the insulin era (Bergqvist 1954, Worm 1955, Post and White 1958) and was still present even in more recent years (Pinget et al. 1979, Burkart et al. 1989, Gens and Michaelis 1990, Kjaer et al. 1992a,b).

Other Factors Regarding Maternal Age

A credible analysis of the influence of maternal age on the PNM rate and its temporal shifts in diabetic pregnancy should also involve the consideration of other possible factors. For example, changes in age-specific birth rates, which have occurred in recent years in the US and western European populations and have been credited with some share in the decreased overall infant mortality rate, might also have had a part in the decreased PNM rate in diabetic pregnancy (Gendell and Hellegers 1973, Morris et al. 1975, Meirik et al. 1979). Such changes could not be evaluated, however, because of the inadequacies of the reported data.

Examination of parity or birth order, also known to be associated with perinatal death, was more productive. Because parity is closely tied to maternal age, its separate relation to PNM is much debated (Golding 1991). Nevertheless, its possible involvement was examined by using the only parity data that were presented in reports of diabetic pregnancies, that is, the proportion of women who were primigravid.

Information regarding the age at conception of pregnant diabetic women was more often reported in older than in more recent publications, perhaps because the greater general interest of past years has given way to the the narrower ones of today. But at all times the information was limited and fragmentary, consisting of age range, mean age (stated or calculated from the facts given), or gravidity proportions.

Data regarding age range, stated in a fair number of reports, revealed little that was definitive, perhaps pointing only to a slight but not clearly defined shift to a younger span over time. Data concerning age, stated in a fair number of reports, gave a clearer but puzzling picture. Mean age at pregnancy hardly changed over the first 50 years of the insulin era, hovering at about 28–29 years. Later, a small change seems to have occurred, with a decrease to about 27 years. This small reduction can scarcely be credited with any but the most minor part in the lowering of the diabetic PNM rate, which began earlier than did the maternal age shift. A direct indication of the apparently negligible effect of maternal age was given by a few comparisons of younger and older women (Andersson 1950, McCain and Lester 1950, Möllerström 1950, Jokipii 1955, Gellis and Hsia 1959, Malins 1968).

The difference between the earlier mean age of diabetic women at pregnancy—28–29 years—and the contemporary overall population mean age—25.7 years in 1962 (Anon 1963) may partly clarify the excessive mortality rate, whereas the closeness of the later diabetic mean of 27 years to the overall 26.7 occurring in 1992 perhaps says something about the mortality rate having approached that of the general population level (Ventura et al. 1992). (Interesting at the same time is the incidental revelation that the continually lowered overall record has not been disturbed by the increase that has taken place in the mean maternal age of the entire population.) Regarding the situation in the earlier era, Lavietes et al. (1943) went so far as to say, "on the basis of age alone it hardly seems proper to compare this group of pregnancies [they found a mean age of 31 years in their patients] with the data on the general population."

Authors of two reports (most unusually) compared maternal age data for diabetic and overall births in their institutions. In Pittsburgh, Rike and Fawcett (1948) found a mean age of 31 years in diabetic births and 23 years in all births for 1936 through 1946, and in a New York City hospital, Frankel (1950) found a mean age of 32 years for diabetic births and 24 years for overall births for 1940–1949. These few data thus indicate that the mean age of pregnant diabetic women was greater than that of nondiabetic pregnant women. However, a quantitative analysis of the contribution that this difference made to the increased PNM rate in diabetic women in those days was virtually impossible.

The rate of primigravidity, a possible measure of average conception age, was less informative, since it varied over time in an apparently haphazard way and did not correlate with maternal age. All in all, this statistic seems irrelevant to the mortality in question. It may be recalled that years ago Gellis and Hsia (1959) examined their own results and those of two other studies and found no indications that the PNM rate was different in multiparous diabetic women from that in primiparous ones.

Various data indicate that insulin-dependent diabetic women did not became pregnant as readily as nondiabetic women earlier in the century and perhaps even more recently, and hence that their mean age during pregnancy was greater than that of nondiabetic women. But these disparities probably accounted for a small percentage of the manyfold increase in the PNM rate the pregnancies of diabetic women once experienced. It may therefore be safely concluded that any deleterious effect of advanced maternal age of diabetic women on perinatal survival was obscured by that of the diabetes itself.

PERINATAL MORTALITY IN THE EARLY INSULIN ERA

The rate of offspring death in the few diabetic pregnancies noted in years before insulin was discovered was incredibly high—about 50% died in utero and during labor and 80% of the remainder in the first days after birth (Chapiet 1907, Lambie 1926). The deaths were ascribed mostly to hydramnios, hypertrophy of the fetal pancreas, neonatal hypoglycemia, and excessive fetal size, making for difficult labor (Lambie 1926).

Although insulin soon brought about a significant improvement in the fertility of diabetic women, it did far less to reduce the high PNM rate, which continued to be high for 20 years or more (Henley 1947).

The first reports of insulin given to pregnant diabetic women came from physicians describing the course of the illness and pregnancy in their patients. A summary of many of these earliest pregnancies illustrated the continuing seriousness of the diabetes for the offspring. In 28 cases of clearly pregestational diabetic pregnancies continuing to the later months of pregnancy (gleaned from American and European medical periodicals), the PNM rate was 39.3% (Wilder and Parsons 1928). This was an appreciable improvement over the pre-insulin record, but far short of the level in the overall US population—7.7% in the 1920s (U.S. Bureau of the Census 1960, p. 25)—which this new miracle medicine must have been expected to equal.

The number of diabetic pregnancies rapidly increased from the 1920s through the 1940s as, of necessity, did the number of American and European hospitals and centers caring for pregnant diabetic women. But the new medical facilities and specialties failed to make substantial dents in the mortality rate of their children. The poor record (called "simply dreadful" by Brandstrup and Okkels 1938) stubbornly persisted into the 1940s, being about 25% in American series and 35% to over 40% in European ones, despite the efforts of clinicians to understand and overcome this intractable impasse (Table 4.1).

Table 4.1 was derived from reports of hospitals and other medical facilities of diabetic pregnancies that included PNM data. The table shows that the number of series generally expanded over the decades, especially in Europe. If it did not increase in the most recent period, it was because the number of articles reporting mortality data were fewer—undoubtedly because there were often none to report. Thus, the figures in the table for the most recent period are probably overestimates, but to what extent it is impossible to say. I urge that omission of this information be corrected so that the present lowered PNM rate be clearly documented. This great accomplishment was recapitulated, and the roles of several of its causes, especially since the 1970s, were enumerated by Kitzmiller (1993).

The mean annual number of diabetic pregnancies cared for has varied greatly from facility to facility, no doubt largely reflecting the variation in their size and

Table 4.1 Perinatal Mortality in Diabetic Pregnancy From Earliest Years of Insulin Era to Recent Times

Era	Series (n)	America	Series (n)	Europe
1920s + 1930s	21	135/483 (28.0)[a]	13	172/397 (43.3)[a]
1940s	18	412/1730 (23.8)	16	497/1463 (34.0)
1950s	26	535/2674 (20.0)	40	904/3751 (24.1)
1960s	15	337/2325 (14.5)	40	730/4730 (15.4)
1970s	34	170/2496 (6.9)	43	421/5613 (7.5)
1980 to late 1990s	27	80/3095 (2.6)	44	227/6211 (3.6)

Data extracted from articles concerned primarily with pregestational diabetic patients.
[a] Perinatal deaths/births (% deaths).

specialization status. For example, in the 1930s in the US the number ranged from 1.2 to 12.1 pregnancies per year. How this affected PNM will be seen below.

Perinatal Mortality in Two Forms of Diabetes

Most diabetic pregnancies reported in the early decades of the insulin era involved women with pregestational diabetes. Later reports increasingly included diabetes that first occurred or was diagnosed during pregnancy (gestational diabetes), but often did not present the outcomes for the two forms of the disease separately. This is unfortunate because the PNM rate in the two forms, not very different in the earliest years, greatly diverged, with improvement in the pregestational form greatly lagging behind the other. Thus, the failure to separate the progressively differing outcomes further complicated the study of trends in the mortality rate associated with the pregestational disease.

Perinatal Mortality and Facility Size

The excessive diabetic PNM rate might be expected to have been mitigated by excellent maternal care, and therefore the larger medical facilities, where such care was more likely provided, would be predicted to have the better record in this regard. To learn whether in the early years facility size, as denoted by patient load, had such an effect, the series reported in each decade were divided into those caring for more and those caring for less than the annual median number of pregestational diabetic pregnancies, the median being chosen because of the frequently very skewed distribution of patient numbers.

Medical facilities with larger patient loads invariably had lower PNM rates than did the smaller ones, but with erratic statistical significance (data not presented) Even this advantage largely faded away after the 1960s, as the steady reduction in the PNM rate in diabetic pregnancy all but wiped out this differential.

The lower mortality frequencies experienced by the larger facilities from another perspective are surprising, because the better care they offered would have been offset to some extent by the patients they served, who were mostly referred and hence more severely diabetic. As Jones (1952) recognized, the larger centers were attended by selected patients but who were "cooperative and superbly supervised." The importance of maternal motivation was also early noted by a commentator (Anon 1954), who remarked that "the experience at the Chicago Lying-in Hospital has been that whenever patients are cooperative the results for mother and baby are better." The argument depends on the relation, if any, among severity, care, and outcome. Only at a later time, when somewhat objective schemes of classifying severity of diabetes in pregnancy were formulated, could some of these questions be addressed.

Stillbirth and Neonatal Death

The composition of PNM in diabetic pregnancy is most relevant. Reports presenting analyzable data made it clear that the rate of stillbirth in the early years was always greater—usually considerably so—than that of neonatal death (Table 4.2), constituting 60–65% of all perinatal deaths. This contrasted with the 50–55% stillbirth rate that occurred in overall hospital pregnancies during these decades and was a clear demonstration of the pathologic effect of maternal diabetes on fetal viability.

It is thus understandable why attention was especially directed toward stillbirths. (Another reason, discussed on p. 34, is that there seemed to be an easy means of forestalling these deaths.) Whether or not this attention corrected the early disproportion will be considered in the following pages, but undoubtedly time brought the diabetic stillbirth picture into line with that of the overall population level.

Most neonatal deaths in diabetic pregnancies happen within 1 week of birth, and most of these within the first couple of days of life (Peel and Oakley 1949, Oakley 1953, Neave 1967). In the early insulin years, this percentage was 80% to

Table 4.2 Stillbirth and Neonatal Mortality Rates in Diabetic Pregnancy From the Earliest Insulin-Era Decades to the Present

Era	Stillbirth (SB)[a]	Neonatal Death[a]	% SB
		America	
1920s through 1940s	477/2791 (17.1)	261/2314 (11.3)	60.2
1950s and 1960s	341/3947 (8.6)	258/3606 (7.2)	54.4
1970s to mid 1990s	162/9065 (1.8)	120/8826 (1.4)	56.2
		Europe	
1920s through 1940s	417/1518 (27.5)	160/1101 (14.5)	65.2
1950s and 1960s	688/6675 (10.3)	552/5987 (9.2)	52.8
1970s to mid 1990s	219/8321 (2.6)	162/7281 (2.2)	54.2

Rates taken from publications presenting stillbirth and neonatal death separately.

[a] The stillbirth rate is based on the total number of births, the neonatal death rate on the number born alive.

nearly 100% as it continued to be thereafter. But this figure is not unusual, since it is also true of neonatal deaths in the general population. For example, 87% of neonatal deaths in the US in 1950 occurred during the first week of neonatal life; in 1980, it was 84% despite the great overall reduction in the neonatal mortality rate in the intervening years (Powell-Griner 1986). This fact reinforces the idea that most deaths in this earliest period of infancy have a largely prenatal basis.

Comparison With the General Population

To be seen in perspective, the PNM rate in diabetic pregnancy and its composition and changes over time must be judged against those occurring in overall hospital-based births. Appreciable numbers of such reports were published beginning only in the 1940s and 1950s. Compared with the still sparser earlier ones, these reports supported the demographic record showing that a marked improvement had occurred. Summing up such data from the 1930s gave a mean PNM rate of about 5–6%, and from the 1940s, about 3–3.5%.

Confounding the picture somewhat was the variability among hospitals, part of which may have been due to differences in offspring gestational age, weight, or size criteria used for inclusion in the reports. Far more important were regional differences within the larger areas. For example, in the US in the 1940s, the mean PNM rate for four hospitals in the northeast quadrant was 3.5%, and for five hospitals outside this region it was 2.6%. Such differences were also conspicuous in Europe: in five hospitals on the continent the mean rate was 4.1%; in six hospitals in Great Britain, it was 5.4%. Within Great Britain, in England it was 4.9% and in Scotland 5.7%.

These facts make it obvious that PNM rate in diabetic pregnancy must also be examined regionally for valid comparison and analysis. Meanwhile, the figures just cited make it evident that PNM in diabetic pregnancies in these years was about 8- to 12-fold greater than in overall births.

Regional Differences in Diabetic Perinatal Mortality

In many instances, appreciable regional differences existed in the rate of PNM in diabetic pregnancy and have largely persisted through the decades. These variations are most clearly seen where the diabetic pregnancies were most amply documented. The best record for Europe in the earliest years was held by the United Kingdom and Ireland, an advantage that seems to have been lost in recent years (Table 4.3). This appears to contradict the poorer overall PNM score in Great Britain compared with other countries in Europe in the earlier years. This can perhaps be explained by the relatively early establishment of clinics for the care of pregnant diabetic women in England and Scotland. In time, the performances of the European regions converged, and by the 1980s all had come to share fairly uniform incidences of PNM.

In America, distinct interregional patterns of PNM had not emerged in the earliest years because of limited numbers of patients in some regions. Still, some regions apparently showed an early higher rate, which has been maintained

Table 4.3 Regional Variation in PNM in Insulin-Dependent Pregestational Diabetes in America and Europe Since the Introduction of Insulin

Era	Region[a]			
	1	2	3	4
		America		
1920s through 1940s	449/1860 (24.0)	42/124 (33.9)	46/201 (22.9)	10/28 (35.7)
1950s and 1960s	644/3798 (17.0)	83/362 (22.9)	129/724 (17.8)	16/115 (13.9)
1970s to mid 1990s	92/1934 (4.8)	53/557 (9.5)	27/245 (11.0)	83/2453 (3.4)
		Europe		
1920s through 1940s	269/844 (31.9)	320/795 (40.2)	57/165 (34.5)	20/56 (35.7)
1950s and 1960s	417/2601 (16.0)	554/2601 (21.3)	436/2330 (18.7)	220/949 (23.2)
1970s to mid 1990s	180/3159 (5.7)	135/3090 (4.4)	140/2156 (6.5)	133/1856 (7.0)

[a] The regions for America roughly correspond to (1) northeast, (2) southeast, (3) northwest, and (4) southwest quadrants, respectively, including Canada in the northeast and northwest quadrants. For Europe, region 1 is the United Kingdom and Ireland, region 2 is Scandinavia and Finland, region 3 is The Netherlands, Germany, Austria, Czechoslovakia, and Switzerland, and region 4 is Belgium, France, Italy, and Spain.

through the years. As in Europe, these differences have recently leveled off, but not vanished.

The possible reasons for regional differences in PNM are legion, but none is well documented. Based on the facts just discussed, one conspicuous possibility is the contribution of specialized clinics to improving the standing of a region, such as the Joslin Center in Boston with a record low mortality rate for that time (White 1950). Analysis of this possibility, through comparison of the annual mean number of diabetic pregnancies, revealed an overall consistent inverse relation between facility patient load and mortality rate. How much of the interregional variation this factor may have accounted for is difficult to determine, and the limited data from some areas precluded an attempt to answer this question by examining the within-region variation.

There may be additional reasons for the regional variations, whose importance cannot be minimized. This subject is taken up again and later more fully probed when trends in diabetic PNM over the entire period since the discovery of insulin are discussed.

CAUSES OF PERINATAL MORTALITY IN DIABETIC PREGNANCY

The Background

The persistently high perinatal death rate in diabetic pregnancy in the earliest insulin decades was baffling. Its possible determinants were numerous, and each had its own adherents. First, a review of what was generally known about the causes of PNM in those years is advisable.

The medical literature shows that deaths in the overall fetal and infant population were not well understood, despite valiant attempts to pin labels on them. In fact, honesty dictated that many deaths could not be attributed to any cause. An early attempt at such delineation was made in Sheffield, England, by Tingle (1926), who divided 160 stillbirths and first-week deaths into maternal, placental, and fetal causes. But the main culprit—fetal trauma—fit into none of these categories. Dippel's (1934) findings in Baltimore were unusual in that 42% of stillbirth records he examined were attributed to syphilis. Of the others, more typically 27% were due to toxemia, and 44% had no known cause.

Other contemporary reports substantiated the vagueness of the knowledge of this subject. Baird (1942), citing the Registrar-General's report for Scotland for 1939, noted that 37% of stillbirths were of ill-defined or unknown cause, 14% were due to difficult labor, 13% to fetal deformities, and the remainder to hemorrhage, toxemia, and general diseases. McNeil (1943), in Edinburgh, reported a common situation, namely, that many babies dying perinatally were "premature" (weighed <1000 g), but he regarded prematurity as "not of itself a cause of death" and that the main lethal factors remained the same as those in mature babies—asphyxia, trauma, congenital malformation, and infection.

The same general theme keeps recurring in publications during the 1940s and early 1950s with the important addition that a significant proportion of PNM could be attributed to toxemia and other maternal illnesses (Potter and Adair 1943, Labate 1947, Arey 1949, Sutherland 1949, Baird et al. 1954). Nevertheless, many deaths were still due to vague and ill-defined "physiological" conditions (Sutherland 1949, Duncan et al. 1952) with autopsy failing "to reveal the cause of stillbirth and first week death in a large proportion of cases" (Baird et al. 1954). We dare not find fault with these early investigators, since even today, in 2000, the delineation of causes of PNM remains fairly rudimentary (Golding 1987, Pauli and Reiser 1994, Incerpi et al. 1998).

The causes of PNM in diabetic pregnancy and their relevance to the general findings can now be examined. Many writers during the 1940s gave their opinions on this vexing question. Lawrence and Oakley (1942) named the four main causes of PNM as they viewed them: fetal overgrowth, due to growth hormone excess, neonatal hypoglycemia, congenital malformations, and maternal toxemia. Miller et al. (1944) considered poor care in regulating the maternal disease as the main culprit. At first, White (1935) pointed to "...a direct agent, active in the last four weeks of pregnancy;" later to a defective ovum, which included congenital anomalies, disturbed chemistry of diabetes, and hormone imbalance during pregnancy (White and Hunt 1943). Obstetric and placental causes were later added to this list (White 1946), and the picture was summed up as follows: "...fetal fatalities have been influenced in varying degrees by (1) poor control of maternal diabetes, (2) the occurrence of congenital defects, (3) the degree of maternal vascular disease, (4) prematurity, (5) duration of diabetes, (6) its age of inception and (7) the imbalance of the sex hormones of pregnancy" (White 1949). In some of the latter, White showed extraordinary foresight; in others, time showed her to be off the mark.

Consensus coalesced in the 1950s as time and the greatly increased numbers of diabetic pregnancies allowed for broader overview and seasoned judgment. It was by then well seen that stillbirth was often accompanied by maternal vascular disease, hypertension, acidosis, toxemia, hydramnios, and fetal anomalies (White 1950, Jones 1958), but most such deaths still had no satisfactory explanation. Even extensive postmortem examination, such as that by Warren and LeCompte (1952), did not clarify this. Little progress has been made in discovering the true causes of stillbirth, since even today, the "precise cause of the excessive stillbirth rate..." in diabetic pregnancies "...remains unknown" (Landon and Gabbe 1995).

Better knowledge of the proximate causes of neonatal death has been helpful. Most deaths were characterized by a combination of chronological but not developmental prematurity (ie, of date, but not size), respiratory difficulties, pulmonary atelectasis (all three associated with each other), generalized cardiac enlargement, overall excessive size—often followed by traumatic injuries secondary to difficult delivery—congenital defects, and so on (Given et al.1950, Hall and Tillman 1951, Hagbard 1956, Miller 1956).

Little was really new in most of the latter observations. For example, poor maternal care had early been said to be a factor in the high mortality rate, and the common triad of prematurity, asphyxia, and atelectasis had been recorded years earlier (Sisson 1940), and respiratory distress is still a problem in diabetic pregnancy (Robert et al. 1976, Bye et al. 1980, Cunningham et al. 1982, Allen and Palumbo 1987, Piper and Langer 1993).

Inadequate Prenatal Care

Quality of prenatal maternal care had been considered to be important in combatting fetal mortality since the 1930s. It was an early and enduring belief that the care that the pregnant diabetic woman received in regulating her disease, through medical and dietary management, was the most important ingredient in mitigating the unfavorable effects of diabetes on the fetus and infant. Some clinicians felt good prenatal care was efficacious "especially if it be instituted early" (Ronsheim 1933), whereas others thought care was most important in the last months of pregnancy (Skipper 1933).

The quality of the care given to pregnant diabetic women has throughout the years continued to be regarded of paramount importance in combating PNM, in distinction to the passing attention given to almost all of the other imputed causes discussed in the following sections.

Macrosomia

A feature continually implicated in poor fetal survival in diabetic pregnancy was macrosomia, that is, significantly increased neonatal length and weight. This is usually defined as 4.0 kg or more, resulting not from prolonged gestation but from fetal overgrowth, especially in the last trimester of pregnancy, producing, as known in the modern parlance, babies large for gestational age.

In the old days, diabetic women frequently had big babies (Hsia and Gellis 1957). Pedowitz and Shlevin (1952) found that one-third of births to diabetic women resulted in such children. In Copenhagen, newborns of diabetic mothers were 18.1% heavier and 2.9% longer than those of a matched control group (Pedersen 1954b). Even more recently, large centers reported 25–42% large babies

(Kitzmiller 1986). Yet, according to certain developmental criteria, such infants could be considered growth-retarded (Pederson and Osler 1958, Gruenwald 1966).

Time has reduced the frequency of these big babies. In the 19030s and 1940s, diabetic mothers had excessively large babies nine times more often than did non-diabetic mothers (Nathanson 1950); 30–40 years later, diabetes only doubled the risk of infant macrosomia (Boyd et al. 1983). But there was never anything new about these babies (has anything ever been new?). The very first baby known to be born to a diabetic mother was huge (Bennewitz 1824), and many articles noting such giant infants of diabetic mothers were already summarized by the 1930s (Fischer 1935).

Heavy babies frequently had a difficult birth and thus were subject to skeletal and neurologic injuries and sometimes death (Given et al. 1950, Pedowitz and Shlevin 1952). But the question remained whether big babies were at increased risk for stillbirth. There is evidence that the PNM rate of excessively large babies in general is at least twice that of normal-sized babies (Stevenson et al. 1982). However, the answer is uncertain as far as diabetic births are concerned (Kitzmiller 1986).

The importance of macrosomia has been sidestepped by the great decrease in the PNM rate in diabetic pregnancies and the lowered risk of trauma in diabetic births (Mimouni et al. 1992). In the past, macrosomia was found even in "cases with excellent control of diabetes throughout pregnancy" (Lavietes et al. 1943, Gilbert 1949), and it occurs today even in well-controlled pregnancies (Knight 1983, Dandona et al. 1986, Berk et al. 1989, Hunter et al.1993, Hare 1991), and it is still not well understood (Kitzmiller 1986, Fenichel et al. 1990). Macrosomia is further discussed in the sections that follow dealing with prediabetes and gestational diabetes.

Sex Hormone Imbalance

An early theory, taken very seriously by many clinicians for 20 years or more, was one that proposed maternal sex hormone imbalances to be responsible for perinatal deaths (White et al. 1939). Such hormonal abnormalities had often been found in toxemic diabetic pregnant women, whose pregnancies were also known to be associated with increased PNM (Murphy 1933, Smith and Smith 1934). The reasoning was that replacement therapy given to patients with abnormal hormone patterns would reduce the incidence of toxemia and result in great improvement in offspring survival rate. The results of hormone therapy, when applied with other, more usual sorts of management of the disease and pregnancy, were claimed to support this belief. (White and Hunt 1943, White 1949, Nelson et al. 1953, White et al. 1956).

The theory began fading when other investigators expressed skepticism, noting the imprecision of the means of assaying these hormones (Reis 1956) and finding that hormone therapy provided no significant advantage, and since just as favorable results were obtained simply by careful supervision of pregnancy (Medical Research Council 1955; Miller 1956, Reis et al. 1958, Gellis and Hsia 1959). Thus, cruel facts, as they will, rapidly vanquished a long and widely held theory.

Nevertheless, belief in the efficacy of hormones in diabetic pregnancy persisted locally a while longer (White 1965).

Disease Severity

Greater promise of clarifying the problem was offered by examining the relation of PNM to severity of the maternal disease. But the difficulty was that there was disagreement about what constituted "severity" and how it was to be classified (Jones 1956). A conflict developed during the early 1950s between two seemingly irreconcilable views—whether severity was to be judged by "historical" or by metabolic criteria. According to the historical view, judgment of disease severity was based on age at onset of diabetes, its duration at the time of pregnancy, and the degree and extent of maternal vascular pathology. According to the metabolic view, it was based on the metabolic state of the diabetic patient, as indicated by insulin requirement during pregnancy—in other words, by the difficulty of management (Given et al. 1950, Tolstoi et al. 1953, White 1949, Nelson et al. 1953). Attempts to classify severity by the use of these criteria were confused, however, because their correlation with fetal loss was inconsistent (Hurwitz and Higano 1952, Oakley 1953).

From the neutral standpoint of a present-day observer, the two apparently divergent approaches (historical and metabolic) can actually be seen to be complementary and should both have had value as indicators of mortality risk if severity were associated with that risk. These indicators might have been especially useful because they were quantitatively classifiable and statistically evaluable and because ample unambiguous data regarding them had been accumulated (though not very systematically) during the previous couple of decades.

Therefore, severity was estimated or classified by two general sets of criteria: by age, duration, and extent of vascular disease, or by insulin requirement. My analyses of the extensive data from the 1930s to the 1950s found that earliness of diabetes onset and duration of the disease were not conclusively related to risk of offspring survival, and not more informative were analyses of severity as gauged by insulin dose. Adding to the difficulty is the fact that disease duration and insulin dose were significantly though barely correlated, whereas this was not always true for age of onset and duration (data for the assertions in this paragraph are not presented).

In contrast, PNM and the quality of control of diabetes during pregnancy were decisively positively related. Although control or supervision of the disease was not always explicitly defined, Lawrence and Oakley (1942) spelled out what it meant for them. For these authors, the degree of completeness of supervision referred to the earliness and regularity of the diabetic woman's being seen by a physician during pregnancy, and her treatment being adjusted as needed. It was such individualized management of pregnancy, apparently not in itself equivalent to insulin dosage, that was associated with the markedly improved PNM rate that my analysis detected (Table 4.4). However, such a favorable outcome was not invariable (eg, see Given and Tolstoi 1957, for disappointing results). Nevertheless, such favorable outcomes guided and foreshadowed the future emphasis on maternal glycemic control that is of paramount importance today (Kitzmiller 1993, Hare 1994.

Table 4.4 Perinatal Mortality and Diabetes Control in the Early Insulin Decades

Reference	Diabetes Control[a]		
	Good	Fair	Poor or None
Skipper 1933	13/80[b]	38/56[b]	20/22[b]
White 1935	4/39	–	3/14
Barns 1941	4/7	–	2/3
Lawrence and Oakley 1942	6/37	2/4	8/11
Pedowitz and Shlevin 1952	5/18	3/16	4/16
Whitely and Adams 1952	3/18	2/16	1/16
Pedersen 1954a[c]	13/109	56/176	–
Hagbard 1956	10/32	80/178	8/10
Total	58/340 (17.07%)	181/446 (40.6%)	46/92 (50.0)

Good vs not good: $P \ll .001$
[a] Complete—partial, or no supervision or its equivalent.
[b] Deaths/births.
[c] Long or short treatment.

Other Alleged Causes

Numerous other causes of offspring death, especially intrauterine ones, were alleged. For example, a direct lethal factor was possibly associated with the toxemia and preeclampsia experienced in the last 4 weeks by many diabetic women (White 1935). There were various other maternal and fetal dangers—ketoacidosis, hydramnios, premature labor, macrosomia, hypoglycemia, developmental immaturity, and congenital malformations (Eastman 1946, Bachman 1952, Miller 1956, Stevenson 1956). But the associations between these features and PNM were illusory or far from consistent (Kyle 1963).

Studies extending over more than 20 years indicated that toxemia was not important (Table 4.5). But another study found fetal mortality rate to be significantly greater in pregnancies of insulin-treated women with various complications than in those without them, whereas there was no such difference in women not requiring insulin (Miller et al. 1944). Clearly, the relation of toxemia to PNM, if any, was complex, and was made even more so by variable standards and definitions of toxemia (Lawrence and Oakley 1942, Peel and Oakley 1949, Hagbard 1956). Even lately, the survival rate of infants from diabetic pregnancies complicated by nephropathy, preeclampsia, and so on, has not always reached that of the general population (Garner et al. 1990, Kitzmiller and Combs 1993).

One concomitant factor of PNM that has received much attention is congenital malformations. In early studies of PNM in the general population, malformations constituted one of the few elements clearly identified as relevant at all. As the PNM rate decreased with the passing years and many of their causes—infectious, nutritious, social—were overcome or diminished in severity, congenital malformations grew in conspicuousness as they came to be present in an increasingly large proportion of these deaths (Edouard and Alberman 1980, Kalter 1991). Their possible importance in the high diabetic PNM rate will be considered in Chapter 10.

Table 4.5 PNM and Maternal Toxemia in Early Insulin-Era Decades

Author (s)	Toxemia	
	Present[a]	Absent[a]
Peckham 1931	3/6	3/11
Barns 1941	6/11	0/8
Lavietes et al. 1943	3/12	9/19
Rike and Fawcett 1948	3/18	6/30
Pederson 1949[b]	10/27	11/30
Sheumack 1949	2/5	7/15
Given et al. 1950	17/60	15/56
McCain and Lester 1950	6/13	5/10
Reis 1950[c]	1/6	7/53
Hall and Tillman 1951	8/34	14/73
Hurwitz and Higano 1952	12/40	20/100
Jones 1952	22/69	26/93
Whitely and Adams 1952	3/14	9/36
Oakley 1953[d]	48/117	208/612
Buck and Day 1953	10/43	10/48
Boughton and Perkins 1957	6/22	7/29
Total	160/497 (32.2%)	357/1223 (29.2%)

$P > .05$
[a] Deaths/births.
[b] In primiparas.
[c] Slight—moderate toxemia.
[d] Questionnaire and Kings College Hospital series combined.

A MEANS OF PREVENTING STILLBIRTHS

The greatest challenge to physicians caring for pregnant diabetic women in the early insulin-era years was the forbidding rate of stillbirths, which accounted for about two-thirds of all the perinatal deaths (see Table 4.2). Since it appeared to be impossible to avert these deaths, attention was focused on stillbirth, and the neonatal mortality problem was largely set aside.

Because intrauterine death was predominantly a phenomenon of the last weeks of pregnancy, it seemed obvious that many stillbirths could be prevented, or rather circumvented, by performing elective delivery by cesarean section before they could occur (Peel and Oakley 1949, Pedowitz and Shlevin 1955). This strategy was advocated especially by obstetricians, but also by others (Nothmann and Hermstein 1932, Ronsheim 1933, White 1935b, Randall and Rynearson 1936, Titus 1937). Cesarean deliveries soon became a widespread practice 4–5 weeks before expected parturition (Eastman 1946). Nevertheless, there was abundant and reiterated skepticism of the necessity and benefits of this practice (Peckham 1931, Skipper 1933, Hurwitz and Irving 1937, Herrick and Tillman 1938, Shir 1939, Mengert and Laughlin 1939, Hall and Tillman 1951, Sindram 1951, Miller 1956). For example, Hurwitz and Higano (1952) noted that a large proportion of stillbirths had already occurred by the end of the 36th week; hence, very few additional deaths would have been prevented by early delivery.

Sometimes the rescued prematurely delivered infants succumbed at birth and added to the neonatal death toll, an unexpected drawback. As Barnes and Morgan (1949) put it, "...early termination does not alter the outcome of pregnancy, but merely changes the death-bed of the foetus...." Such deaths followed from the difficulty of striking a balance between the need to deliver babies before most intrauterine deaths occurred and not delivering them so early that neonatal deaths might occur because of respiratory immaturity (Hurwitz and Higano 1952, Gellis and Hsia 1959). To thwart most of the intrauterine deaths and also minimize the neonatal problem, the preferred time of delivery was selected to be about the 35th to 38th weeks of gestation. This compromise appeared to lead to the hoped-for outcome.

Bachman (1952), in summarizing several findings, found that the stillbirth rate was reduced by 50% or more and that the one unfavorable by-product—a slightly increased neonatal mortality rate—did not tarnish the overall improved result. Miller (1956) later noted that this optimistic appraisal was marred by statistical nonsignificance. My summary of the reports of an even larger number of

Table 4.6 Effect on PNM of Preterm Pregnancy Intervention: Cesarean Section vs Vaginal Delivery

Author (s)	Vaginal Delivery[a]	Cesarean Section[b]	*P*
Titus 1937	3, 3/19	3, 5/29 ($7\frac{1}{4}$–$8\frac{1}{2}$ mo)	
Barns 1941	9, 0/16	0/6 (end 36 w)	
Lawrence and Oakley 1942	8, 2/23	3, 5/29 (79% 36–38 w)	
Gaspar 1945	18, 6/40	1, 0/9 (89% 34–36 w)[c]	
Randall 1947	5, 3/22	0, 1/26 (73% 36–38 w)	
Paton 1948	6, 3/29	0, 1/9 (35–37 w)	
Rike and Fawcett 1948	7, 2/34	0/14 (?)	
Peel and Oakley 1949	50, 39/286	3, 31/213 ("many ... at term")	
Andersson 1950	12, 5/34	0, 1/10 (8–$8\frac{1}{2}$ mo)	
Crampton et al. 1950	1, 2/4	2, 3/20 (?)	
Frankel 1950	4, 1/14	1, 0/5 (?)	
Harris and Fisichella 1950	4, 0/9	0, 2/8 (75% 35–39 w)	
Zilliacus 1950	5, 21/21	0, 3/4 (?)	
Pease et al. 1951	2, 0/16	0/9 (34–36 w)	
Jones 1952	15, 12/103[d]	1, 0/19 (≥ 36 w)	
Pedowitz and Shlevin 1952	24, 4/104	1, 4/52 (36–38 w)	
Whitely and Adams 1952	3, 1/25	3, 5/25 (76% 36–38 w)	
Rolland 1954	10, 2/28	1, 3/43 (35–38 w)	
Buck and Day 1955	11, 5/40	1, 3/51 (avg. 23 d early)	
Stevenson 1956	20, 4/50	2, 5/63 (mostly 36–38 w)	
Total	217, 96/917	22, 72/644	
% Stillbirth	23.7	3.4	« .001
% Neonatal death[e]	13.7	11.6	> .05

[a] Stillbirths, neonatal deaths/total born.
[b] Time of delivery.
[c] A "monster."
[d] 19 of 27 were recognized intrauterine deaths or malformed.
[e] Neonatal deaths/liveborn.

pregnancies mostly during the 1930s and 1940s supported the optimistic outlook respecting stillbirths (Table 4.6) and found no worse neonatal mortality rate.

Flaws Involving Patient Selection

Favorable results were much weakened by several flaws. The first concerns patient selection. Women chosen for cesarean section delivery presumably were those who had supposed indications of impending intrauterine death—obstetrical history, fetal oversize, uncontrolled diabetes, and so on (Kyle 1963). In some cases, cesarean section delivery was also carried out at or near term when emergencies in pregnancy necessitated them (McCain and Lester 1950, Hall and Tillman 1951). Many such indications, however, were not helpful in distinguishing women at risk (Whitely and Adams 1952). As Stevenson (1956) admitted, "The factors which influenced the obstetrician to induce labour or await spontaneous onset rather than deliver by cesarean section are not always clear..."

Other biases were also entailed in the act of selection. Women who underwent cesarean section probably received medical attention earlier in pregnancy, more frequently, and with more continuity than those delivering at term. Since maternal care was an important element in mitigating the PNM rate, this factor may have been a source of some of the improved stillbirth record in cesarean section deliveries.

Deaths in Utero

The results were also made more favorable by the practice of allowing fetuses already known to be dead in utero to be delivered at term. The proportion of stillbirths and neonatal deaths in such deliveries could not legitimately be compared with that of cesarean section deliveries (Reis et al. 1950). Only by excluding the stillborns could this be done. As Jones (1952) pointed out, when the recognized intrauterine deaths were omitted from the calculation, the fetal loss in vaginal deliveries was reduced to a level that would not have been bettered by additional cesareans.

But Gellis and Hsia (1959), in comparing neonatal deaths in vaginal and cesarean section deliveries reported by several studies, noted a slight but statistically significant advantage of cesarean deliveries. This was influenced, however, by misleading data from deliveries before the 33rd week, vaginal or cesarean. When all such early deliveries were excluded from their own data, no significant difference was seen in the rate of neonatal death in the two types of delivery. This demonstration plus the good results that were achieved simply by diligent care during the last weeks of pregnancy (Nelson et al. 1953, Pedersen and Brandstrup 1956) confirmed the opinions of those who throughout had regarded the routine cesarean section delivery practice skeptically.

THE WHITE CLASSIFICATION AND PERINATAL MORTALITY

What had partly hampered the study and management of pregnancy in the first 25 years or so of the insulin era was the lack of an objective system of grading the seriousness of the overall diabetes disease state. Such a system might also have had an important use as a possible indicator of the extent of fetal risk and, if found predictive, might have permitted preventive measures where they were most called for. Some of the need for a new focus also came from the growing recognition that the benefits of close management of pregnancy meant that at least some of the causes of the excessive prenatal mortality rate resided in the mother.

Such considerations may have been the rationale for the new system of classification of diabetes in pregnancy offered by White (1949). This system is one of the most important and certainly the most durable of her many contributions to the study of diabetes in pregnancy. It consisted of an integrated method of grading the "pre-pregnancy" maternal state—disease onset age and duration plus intensity of vascular pathology—into increasing levels of severity, classes A through F. (The scheme is described and discussed in Chapter 7.)

The White system, although soon accepted by many investigators, at first had its critics. For example, Long et al. (1954) noted the difficulty of applying it to patients in a general hospital, because of the need to make certain assumptions when classifying patients who were first seen during pregnancy by a system based on prepregnancy criteria. Dampeer (1958) complained that it "did not take into account insulin amount needed or ease or difficulty of maintaining control." Whether justified or not, these complaints apparently were not widely shared, because the White system was soon broadly applied and said to have been accorded "virtually semiofficial status" (Jones 1956), at least in the US.

In Europe, some investigators felt that an entirely satisfactory system of classifying severity of diabetes in pregnancy was still to be formulated, since relations between the variables proposed by the White system and pregnancy outcome were inconsistent (Oakley 1953, Pedersen 1954a). Pedersen, an early critic of the White system, nevertheless tentatively accepted it while awaiting the perfect one. Some years later, he proffered an alternative classification, which was believed to be better able to predict diabetic pregnancy outcome (Pedersen and Mølsted-Pedersen 1965). It was an individualized scheme, which relied on "prognostically bad signs" appearing during pregnancy. In combination with the White system, it seemed to be a useful adjunct, but it never caught on and has rarely been used outside of Copenhagen (Pedersen et al. 1974).

A greatly simplified scheme of classifying diabetes in relation to pregnancy was proposed still later (Essex et al. 1973), but its purpose, and that of its modifications (Jovanovic and Peterson 1982), was less to predict and prevent harmful fetal outcome than to aid in management of pregnant diabetic women.

The increasing number of patients supervised by individuals applying the White system in the years after its promulgation firmly established its usefulness in relating disease severity to PNM (Kyle 1963). Other indicators, as noted, also did this, but the superiority of the White system was that it could be put to the practical use of estimating the fetal risk prenatally or early in pregnancy, thus possibly helping to avert the threat of fetal death. The continued fairly close relation through the years between diabetes severity as graded by the White system and the PNM rate (even as the PNM rate dropped precipitously) is noteworthy—more so in recent years in America than in Europe (Table 4.7).

The good overall correlation of disease severity and fetal risk masked some disagreements. For example, there were differences between individual medical

Table 4.7 Perinatal Mortality and the White System of Classifying Pregnancy in Diabetes

Era	White Class				
	A[b]	B	C	D	> D
			America		
1940s[a] + 1950s	40/484 (8.3)	263/1668 (15.7)	232/1245 (18.6)	181/843 (21.5)	92/289 (31.8)
1960s	35/1046 (3.3)	67/515 (13.0)	42/396 (10.6)	66/601 (11.0)	25/127 (19.7)
1970s	22/1062 (2.1)	39/807 (2.6)	29/376 (7.7)	11/198 (5.6)	5/60 (8.3)
1980s to mid 1990s	15/2064 (0.7)	5/201 (2.5)	12/170 (7.0)	6/62 (9.7)	1/32 (3.1)
			Europe		
1940s + 1950s	4/72 (5.6)	120/679 (17.7)	42/347 (12.1)	78/361 (21.6)	64/338 (18.9)
1960s	49/964 (5.1)	278/2002 (13.9)	207/1324 (15.6)	224/1300 (17.2)	69/324 (21.3)
1970s	24/816 (2.9)	46/726 (6.3)	63/704 (8.9)	61/618 (9.9)	10/141 (7.1)
1980s to mid 1990s	5/107 (4.7)	10/151 (6.6)	7/128 (5.5)	7/111 (6.3)	2/35 (5.7)

[a] White system applied retrospectively.
[b] Deaths/births (%).

facilities in the mean disease severity of their patients, as denoted by the White system, and in the sometimes poor relation between severity and pregnancy outcome. The Lying-in Hospital in Providence, Rhode Island, had a distribution, relative to the mean of all the examples, of less severe cases of diabetes but a higher PNM rate (Jones 1958). In contrast, patients seen at the Joslin Clinic and delivered at the Faulkner and Lying-in Hospitals in Boston were more severely affected but had a lower PNM (Gellis and Hsia 1959). Could such disparities have been due in part to differences in quality and earliness of patient care and in medical skill and experience? Was recognition of the efficacy of such resources—perhaps subtle and nonspecific—the predominant reason for the improvements in PNM in later years? These are all possibilities.

5

PREDIABETES

The term "prediabetes" refers to two separate areas of study, similar yet different: an earlier one, now passé and largely forgotten, and a current one, in a state of lively development. Both are similar in the focus of their attention, the period preceding the onset of overt diabetes, and in the purpose of their investigation, the discovery of elements leading to full-blown diabetes, in order to forestall its manifestation. They differ, however, in the phenomena studied: the older area, adverse outcomes of earlier pregnancies, and today's area, foregoing pathophysiological processes (Leiva 1996).

In any case, what should not be neglected by present-day searchers for the basis of the causation of diabetes is that this is an old quest. Thus, Joslin, in 1928, noted that "He [Naunyn] sees in heredity the common bond which unites the different forms, or as he says, 'to speak more exactly, the heredity of the diabetic tendency.'...Almost any illness or injury...may serve as the cause."

INTRODUCTION

This chapter is concerned with the first area of study, a virtually forgotten chapter in the saga of diabetic pregnancy, and recounts the years of intense study of what came to be realized was a "disease" that did not exist, or as Pyke (1962) put it, "...a unique disease. No one has ever suffered from it." What students of this condition studied were adverse outcomes of pregnancy occurring in the prediabetic period, outcomes thought to be premonitory of manifest diabetes and whose study, it was hypothesized, would yield an understanding of the processes leading to it (Camerini-Dávalos 1964). This they would do since they were taken as signs of a life-long process (Jackson 1959, Conn and Fajans 1961) that eventuated in the emergence of the overt disease—as stated by Krall (1965) "Diabetes doesn't occur overnight but starts at birth or earlier...," astutely foreshadowing present ideas of a genetic etiology of diabetes.

The adverse outcomes were the familiar ones: perinatal mortality and congenital malformation, plus one other (Jackson 1959). In fact it was the last—excessive offspring birth weight or macrosomia—that was considered the hallmark of prediabetes, and belief in which as an indicator of potential diabetes was most durable.

This macrosomia is an old phenomenon. It was present in the very first documented instance of a birth to a diabetic woman (Bennewitz 1824), the subject of a thesis in which the comment appeared, as translated from the Latin text, that there had been a "child…Hercules weighing twelve civil pounds…" (Hadden and Hillebrand 1989). Fifty-eight years later, in a survey of the few diabetic births that had been recorded in the interval, another such outcome was noted by Duncan (1882) who was impressed by a "dead foetus…described as enormous…its weight…extraordinary…." Death, it seems, was generally the fate of these large babies, so much so that they were expressively depicted (Fournier, cited by Lambie 1926) as "giant babies with feet of clay, unfit for life" [my translation].

As pregnancies of women with overt diabetes became more common during the early insulin years, reports of large babies born to them also became more common, but not to a clear extent. One author found that they occurred in 15–25% of births (Eastman 1946); another found it far more frequently, 45–75% (Bachman 1952), the sort of disagreement that perhaps delayed understanding of the phenomenon.

MACROSOMIA IN PREDIABETIC PREGNANCY

It was soon discovered that diabetic women often had very large babies not only in the years after but also in the years before developing the disease. What undoubtedly enabled this discovery was the mounting number of diabetic women living to mature ages (eg, Pedersen 1952), which permitted investigation of the outcome of their prediabetic pregnancies.

In what appears to be the first such report, Bix (1933) in Vienna identified 155 women who had developed diabetes in middle or later life and who recalled the birth weights of 608 of their babies of earlier pregnancies. Nearly 11% weighed 5 kg (11 lb) or more, in contrast with only 0.3% in a large group of overall births. Earlier though inconclusive reports of excessive neonatal weight were cited by Skipper (1933), who nevertheless said "It is no exaggeration to state that the birth of a child of excessive size always suggests the advisability of investigating the mother for diabetes."

Allen (1939) added another dimension when he presented evidence that giant babies were often born many years before clinical diabetes became manifest, a suggestion whose scope became clearer when corroborative reports started pouring forth. The first of these (Miller et al. 1944), which in several ways set the pattern for its successors, noted that 3.9% of 256 prediabetic babies weighed over 5 kg (a much lower percentage than Bix noted, perhaps because hospital records, not maternal memory, were relied on), but even so much greater than the control 0.07%. The latter was close to the 0.13% of full-term infants born in 1932–47 in a New York hospital (Nathanson 1950).

Miller et al.'s (1944) data also sustained Allen's (1939) preliminary finding that excessive birth weight occurred as long as 10 years before diabetic symptoms appeared. Another important point, whose possible meaning was not immediately appreciated, was that the frequency of excess birth weight seemed to increase with closeness to the time of onset of the diabetes (Miller 1946). In the next 10 years or so, many articles appeared that to one extent or another supported these general findings (eg, Kriss and Futcher 1948, Reis et al. 1950, Kade and Dietel 1952, Marquardson 1952, Moreau et al. 1955). Confirmation was not universal, however, others (eg, Barns and Morgans 1948) finding no significant difference between the mean birth weight of children of prediabetic women and the control or normal value.

The positive findings, while more convincing, varied in several respects, a major one still being in the frequency of big babies. This was due not only to variable weight criteria and uncritically accepted maternal memory (see Pyke 1962 for a discussion of this point), but probably mainly to differences among studies in various maternal attributes, whose association with birth weight was apparently not yet well recognized.

The trend of big babies before diabetes onset also differed among studies. Some saw no clear indication that big babies occurred earlier than in the years immediately preceding onset (Paton 1948; see Pirart 1955 for further references); others saw an increasing frequency, apparently throughout the prediabetic years (Moss and Mulholland 1951, Jackson 1952, Hagbard 1958); some the opposite, that generally the frequency of big babies decreased (Peel and Oakley 1949, Malins and FitzGerald 1965); and still others an elevated but constant level over most of the prediabetic period (Futcher and Long 1954, Rolland 1954, Pirart 1955). In fact, it was Pirart's (1955) finding of the last pattern that led him to suggest that the macrosomia was a constitutional feature of the prediabetic period and thus to call attention to the role of other factors as well as or even rather than the potential diabetes in its occurrence.

One of these was maternal obesity, whose frequent presence in the prediabetic period and whose possible association with neonatal macrosomia had been mentioned by several authors. Some thought it irrelevant (Miller 1945), but others found definite evidence of the association in retrospective studies (Futcher and Long 1954, Pirart 1955, Pomeranze et al. 1959) and in others of a different variety, discussed below.

PERINATAL MORTALITY IN PREDIABETIC PREGNANCY

Prediabetes was also believed to be associated with increased PNM. White (1935) was the first to mention this, in an incidental tabular entry, without further explanation, to the effect that 19% of 142 pregnancies of her patients ended in stillbirth, "prior to the onset of diabetes," in contrast with 6% in a contemporary series of unselected consecutive births. This received much attention and was followed over the next 25 years by many such reports (Mengert and Laughlin 1939, Miller et al. 1944, Barns and Morgans 1948, Rike and Fawcett 1948, Patterson and Burnstein 1949, Peel and Oakley 1949, McCain and Lester 1950, Zilliacus 1950, Moss and Mulholland 1951, Jackson 1952, Pedowitz and Shlevin 1952, Rolland 1954, Jokipii 1955, Moreau et al. 1955, Hagbard 1958).

Increased mortality also sometimes made its appearance years before—as many as 15 or more years before—the onset of diabetes, though it was most or only evident in the preceding 5 years (eg, Malins and FitzGerald 1965). This paralleled the common finding of macrosomia in the immediate years before the onset of diabetes. But there were also a large number of equivocal or negative findings, that is, of mortality frequencies in the prediabetic years similar to contemporary overall population levels (Palmer and Barnes 1945, Herzstein and Dolger 1946, Imerslund 1948, Reis et al. 1950, Kade and Dietel 1952, Marquardsen 1952, Pirart 1955).

Interestingly, it was agreed by all, even by some of those reporting an increased PNM rate, that spontaneous abortion defied this hazard, that its frequency was unaffected in prediabetic pregnancies (White 1935, Herzstein and Dolger 1946, Imerslund 1948, Paton 1948, Barns and Morgans 1948, McCain and Lester 1950, Moss and Mulholland 1951, Marquardsen 1952, Rolland 1954, Jokipii 1955, Moreau et al. 1955, Hagbard 1958). Much of the literature on these and other facets of the subject were adequately reviewed (Bachman 1952, Kyle 1963, Pedersen 1977).

Any attempted analysis of the association between prediabetes and harmful pregnancy outcome raises the question of the possible confounding role of numerous variables. But of far greater importance is the fundamental question of what was meant by prediabetes. Authors addressing this matter usually agreed that the term referred to the period preceding "known" diabetes or the "discovery" or the "clinical manifestation" or the "recognition" of diabetes. But it was not long before it was widely admitted that time of disease onset defined in this manner was far from precise.

This murkiness had been alluded to even during the first decades of the insulin era. For example, White (1935) admitted that some prediabetic pregnancies probably included cases of undiagnosed diabetes, and Herzstein and Dolger (1946) also not only conjectured that there was an "inability to determine the exact date of onset of diabetes," but reasoned that this "probably led to the inclusion of instances of existing diabetes...." Many others soon echoed this doubt (Reis et al. 1952, Hagbard 1961, Kyle 1963, Malins and FitzGerald 1965).

Understandably this fatally weakened the legitimacy of the concept of prediabetes, and made its supposed effects on pregnancy outcome doubtful. In fact the conclusion became inescapable that the evidence gave "very little support to the notion that the prediabetic state produces untoward effects on the fetus or infant" (West 1978, p. 343), and that all of the infelicitous outcomes attributed to prediabetes must actually be imputed to association with very early as yet unrecognized stages of diabetes itself. But this was not the whole story.

AN INSIDIOUS FORM OF DIABETES

The studies of prediabetes just discussed obviously were all made retrospectively. Starting with frankly diabetic women they looked back to adverse events occurring before the onset of the disease. But the significant fact noted in nearly all these reports was that diabetes onset was at advanced maternal ages (Miller 1945, Herzstein and Dolger 1946, Kriss and Futcher 1948, Paton 1948, Gilbert and Dunlop 1949). That is, most instances of the disease appeared near the end of the reproductive years or even postmenopausally; and furthermore were not insulin dependent. As was later better realized the form of diabetes that followed this precursory span was what came to be known as non–insulin-dependent or type 2 diabetes, a form mostly of late adult onset. Even then it was understood to become "manifest over a longer period" (Kirk et al. 1985) and frequently to have an "insidious or asymptomatic onset" (Knowler et al. 1983). The distinction between the late-occurring form of diabetes and the insulin-dependent early-onset variety, although explicitly enunciated only quite recently (Larsson et al. 1986, Orchard et al. 1986), was already recognized a century and more ago, when Lecorché (1885) wrote "Le diabète s'observe surtout chez elle au deux périodes extrême, avant la puberté, après la ménopause," and two generations later when Barns (1941) reiterated "...diabetes is much commoner in women during the latter part of the child-bearing period...which is largely responsible for the comparative rarity of pregnancy in the diabetic."

What can be called the initial phase of the story of prediabetes can be summarized as follows. It came to be widely believed that the prediabetic period was characterized by several untoward outcomes of pregnancy, especially excessive birth weight and increased perinatal mortality (Malins and FitzGerald 1965). But it was soon perceived that the bad outcomes happened mostly or only in the years immediately preceding diabetes onset, at a time when diabetes might already have been present, but undiscovered. This made for the realization of the virtual impossibility of establishing the "end" of the prediabetic period, which, combined with the accumulating negative evidence regarding the impact on perinatal mortality, led to abandoning further attempts to associate increased perinatal mortality, at any rate, with prediabetic pregnancies.

More persistent, however, was the belief that babies born during this period were often very heavy. That such occurrences were auguries of, or as they would be termed today, risk factors for potential diabetes was much weakened however, not only by the difficulty of clearly establishing the time of diabetes onset, but also by early indications of the complex entanglement of giant babies and potential diabetes with other factors, such as maternal predisposition to obesity (Futcher and Long 1954, Pirart 1955, Pedersen 1977). It was only in later studies that these confounding elements were to some degree disentangled. But explanation of the births of these big babies during the prediabetic period was still called for.

THE PROSPECTIVE APPROACH

The subject of prediabetes would seem to be far removed from the main strands of this work, pregestational and gestational diabetes. Nevertheless this topic, aside from its intrinsic interest, is being considered because, by a trail we shall be following, it eventually led to areas that are directly relevant.

It may have been doubt about the validity of retrospective studies that turned investigators to using a prospective approach. But the new studies in their turn raised other questions. In the latter type of study women whose reproductive history contained features indicating a risk of developing diabetes were glucose-tolerance tested (for more about this test, see Chapter 6 under "Establishing Blood

Glucose Standards") and an abnormal test response was taken as possible evidence of this potentiality.

At first the risk factors were mainly unexplained perinatal death and macrosomic babies, features held to be germane because they had been noted in studies of the prediabetic period (although by then the concept of prediabetes was largely discredited!). Diabetes in close family members and other features were added later (Hare 1985).

Many investigators now turned to the prospective approach and found that a sizable proportion (usually 20–40%) of such at-risk women, especially those who had had big babies, responded abnormally to the glucose tolerance test (summary of many citations will be found in Engleson and Lindberg 1962). The latter authors, as well as others, could therefore be excused for conforming to the prevailing opinion in considering that an aberrant test response in these cases "can be a sign of prediabetes in the mother, with risk of subsequent manifest diabetes." Except that this simplistic notion had already begun to be discounted.

As alluded to above, some maternal attributes had been found to be associated with big babies in prediabetic pregnancies. Complexities had already turned up in what may have been the first such prospective study, with one of the major ingredients, as previously suspected, being maternal obesity (Gilbert 1949). Many other variables, confounding the analysis, were discovered later. The full and numerous list was recorded by Larsson et al. (1986).

To put the situation in a nutshell, many mothers of big babies were obese, and obese mothers often had typically diabetic glucose-tolerance responses; but to take a foreglimpse, the diabetic fate of persons with such abnormal responses was still unclear. That is, the three elements—big babies, maternal obesity, and abnormal carbohydrate metabolism—were all closely correlated, but their causal relations were uncertain. The existence of this tight triadic state was often confirmed in succeeding years (Kritzer 1952, Lund and Weese 1953, Cretius 1957, FitzGerald et al. 1961, Mickal et al. 1966, O'Sullivan et al. 1966, Lunell and Persson 1972, Pehrson 1974, Horger et al. 1975, Jarrett 1981, Larsson et al. 1986). But in the final analysis none of the parts of the complex was found useful in predicting diabetic outcome in any one individual.

A multifactorial analysis of the entwined ingredients associated with excessive birth weight in pregnancies of women ostensibly at risk for development of diabetes may have made it possible to say whether big babies presaged its appearance. A few analyses were attempted, but consensus was not reached as to any one best prediabetic notifier (O'Sullivan et al. 1966, Lubetzki et al. 1973, O'Sullivan and Mahan 1966). There was little doubt, however, that a big baby alone was a very poor predictor of the risk of developing the noninsulin dependent form of the disease (Larsson et al. 1986). Thus, although prospective study of risk factors was capable to an extent of characterizing populations, when faced by the familiar hindrance of the principle of indeterminacy, it was powerless to predict the fate of individuals. Whether part of the difficulty was related to the uncertainties of estimating gestational blood glucose level (a subject discussed in Chapter 6) is unclear (Victor 1974, Larsson et al. 1986, Harlass et al. 1991, Phillipou 1991).

Despite the seeming fruitlessness of these many years of study by devoted researchers something of positive value emerged. The glucose tolerance testing of pregnant women with the risk features mentioned above led investigators to stumble onto the fact that a considerable proportion of all pregnant women have aberrant responses to such testing. In all fairness, this revelation was preceded (but not well appreciated) by a study that noted frequent abnormal responses in normal pregnant women, a study that was prompted by recalling that preexisting diabetes may be worsened by pregnancy (Hurwitz and Jensen 1946). This discovery opened up a new area of concern, carbohydrate disturbance exhibited during pregnancy, or gestational diabetes, and a new school of research, to which Chapter 6 is devoted.

PREDIABETES AND CONGENITAL MALFORMATIONS

A considerable number of reports noted the birth of congenitally malformed children during the prediabetic period, which were said or inferred to have been due to this state. These were roughly of two kinds, single cases and surveys. Both suffered from the same deficiencies: the abnormalities were without consistency or pattern, the pregnancies producing them preceded the onset of diabetic symptoms by months to years, and so on.

The following few examples of case reports give an idea of the looseness of thinking about what constituted proof of prediabeticity. The earliest such report was of a child with congenital heart disease born 6 months before the clinical onset of diabetes (Barns 1941). The next was a hydrocephalus in a big baby whose mother was identified as prediabetic either because she had previously had a big baby or an abnormal glucose tolerance response in the index pregnancy (Lund and Weese 1953).

Like instances were cited by Hoet (1954): three infants with spina bifida and meningocele of a woman considered to have been prediabetic at the time of these pregnancies because 3 months after the third one she displayed a typical abnormal glucose tolerance curve. This was corroborated by the fact that her grandmother was a diabetic and had 6 neonatal deaths in 14 pregnancies and that in her fourth pregnancy she received insulin and had a perfectly normal child. Hoet et al. (1960) later mentioned other convincing examples of this sort.

Further cases concerned children with skeletal abnormalities, one with lower-limb defects whose mother became diabetic 6 years after the birth (McCracken 1965), one with lumbosacral absence whose 38-year-old mother was discovered to have a high blood glucose level 1 year after the birth (Kalitzki 1965), and another with a similar condition whose mother had an abnormal glucose tolerance on the second day postpartum (Thalhammer et al. 1968). Incidentally these three children were almost certainly brought to attention by the then-recent reports of similar abnormalities in children of diabetic women (Lenz and Maier 1964, Kučera et al. 1965, Passarge 1965), discussed in Chapters 9 and 14. Even quite recently the same allegations were made, namely, that women with children with various defects who had "slightly elevated blood glucose levels" and a family history of type 2 diabetes were "at risk for diabetes" (Van Allen and Myhre 1991, van der Wal and Mulder 1993).

Survey studies also led to such conclusions. A report of 3.2% malformations in offspring of prediabetic pregnancies was contrasted with 0.5% in nondiabetic pregnancies (Kade and Dietel 1952), an early example of an erroneous deduction based on a gross underestimate of the background malformation frequency, not infrequently committed in later years as well. Hagbard (1958), making the same mistake, reported 4.0% of "serious" malformations compared with 1.7% in controls, but giving the finding a logical basis, believed that it was probably due to "transient unrecognized diabetes during pregnancy." Carrington (1960) made the interesting comment that her findings were similar to Hagbard's, about 4%, but only if minor malformations were also considered. It should be recalled that malformation frequencies reported in these prediabetic pregnancies were close to that of major malformations ordinarily noted in the general population (Kalter and Warkany 1983).

Turning things around, several studies examined the frequency of prediabetes (ie, of the usual features considered indicative of diabetes risk) in mothers of infants with specific malformations or malformations in general. Downing and Goldberg (1956a,b) found that 20–30% of operated children with cardiac septal defects had immediate family members with diabetes, but not any of their mothers, who ostensibly were considered latent diabetics. This investigation lacked controls, however, whose importance was clearly pointed out by a similar study that failed to find a difference in the frequency of diabetes in the relatives of children with and without congenital heart disease (Fraser 1960).

Other surveys of infants with various specific malformations had similar findings (López-Quijada and Carrion 1974, Goldman 1976), including one in which 75% of children with Down syndrome had mothers with evidence of prediabetes (Navarette et al. 1967)! Such evidence, in the form of increased immunological antagonism to insulin, in otherwise asymptomatic individuals, was found in many mothers of children with certain defects (Wilson and Vallance-Owen, 1966, Vallance-Owen et al. 1967). In studies 20 years later, of insulin immunogenicity in pregnant diabetic women and their fetuses, higher anti-insulin antibody level was not associated with spontaneous abortion, perinatal mortality, or major and minor congenital malformation (Mylvaganam et al. 1983).

Several surveys with negative findings deserve to be mentioned. Wilkerson (1959) and Barnes (1961) found no significant difference in malformation frequency in children of mothers with abnormal glucose tolerance and control mothers; Neave (1967, 1984) found a statistically insignificant difference between the control malformation frequency and that in infants of mothers diagnosed as diabetic after 35 years of age and thus prediabetic when pregnant.

This chapter can fitly be closed with a quotation from Hadden (1979): "Untreated asymptomatic diabetes does not often progress to frank diabetes. This...casts some doubt on the whole concept of a pre-diabetic phase...."

6

GESTATIONAL DIABETES

Gestational diabetes was "discovered" only 39 years ago—in the sense that it was not until 1961 that it was given a name and thus became a definite entity. This late emergence into specificity should be surprising, since the condition was noted over 100 years ago. But its long relegation to the sidelines is understandable because it was only fairly recently that some of the demanding problems presented by overt diabetes in pregnancy began to relent and allow some attention to be turned elsewhere.

Compensating for this early neglect, the last 39 years have seen a great surge of interest in the condition and an outpouring of writings devoted to it—so much so that this minideluge was derided by a long-time worker in this vineyard. Using the current jargon in a paper that appeared soon after his death, he commented, "Studies relating to gestational diabetes constitute a growth industry and the many publications flowing therefrom have done little to clarify our thinking" (Drury 1989). So, this chapter opens by asking how this proliferation came about and why clarification has been long frustrated.

WHAT IS GESTATIONAL DIABETES?

As has been known for a long time and is ritually recalled every so often, diabetes and pregnancy can be associated in two ways: pregnancy can occur in a woman who is already diabetic, and diabetes can occur in a woman who is already pregnant. This sometimes newly recalled distinction is an important one.

The latter—diabetes appearing or discovered for the first time during pregnancy—has been called gestational diabetes since O'Sullivan (1961) coined the term. He explained that it referred to an asymptomatic condition signaled by a range of concentrations of blood glucose lying between a borderline area at the upper reaches of normality on the one hand and unequivocal diabetes on the other.[3] The

3 Before the term was introduced, pregnancies of diabetic women not requiring insulin, which is the case for most gestational diabetics, were designated White class A, even though it was not stated whether in many of them the condition conformed to White's (1949) original intent that this denotation referred to diabetes of pregestational origin. Calling such pregnancies class A continued after 1961, but less and less so, until it was just about replaced by the newer term. In this section, regardless of how named in the various publications, all pregnancies that could possibly be identified as such are subsumed into the category gestational diabetes.

fundamental problem in studying this phenomenon has been to define the nebulous state "normality" in order to know where to draw the line separating it from that which lies even just beyond. The primary tasks—of coming to some agreement about definition and classification—took time to accomplish and even now are not fully resolved. But in the beginning there was another problem.

Early Difficulties

The earliest difficulty was in agreeing that diabetes sometimes had an onset during pregnancy at all. Duncan (1882), summing up the 20 or so cases of diabetes associated with pregnancy that he had personal or other knowledge of, stated—the soon-to-become truism—"Diabetes may come on during pregnancy...[and] pregnancy may occur during diabetes." The first of these possibilities was brought to his attention by about half these cases, it can be construed, being of intragestational origin.

Questions about Duncan's interpretation soon arose.[4] Stengel (1904) suspected that in some instances of diabetes developing during pregnancy, it was only its "earliest manifestations [that] were discovered during that condition." Eshner (1907), voicing other hesitations, reasoned most sagaciously that when such occurrences were recognized in the first half of pregnancy, the diabetes may have existed before it was detected.

Williams (1909) concurred and, going even further, held that the apparent infrequency of diabetes with onset before pregnancy was an illusion resulting from the failure to detect preexisting mild or inapparent instances of the disease; and supported this contention with a collection from the literature of 66 "definite" cases of diabetes in pregnant women, 55 of which he considered were present before conception and persisted afterward. The contrary belief, that diabetes frequently arose during pregnancy, was due, he claimed, to the difficulty of distinguishing between diabetes and the physiological glycosuria of pregnancy.

Before turning to this glycosuria, which confused the early students of diabetes, a brief discussion is called for of a common feature of the form of diabetes that first appears during pregnancy.

Maternal Age in Diabetic Pregnancy

In commenting on the general scarcity of diabetes in pregnancy, Eshner (1907), making an observation that, as has so often been the case, would be repeated years later, noted that it was so "principally because diabetes occurs as a rule at a later period of life than pregnancy usually takes place." Or, as Williams (1909) put it, "because the disease usually occurs after menopause." Diabetes appearing in later age had already been recognized some years before, when Lecorché (1885) remarked that in his experience of 114 cases of diabetes in women, 70 of them

4 Such questions were resurrected in later years and continued to arouse debate, as will be seen later in this text.

developed after menses had ceased; furthermore he described these instances—again with a prevision that would not be overtaken for several generations—as having (translating as literally as possible) a static manner, an attenuated form, and a slow course, characteristics of what is today recognized as noninsulin-dependent diabetes, in distinction to the type that occurs at younger ages, which is overt and serious.

Glycosuria

This admixture of diabetes types—earlier or later appearing, predating or occurring during pregnancy—was further complicated by questions raised by the phenomenon of glycosuria. It had been shown half a century earlier that appreciable amounts of sugar may be found in the urine of pregnant women (Blot 1856), but the nature of its presence was uncertain. Various interpretations had been given, some regarding it as indicative of mild diabetes or even presaging worse (Williams 1909). This dire outlook, incidentally, continued for a long time (Allen 1939, Hoet 1954).

One of the lesser sources of the confusion, hardly ever absent from human affairs, was merely semantics. One example: in an article obviously mistitled "glycosuria gravidarum" Ruoff (1903) listed the symptoms supposedly to be found in this condition: polyuria, great thirst, emaciation, vulvar pruritus, maternal mortality of nearly 50%, frequent fetal and neonatal death, as well as sugar in the urine. This list makes it clear that Ruoff's paper was really concerned largely with true diabetes. Nevertheless he persisted in ignoring the significance of his having been able to collect from various sources relatively few pregnancies with such symptoms, and noted irrelevantly that others had found that as many as 50% of pregnancies were affected by glycosuria.

It was understood, of course, that there could be no mistaking the diagnosis of diabetes if the glycosuria was excessive, was accompanied by definite diabetic symptoms, or persisted after delivery. Otherwise glycosuria still presented a puzzle, and despite considerable study in the ensuing decades (Eastman 1946), some could still ask at a relatively late date "is it diabetic or non-diabetic?" (King, discussion following Selman 1932).

On the whole by the mid-1920s, this uncertainty seemed to be dissipating. By then it was fairly well established that trace amounts of glucose could be found in urine quite frequently during uncomplicated pregnancy (Wiener 1924, Crook 1925, Lambie 1926). It was generally accepted that it occurred most often in the absence of elevated blood glucose levels, first appeared during the last trimester of pregnancy, and disappeared rather abruptly soon after delivery. These characteristics were further substantiated over the years, especially by the use of chromatographic methods (Rowe et al. 1931, Flynn et al. 1953, Davison and Lovedale 1974).

This state has been called "nondiabetic mellituria"(Marble 1985), a term used as early as 96 years ago (Stengel 1904), affirming the realization that it was asymptomatic and unrelated to the disease diabetes. At present there are different opinions about its basis; it may be due to the markedly increased glucose load presented to the kidneys by the increased renal plasma flow that normally accompanies some pregnancies or to increased glomerular filtration together with impaired tubular reabsorptive capacity for filtered glucose (Cunningham et al. 1993).

Diabetogenicity of Pregnancy

This glycosuria is a spontaneous or physiological state and occurs far from universally in pregnant women. But there is another kind as well. Late in the 19th century, it was discovered that glycosuria is induced in virtually all pregnant women upon ingesting a large amount of carbohydrate (see Höst 1925); so constant was this response that it was even regarded as a possible way of detecting pregnancy. Much study of this artificial condition during later years led to the finding that it was preceded by hyperglycemia (Ehrenfest 1924).

In the light of this finding, it is not surprising that a blood glucose test devised some years earlier was soon adapted to the diabetes arena,[5] and that, at a time when some difficulty of differentiating glycosuria from diabetes still lingered, it was found that this task could be made more manageable by determining the glucose content of blood, whose aid in this diagnosis, it was said in the heartfelt words of another age, "conduces to peace of mind" (Joslin 1923). By not long thereafter, it could be asserted that the ability to make such estimations had eliminated diagnostic uncertainty (Walker 1928).

Side by side with the application of this newly devised tool for the diagnosis and care of pregnant diabetic women were numerous studies that attempted to characterize and quantify the attribute of blood glucose level during pregnancy in general. Many such efforts were made over the following 20 years or more, but when summarized by Cobley and Lancaster (1955) they were judged to be "confusing" in their inconsistent findings overall and especially in describing variations at particular times during pregnancy. Like many others, these authors found no evidence of hyperglycemia in their large and relatively unselected sample of pregnant women, but as had also been noted previously they did find that the pregnant state exerted certain distortions on carbohydrate metabolism. A main finding was that blood glucose elevation following glucose ingestion was sometimes delayed in returning to the basal level and that this unusual response occurred especially during the last 2 months of pregnancy.

Many earlier observations of disturbances of carbohydrate metabolism first being clinically manifested during pregnancy and all of their signs and symptoms disappearing after delivery were also often interpreted as indicating that pregnancy had a diabetogenic effect (Berkeley et al. 1938; see Hagbard 1956 for additional reports of such observations).

Such findings soon became intertwined with questions regarding carbohydrate metabolism during pregnancy. For example, Hoet (1954), in reviewing the then current understanding of the "disturbances in carbohydrate metabolism" that can appear during pregnancy, especially late pregnancy, offered the explanation that

---

5 The year 1917 saw the introduction of the oral glucose tolerance test simultaneously by Hamman and Hirschmann (1917) in the US and by Jacobsen (Lundbaeck 1962) in Denmark.

pregnancy imposes a "functional burden," which is further intensified by a diabetic tendency. To this, Jackson (1961) added the qualified concurrence that there was no evidence that normal pregnancy was "diabetogenic," except temporarily when combined with a situation such as prediabetes. This was a twist on his earlier view that somewhat increased blood glucose levels late in pregnancy were a "warning of prediabetes" (Jackson 1952).

A cautionary note was injected into all this by Burt (1960), who advanced the possibility that the unusual glucose tolerance responses noted in some pregnant women were due to variables introduced by the intestinal absorption of the orally administered glucose. Nevertheless he was of the opinion that pregnancy is diabetogenic, at least as expressed by a loss of reactivity to insulin in late pregnancy (Burt 1956), a fact now well established (Cousins 1991a).

The evolution of the disputatious question of the so-called diabetogenicity of normal pregnancy is intertwined with the even more contentious one of prediabetes, which must be returned to briefly. After years of the fruitless examination of the earlier records of pregnancies of individuals who had later developed diabetes, it became obvious that the nearly unanimous belief that such prediabetic pregnancies were particularly subject to adverse outcome was erroneous (see above). But before the idea of prediabetes became entirely discredited, it was discovered, almost fortuitously, that "disturbances" of carbohydrate metabolism were common during normal pregnancy.

In time, this disturbance—mild glucose intolerance—was accepted as a "part of normal pregnancy" (Freinkel et al. 1985). The question then followed, as these authors framed it, "How intolerant does the pregnant women have to become to be deemed abnormal?" However this excess blood glucose level is defined, which was and apparently remains undecided (West 1975, O'Sullivan 1980, Schwartz and Brenner 1982, Naylor 1989), such an excess labels a women as having gestational diabetes.

The range of prevalences of gestational diabetes in various populations, races, and groups with several exceptions (Beischer et al. 1991, Coustan 1991, Berkowitz et al. 1992), has proved to be fairly narrow. Depending on the factors influencing it—the limit assigned to normality, the character of the population surveyed, and so on—usually about 1–5% of unselected pregnant women have been found to be hyperglycemic during the last half or third of pregnancy (Sepe et al. 1985, Cocilovo 1989).

Establishing Blood Glucose Standards

Investigators in the 1940s and 1950s were aware that carbohydrate metabolism was frequently mildly disturbed during pregnancy, a situation called the diabetogenic effect of that state. But they were unsure whether or not it was merely a physiological by-product of pregnancy itself.

Thus, it is not clear when the entity gestational diabetes was first "discovered," especially since earlier investigators may not have had the same concept in mind as O'Sullivan (1961) did in coining the term. For example, Hurwitz and Jensen (1946) called the diabetes that often began during late pregnancy "true diabetes," though in some of their patients the blood glucose curve returned to normal some time after delivery (Hurwitz and Irving 1937).

It was also remarked that following glucose ingestion by normal pregnant women, blood glucose was often elevated in the later trimesters, but mostly only at 2 hours thereafter (Hurwitz and Jensen 1946), which prompted the proposal that such high levels be considered diagnostic only if they persisted for 3 hours (Hurwitz and Higano 1952). This was an early hint of the complexities that would necessitate the establishment of arbitrary criteria for the diagnosis of this entity. (Time and time again one finds that older studies have been forgotten and that their findings are echoed later as novel revelations. Conspicuous in this respect are unknowing or unacknowledged repetitions of many of the findings described just above, eg, by Lind et al. 1991).

A stab at setting up such diagnostic standards was made by O'Sullivan (1961) in the first of his many influential papers. The merit of his approach was that he clearly spelled out what he considered gestational diabetes to consist of, beginning with the subtitle of his paper, "Unsuspected, asymptomatic diabetes in pregnancy." Two criteria for this judgment were specified: first, a concentration of blood glucose must be present that "removes it from the borderline areas that are subject to disagreement;" and second, as the term indicated, not only must it arise or first be detected during pregnancy, but be "temporary" or "transient," that is, disappear when pregnancy ended. That this sort of diabetes was indeed overwhelmingly transitory was shown by a very large proportion of cases reverting to normal soon after delivery (eg, O'Sullivan 1979), regardless of what later studies found it may indicate for the future. Although postpartum remission has been considered a sine qua non (eg, Hadden 1979, Hare 1989), it will be seen later that difficulties arose with this rule and attempts were made to give it less weight.

Vagaries of Blood Glucose Level

Since the glucose tolerance test plays so major a role in the story of gestational diabetes, what it consists of and what its shortcomings are must be described and discussed. The need for a clinical test to evaluate carbohydrate tolerance led about 75 years ago to devising such a procedure. Over the years several variations of the test were introduced, most commonly oral and intravenous tests, which, despite both being flawed (Moyer and Womack 1950), vied for acceptability. In time the oral test won out and obtained the imprimatur of the Second International Workshop Conference on Gestational Diabetes (1985).[6]

Nevertheless, the test is controversial and complicated by three sources of difficulty: the procedure itself, the criteria for selecting those to be tested, and

6 The test consisted of the following: after eating a diet containing 250 g carbohydrate daily for 3 days and then fasting overnight, registrants consumed 100 g of a glucose solution. Blood glucose levels were determined soon after the fasting period and 1, 2, and 3 hours thereafter. Excluding women with previously known diabetes, classic diabetic symptoms, and blood sugar levels exceeding 300 mg/dL, those with or exceeding one or more levels of 110, 170, 120, and 110 mg/dL, respectively, at the four times mentioned met the criterion for classification as gestational diabetic.

defining abnormality. Attempts have been made to deal with the first; the second, though paid much attention, is unresolved; and the last remains in dispute.

The Procedure

In essence, the purpose of the test is to determine how quickly an induced hyperglycemia is reversed, as a gauge of the presence and degree of a disturbed carbohydrate metabolism. It is done by measuring the glucose content of blood, first after an overnight fast (the fasting or basal level), then at several intervals after oral ingestion of a specified amount of glucose. Clearly, many variables can intrude on this general procedure (Keen 1991, Schmidt et al. 1994, Schwartz et al. 1994): the composition of the food eaten on the several days before the fast, the length of the fast, the component tested (blood, plasma), its source (vein, capillary), the dose of the glucose load and the volume and composition of the liquid containing it, the length and number of intervals at which blood samples are taken following glucose ingestion, ambient temperature, the analytical method used to measure the blood glucose concentration (Schwartz and Brenner 1982, Naylor 1989).

These factors can have a greater or lesser impact on the glucose determination, and obviously it was necessary for the sake of comparison that a standardized procedure be agreed upon. Efforts to reach such agreement were made over the years, and at various intervals newer versions promulgated (Meinert 1972, First and Second International Workshop-Conferences on Gestational Diabetes 1980, 1985, Metzger et al. 1991). For some of the more important variables, this was achieved: the prescribed fasting period is now usually about 12 hours,[7] the measurement is made with plasma, and enzymatic assay techniques are used. One influential variable, the amount of glucose load administered, is still not uniform from place to place, being mostly 100 g in North America, 75 g widely in Europe, and 50 g most commonly in Australia. Authoritative suggestions advocated that 75 g be universally adopted (Diabetic Pregnancy Study Group of the European Association for the Study of Diabetes 1989, Metzger et al. 1991).

The Subjects

Other variables, no doubt at least as significant and usually far less controllable than those just noted, have to do with the subjects themselves and how they are selected for testing. The earliest selection criteria were predominantly the supposed clinical indicators of "potential" diabetes, adopted with little or no

7 Pregnant women are apparently considered to be far less frail today than they once were when it "was found impracticable to make the patients report fasting from the night before, as many pregnant women cannot starve long without feeling faint" (Williams and Wills 1929).

modification from the expiring concept of prediabetes, with the one addition of a preliminary blood glucose test (Wilkerson and Remein 1957).[8]

Analysis revealed that most of the clinical indicators were of little use in identifying individual pregnant women as at risk for gestational diabetes (O'Sullivan et al. 1973), a finding supported by others (eg, Marquette et al. 1985). It was recommended therefore that screening be limited to the most indicative item, the preliminary blood glucose test (O'Sullivan et al. 1973) and this has been widely accepted, especially for economic and other reasons (Carpenter and Coustan 1982, American Diabetes Association 1980, Metzger et al. 1991).

[The question of how extensive the screening of pregnant women for impaired glucose tolerance or gestational diabetes should be still has not been agreed upon, the underlying difficulties apparently having mostly to do with pragmatic considerations (Jarrett 1993)].

The one maternal feature incontrovertibly found to affect glucose tolerance was age, advances in which were associated with increased frequency of gestational diabetes (O'Sullivan et al. 1973), as was found true for glucose intolerance generally (Wilkerson and O'Sullivan 1963, West et al. 1964, Krall 1965, Harris 1988).

Although this association had been noted frequently (Macafee and Beischer 1974, Granat et al. 1979, Marquette et al. 1985, McFarland and Case 1985, Coustan et al. 1989, Jacobson and Cousins 1989), it may be confounded by the often coexistent maternal obesity (Macafee and Beischer 1974), whose separate impact has proved difficult to analyze.

A topic much considered and of particular relevance concerns the optimal time during pregnancy to perform the glucose tolerance test, that is, the time that will identify most gestational diabetics. This is of consequence because of the frequent observation that the blood glucose level varies over the course of pregnancy, generally increasing with advancing time during the last two trimesters (Lind et al. 1973, Merkatz et al. 1980, Jovanovic and Peterson 1985, Benjamin et al. 1986).

Other inherent sources of the variability that make identification of those with aberrant blood glucose levels problematic are factors such as race, ethnicity, geography, and the like (Hadden 1985, Sepe et al. 1985, Cocilovo 1989, Jacobson and Cousins 1989, Berkowitz et al. 1992), and not least of all, emotional factors (Yudkin et al. 1990, Campbell et al. 1992, Monteros et al. 1993) and intraindividual variability (West et al. 1964, McDonald et al. 1965, O'Sullivan and Mahan 1966, Campbell et al. 1974, Beischer et al. 1991, Dooley et al. 1991, Harlass 1991). In the end, as O'Sullivan et al. (1973) confessed, "There is no perfect way of screening for chronic disease entities. Economic, pragmatic, and individual factors are always the final determinants...."

8 Namely, diabetes in the immediate family, a history of having borne a baby weighing 4.1 kg (9 lb) or more, a history of fetal or neonatal death or a child with a congenital anomaly, prematurity, toxemia (ie, excessive weight gain, hypertension, and proteinuria) in two or more pregnancies—all of which it will be readily recognized originated with studies of the phenomenon of prediabetes—plus a novel one: a venous blood sugar of 130 mg/dL or more 1 hour after taking 50 g glucose by mouth.

The Definition

The ultimate difficulty concerns definition, and this is tied to the nature of the blood glucose characteristic itself. Since its distribution in a random sample of individuals in most populations is by and large unimodal[9] (O'Sullivan et al. 1964, Gaspart 1985, Neilson et al. 1991, Tchobroutsky 1991), much as is true, for example, of blood pressure (Roccella et al. 1987) and other physiological characteristics, there is no point on this curve that can be designated as the absolute borderline between the upper limit of normality and the lower one of abnormality.

Thus, the diagnosis for any given woman with a blood glucose level within the region of this vaguely defined borderland is bound to be unclear (Stern et al. 1985). As said years ago, though every diabetic has a high prolonged glucose tolerance curve, not every such curve is indicative of diabetes (Mosenthal and Barry 1950); the same is patently true of the gestational diabetes phenomenon.

How relevant this murkiness can be is indicated by the likelihood that the blood glucose level in the majority of supposedly gestational diabetic women is not "excessive," but lies at the upper end of the normal distribution of this variable in pregnancy (Hadden 1975, 1979, Lind 1984, Buchanan 1991). A way around this difficulty was perhaps to partition gestational diabetes into degrees of severity, as recommended by Beard and Hoet (1982), and to determine whether the frequency of any associated fetal morbidity or mortality is similarly graded. The many problems entailed in grappling with epidemiological aspects of gestational diabetes were addressed in an excellent overview (Keen 1991).

CHANGES IN DEFINITION OF GESTATIONAL DIABETES

Almost simultaneous with the adoption of the term gestational diabetes came elaborations on its concept, based on evidence of differences in its form and degree. Early investigators pointing to such heterogeneity divided pregnant women with abnormal glucose tolerance responses into those with lesser and those with greater degrees of intolerance (a small minority of cases), the former having blood glucose levels that could be restored to normal limits in most cases by dietary means alone and the latter requiring in addition insulin for its accomplishment (Pedowitz and Shlevin 1964). These differences in degree of metabolic aberration, they felt, carried differences in fetal risk—a subject to be considered later in this chapter. Still, in the majority of cases the glucose tolerance in both forms reverted to normal soon after pregnancy ended.

This was the earliest exercise in dividing gestational diabetes into different forms according to expression, severity, natural history, and etiology; and in recommending different courses of medical and obstetric care for them. Later efforts of this sort were all more or less variations on this one, in that they distinguished between the great majority, who had a normal fasting blood glucose level, and could be managed without special effort or by dietary means alone, the remainder, who had an elevat-

9 Exceptions to this unimodality have been found in a few populations with high incidences of type 2 diabetes (Stern 1988).

ed fasting value, which was itself sometimes subdivided according to its degree and need for insulin (Dolger et al. 1966, Zarowitz and Moltz 1966, Stallone and Ziel 1974, Pedersen 1977, pp. 63 et seq., Mestman 1980, Beard and Hoet 1982, Freinkel et al. 1985). Questions later arose about the benefits and safety of insulin therapy in mild cases of gestational diabetes (Hare 1991, Jarrett 1992).

After standing for more than 20 years, the basic definition of gestational diabetes began to undergo change. The first sign of discontent with the standard appeared in an article dealing with an assortment of terminological questions (Hadden 1979). While accepting the two fundamental attributes of the condition—onset or recognition during pregnancy and reversion to normality afterward—the author broadened the definition by allowing the condition to be symptomatic as well as nonsymptomatic. This seems to exaggerate the importance of the few trivial signs that may appear.

This was a minor alteration compared with the modifications introduced next. The summary of the First International Workshop-Conference on Gestational Diabetes Mellitus (1980) omitted what had up to then been considered one of the two hallmarks of the condition—the return to normality of the blood glucose level after parturition. No reason was given for this radical change, but one may hazard a guess that it had a practical basis, namely, to obviate the diagnostic quandary that ensued from patients very frequently not returning to be seen by physicians after giving birth. The Second Workshop (1985) went further and made this feature explicit, by adding the phrase "whether or not...the condition persists after pregnancy." (A participant in the meeting told me that the supposition made above was correct: the purpose of the addition was the pragmatic one of eliminating the necessity of having to wait till after the delivery to be sure of the diagnosis.) The Third Workshop (Metzger et al. 1991) retained this version without further change. Other reasons mentioned for these changes were that it would eliminate "obfuscating variables" and facilitate "worldwide standardization" (Freinkel et al. 1986).

It was inevitable that the upshot of these modifications would be to expand the concept of gestational diabetes and thus gather within its folds a heterogeneous assortment of conditions. It is not surprising that very soon after these changes were made, the inference was drawn that if the "condition"did not return to normal after delivery it probably was of the sort that predated pregnancy (Oats and Beischer 1986). And in fact the inclination of the conferences had anticipated this logical step by also stating that the definition "does not exclude the possibility that the glucose intolerance may have antedated the pregnancy." Lind (1984) had even earlier predicted that such loosening of the definition would lead in this direction, by permitting inclusion of instances of glucose intolerance etiologically different from that of the majority. These might consist of forms more strictly endogenous and hence more likely to be persistent. Gestational diabetes—if little else about it can be agreed upon—is understood typically to be a disorder of late gestation (Hare 1989). On the other hand, examples of the disorder that would be included under the enlarged rubric are those usually first detected early in pregnancy (as was noted long ago by Williams 1909), such as mild glucose intolerance predating pregnancy, unmasked or precocious type 2 or noninsulin-dependent diabetes, and slowly evolving type 1 diabetes (Freinkel et al. 1986, Harris 1988, Buchanan 1991, Hare 1994).

It is a wry comment on the sluggish development of ideas about the phenomenon being discussed here that some of the same confusion about terminology, classification, and definition that investigators, not surprisingly, were attempting to sort out 90 years ago seems still to be befuddling their present-day counterparts. Fortunately, it would appear, the definitional aggrandizement being promulgated, wisely, is sometimes being ignored (eg, Philipson et al. 1985).

The latest American Diabetes Association and World Health Organization definitions of diabetes, which have departed from classification based on extent of insulin requirement and now recommend a pathogenesis-based one, continue to insist that the definition does not exclude the possibility that the glucose intolerance may antedate pregnancy (Wareham and O'Rahilly 1998).

GESTATIONAL DIABETES AND THE WHITE CLASSIFICATION

Beginning with Pedowitz and Shlevin's (1964) division of gestational diabetes by severity, further subgroupings were introduced by various authors with labels such as classes I and II, A1 and A2, A and AB, and so on. It was partly such assignments that engendered the confusion between the mildest degree of gestational diabetes and the category of minimal abnormality of carbohydrate metabolism that White (1949) in her classificatory system called class A. Thus we must now pause to consider her system.[10] Its purpose was to grade the severity of ostensibly overt diabetes according to its chemical, clinical, and pathological features. The mildest degree, called class A, consisted of and was identified by a response to the glucose tolerance test that deviated but slightly from normal and required no insulin and very little or no dietary regulation for its management. As originally formulated, class A, like all the other, more severe, grades of White's classification, explicitly postulated the existence of the condition in the nonpregnant state. In this respect, her class A was clearly distinct from the mild, nonsymptomatic condition arising or diagnosed during pregnancy known as gestational diabetes. (What brought such nonsymptomatic individuals to her attention in the first place was never clarified.)

White was able to devise and use such a "prepregnancy" classification because she worked in the specialized Joslin diabetes clinic, which was attended by patients from very early age and very early in the course of the disease. For example, of the 525 patients seen at the clinic in 1936–1951, 60.5% had the disease from childhood or adolescence, and 53% of the females were nulliparae (White 1952). Other investigators, working in different settings, most often public maternity hospitals, only saw women who were already pregnant and might not know their prepregnancy status.

This pre-/intra-pregnancy distinction was soon greatly blurred or lost, however, since over the years many physicians, ignoring or impatient with the strict application of the term, classified their patients as class A diabetics even though they did not indicate (probably did not know) whether the women had been diagnosed prior to pregnancy or not. This confusion was encouraged by White herself,

---

10 The White system of classifying diabetes in pregnancy is fully described elsewhere (see p. 71).

Table 6.1 Frequency of White Class A in Pregnant Diabetic Women Diagnosed Before or During Pregnancy

Era	America		Europe	
	Total Pregnancies	% Class A	Total Pregnancies	% Class A
1940s + 1950s	4583	15.9	1176	5.0
1960s	2442	25.4	5046	18.5
1970s	2861	47.7	2897	33.2
1980s to mid 1990s	3963	60.9	2313	25.3

Data from publications classifying patients by the White system.

since she soon weakened her definition by sometimes omitting the prepregnancy stipulation or stating that the condition could be diagnosed either before or during pregnancy (White 1952, 1974).

Many authors, failing to recognize the distinction, called attention to the increasing frequency of class A among their diabetic patients, without explaining it (eg, Ayromlooi et al. 1977, Corwin 1979, Mølsted-Pedersen 1984, Olofsson et al. 1984). (This increase is clearly illustrated by contrasting the 5% of White's 1935 patients of childbearing age with onset of diabetes during pregnancy with Gabbe et al.'s 1977 finding that "gestational diabetes constitutes 90% of all diabetes in pregnancy".) The upshot was a continuing increase in the proportion of pregnant diabetic women who were put in class A, although, as Table 6.1 shows, this trend was much more prevalent and grew to greater heights in America than Europe.

The blurring of class A and gestational diabetes is unfortunate. In my opinion the distinction is not merely an academic one, because although sharing secondary, metabolic features the differences between the two is probably meaningful. Thus, gestational diabetes is a response of certain individuals to the pregnant state, regardless of what it may or may not presage, whereas class A diabetes is presumably endogenous and independent of pregnancy or other stimuli.

To get out of this sometimes semantic thicket Pedersen (1977, pp. 61, 64) suggested that the term class A be considered a comprehensive one, subsuming all "diabetes of such a mild degree that treatment with insulin was not felt necessary" and thus comprised cases diagnosed both prior to and during pregnancy. But this did not address the possibility voiced in the preceding paragraph. Even with Pedersen's outlook there was disagreement. Hadden (1979) in his explication of the classification of asymptomatic pregnancy in diabetes averred that White's class A was not identical with asymptomatic diabetic pregnancy, but did not clearly explain his demurral.

Has the class A designation outlived its usefulness? The White system as a whole, right from the beginning, was felt to be confusing and difficult to apply (Pedersen 1954a, Jones 1956). Because the term gestational diabetes has been taken to be equivalent to and used interchangeably with class A (eg, Gabbe et al. 1977, Mølsted-Pedersen 1984) the former less equivocal expression has largely displaced the latter.

But a recent proposal may still rescue it, one that brings the saga full circle and returns it to its original signification. Hare (1989), a quondam colleague of White's, to damp the still existing confusion and try to preserve a place for it, would categorize class A separately from gestational diabetes, stipulating that it should refer, *mirabile dictu*, strictly to diet-managed diabetes of pregestational onset. Broaching new thoughts on the subject, however, Hare (1994) next expressed the opinion that the separate categorization of gestational and pregestational diabetes "diminished the utility of class A," based on the fact that since 1980 no class A patient had been seen at the Joslin clinic, because women with pregestational diabetes invariably needed insulin during pregnancy. As for the entire White classification scheme generally, it too may still be clinically useful, for example, for alerting physicians to the possibility of hypertensive complications and the need for preterm delivery (Greene et al. 1989).

To end this section, the provocative question must be asked, as has been done more or less explicitly by several authors during the last 10–20 years, whether there is in reality a clinical entity gestational diabetes at all (Jarrett 1981, 1993, Beard and Hoet 1982, Drury 1989), and if it does exist, does it have any of the unfavorable effects on pregnancy outcome that have been laid at its feet (to be discussed just below). At its most elemental, the argument for there being no such entity holds that glucose intolerance first discovered during pregnancy is not a unique phenomenon, but is no more than a temporarily disturbed glucose tolerance associated with pregnancy; regardless of whether or not it may foretell a noninsulin-dependent diabetes. If this is so, is it possible—just as the well-known confounding factors of maternal obesity and age are implicated in garden variety impaired glucose tolerance—that the imputed undesirable effects of gestational diabetes are also largely attributable to such confounding influences? The points in defense of this position were succinctly set forth by Jarrett (1993). The final word may have been spoken by Harris (1988), who argued that impaired glucose tolerance is no more common in pregnant than in nonpregnant women.

PREGNANCY OUTCOME IN GESTATIONAL DIABETES

The near-final topic in this chapter, the core topic of this book, deals with the belief—once almost intuitive—that elevated blood glucose levels indicative of gestational diabetes must threaten harm to the conceptus. Initially the most serious of these perceived risks was perinatal death. But this danger progressively abated, partly because of the diligent care gestationally diabetic women have widely received in recent years; but which without doubt has primarily been due to the great improvement in the overall perinatal mortality record (Kalter 1991) stemming from the social and medical advances of the past several decades.

The second type of prenatal damage gestational diabetes was said to cause—congenital malformations—was pretty much invalidated from the start; but its story is nevertheless instructive and will be detailed on pp. 65–66. Effects of this maternal condition still frequently occurring, despite its apparently satisfactory management, which entail harmful consequences to offspring are fetal overgrowth and its concomitants, and neonatal hypoglycemia (Metzger et al. 1991), subjects that will not be dealt with here, being outside the purview of this monograph (except for cardiomegaly).

Spontaneous Abortion

It was never seriously claimed that gestational diabetes was associated with increased spontaneous abortion, perhaps because it was soon realized that this form of diabetes occurs predominantly in the later months of pregnancy, beyond the time it could be responsible for embryonic loss. A possible exception is class A diabetes, which having a pregestational onset could affect early stages of pregnancy. But it was clearly established that neither type of diabetes was associated with a frequency of spontaneous abortion beyond that expected (Kalter 1987), which is well supported by Chapter 3 on spontaneous abortion.

Perinatal Mortality

Early Indications

The widely held belief that prediabetes, like overt diabetes itself, was associated with an increased frequency of perinatal mortality and congenitally malformed offspring, was unhesitatingly transferred to the newly conceived and as yet poorly defined condition, gestational diabetes (Dandrow and O'Sullivan 1966).

It must again be cautioned that these questions are complicated, first by the diagnostic and terminological fluctuations that have been applied over the years to the phenomenon of disturbed carbohydrate metabolism associated with pregnancy, and second, by the ubiquitous socioeconomic, demographic, and other variables often inextricably raveled together with perinatal mortality and abnormalities of prenatal development (Leck 1972, Chung and Myrianthopoulos 1975a, Saxén 1983, Bakketeig et al. 1984).

Even before the term gestational diabetes was invented, the glucose and other tolerance tests had been used as adjuncts to various obstetrical studies. In one of these, from Australia, the earliest report it seems of the outcome of pregnancy in glucose tolerance-tested women (Basil-Jones 1949), it was noted that there were 9 perinatal deaths (including two with unnamed congenital malformations) in 40 viable pregnancies of women with abnormal tolerance curves, and 4 (1 malformed) in 55 with normal curves, that is, an apparently greater rate in the former. But as in many such later studies, questions regarding ascertainment of the women tested, interpretation of the results, and similar questions were not addressed. For example, 23 of the women were tested early in the puerperium; whether the outcome of their pregnancies or other selection factors played a part in their being so tested was left unanswered. Problems of these sorts continued to pervade such studies in later years.

The next study dealing with these questions, if only indirectly, was one examining the glucose tolerance of mothers of babies of excessively large birth weight (Lund and Weese 1953). Six of the 61 such infants born during the interval surveyed died perinatally, and 1 other had hydrocephalus (apparently the only one of the 61 malformed). But the authors neglected to relate how many of these mortalities were borne by the approximately 40% of women that had abnormal tolerance responses. Since big babies then and even later had an increased mortality rate (Hosemann 1950, Nathanson 1950, Saugstad 1981, Wilcox and Russell 1983), the study told us nothing of the possible relation of such deaths to abnormal maternal metabolism.

A large number of occurrences of diabetes with onset during pregnancy was identified during routine examination or by the presence of the classic symptoms of polydipsia, polyuria, and weight loss (Hagbard and Svanborg 1960). Although not entirely conforming to the definition soon enunciated by O'Sullivan (1961), they did so as far as onset time—the single criterion for inclusion in the study—was concerned. About half of the patients had "transitory" diabetic symptoms, that is, the metabolic and other abnormalities disappeared after delivery and nursing; in the remainder, called "permanent," the symptoms persisted and insulin was required. The two did not differ in severity of the symptoms however. Perinatal mortality was only noted in passing—the overall frequency was 40.8% and little different in the transitory and permanent forms (43% versus 38%), fearful consequences that were imputed to late diagnosis and consequent inadequate treatment.

Even before the upsurge of interest the new name gave to the phenomenon, evidence had accumulated that perinatal mortality was increased in such pregnancies. Hoet (1954) went so far as to state that "the fetal loss rate progresses from 20 to 50 percent in proportion to the increasing severity of the disordered glucose metabolism." Although it did not go this far, an early (but flawed) summary of the then-sparse class A data confirmed the impression (Kyle 1963). Data from earlier surveys (Table 6.2) lent further support to the proposition that the perinatal mortality frequency in pregnancies with intragestational onset of diabetes during those years was significantly greater than that occurring in overall American and European hospital births in the 1950s (Kalter 1991), but less than that in the births of overtly diabetic women (see Table 4.1).

The Later Picture

Substantial improvement in the perinatal mortality rate in gestational diabetic pregnancy began as early as the 1960s and soon approached the background level (see Table 6.2). But the full extent of the improvement has no doubt been obscured by recent authors' failure to mention perinatal mortality (eg, Bacigalupo et al. 1984, Algert et al. 1985, Kitzmiller et al. 1988, Pastor et al. 1988, Mazze and Krogh 1992). From this it would appear that this problem has become of such little con-

Table 6.2 Perinatal Mortality in Gestational Diabetic Pregnancy in the Last 80 Years

Era	Series (n)	America[a]	Series (n)	Europe
1920s through 1940s	10	32/146 (21.9)	7	14/62 (22.6)
1950s	10	36/437 (8.2)	15	48/205 (23.4)
1960s	21	110/2674 (4.1)	22	85/1653 (5.1)
1970s	23	34/1833 (1.8)	27	64/2548 (2.5)
1980s to late 1990s	20	41/6480 (0.6)	24	37/3736 (1.0)

Data are from publications giving relevant information.
[a] Perinatal deaths/births (% deaths).

Table 6.3 Perinatal Mortality in Studies of Gestational Diabetes (GD) That Included Controls

Years of Study[a]	GD[b]	Control	*P*
1950–1969	57/1018 (5.6)	60/1410 (4.3)	> .05
1970 to late 1990s	14/2941 (0.5)	26/3374 (0.8)	> .05

[a] Citations (first author only). 1950–1969: O'Sullivan 1966, Hadden 1967, Grimaldi 1968, Lufkin 1984; 1970 to late 1990s: Engelhardt 1976, Weiss 1986, Leikin 1987, Drexel 1988, Jacobson 1989, Langer 1988, Maresh 1989, Nordlander 1989, Roberts 1993, Greco 1994, Sachon 1994, Casey 1997, Garner 1997.

[b] PNM/GD (% PNM).

cern that the absence or scarcity of these deaths has not been thought important enough to record. Obviously, perinatal mortality in gestational diabetes is no longer considered a useful measure of the risks attendant upon such pregnancies, and that attention is now better spent on the various fetal morbidities that continue to occur (Coustan 1988).

What was the reason for this gratifying achievement? Was it due, as Beard and Hoet (1982) and many others thought, in part at least to normalization of blood glucose? This is not the impression gotten from the results of a study that found no significant difference in perinatal mortality rate between untreated and insulin-treated gestationally diabetic women (O'Sullivan et al. 1974), which led to the conclusion that hyperglycemia was not the sole factor responsible for the increased fetal loss in gestational diabetic pregnancy (O'Sullivan 1975). Other such studies led to the same conclusion (Table 6.3). On the other hand, evidence of benefits of insulin treatment were presented by Roversi et al. (1975), who found a lower perinatal mortality frequency in treated pregnancies than in previously untreated ones of the same women, an example perhaps of a risky comparison with a non-contemporaneous "control." Later analyses of untreated and insulin-treated women with glucose intolerance, made primarily to examine the possible benefits of therapy on macrosomia and other persistent undesirable pregnancy outcomes, have come too late to be able do the same for perinatal mortality, since its overall rate is now so low (Coustan and Lewis 1978, Kalkhoff 1985, Thompson et al. 1990 Lurie et al. 1992).

A more probable though perhaps less appealing explanation of the temporal decrease is another that Beard and Hoet ventured, simply that, as already noted, gestational diabetic women have shared in the steadily falling perinatal mortality rate that pregnant women in general now enjoy throughout the Western world; a view shared, for example, by Hadden (1980), who ascribed this beneficial outcome to overall improvements in maternal and obstetric care.

Did Gestational Diabetes Ever Affect Perinatal Mortality?

Just as today's common failure to record perinatal mortality in gestational diabetes has probably led to an underestimate of its current frequency, so it may be speculated that in the past an opposite exaggeration resulted from a different, unsuspected type of selection.

Studies of gestational diabetes in the past, when a greatly increased perinatal mortality rate was the usual finding in such cases, were largely conducted on pregnant women who satisfied one or more risk criteria. These criteria, as discussed, were features that had originally been discovered retrospectively through their association with pregnancies anteceding the development of diabetes—in the so-called prediabetic period—and were thus thought to foreshadow its development.

Even after the prediabetes concept was repudiated and these features as presages of the overt disease were made doubtful, they nevertheless were long thought to identify women who were candidates for developing diabetes ("potential diabetes," as it was called by Hadden and Harley 1967) and long afterwards continued to be used for the purpose of selecting pregnant women to be glucose tolerance–tested.

Ironically, these supposed foretellers of diabetes were some of the very conditions and attributes that are linked, directly or indirectly, to increased perinatal mortality in the general population, some as much so today as previously; namely advanced maternal age, multiparity, and obesity, repeated stillbirth and neonatal death, and fetal macrosomia (Nathanson 1950, Stevenson et al. 1982, Boyd et al. 1983, Bakketeig et al. 1984, Hansen 1986, Kitzmiller 1986, Cousins 1987, Naeye 1990). As a result, these features were unduly present in gestationally diabetic women and may have contributed to the excessive perinatal mortality once apparently characterizing them. Further complicating the situation, it was early revealed that maternal obesity, large babies, and abnormal glucose tolerance were associated with one another (Lund and Weese 1953), and in addition it was found that glucose intolerance was correlated with maternal age and obesity (Wilkerson and O'Sullivan 1963, Gillmer et al. 1980, Spellacy et al. 1985).

Direct examination of the possible influence of such features on perinatal mortality was all but prevented, however, because the subjects of most studies of gestational diabetes were seldom and only sketchily described with regard to relevant aspects like age, parity, and so on, Futhermore, the studies rarely included a control group. One group of investigators who did examine this possibility found that maternal weight and age were of undeniable influence (Dandrow and O'Sullivan 1966, O'Sullivan et al. 1966, 1973).

The findings from this set of studies were suggestive. But how, at this late date, can such suspicions be tested? Perhaps some circumstantial or even negative bits of evidence may be useful in this regard. One possibility would be to compare the pregnancy outcomes of women found to be gestationally diabetic following selection for the supposed risk criteria with those of women of the White class A designation discovered through an overall diabetes program. The former would be expected to be older, heavier, etc, than the latter, and to experience more detrimental effects. There is no way of proving this supposition, however, since such features with regard to class A women were rarely if ever recorded. It happens that the perinatal mortality frequencies in pregnancies of these groups of women in the 1950s and 1960s in America did not differ (4.2% versus 4.5%), so nothing can be proved one way or another by this comparison.

Control data, scarce though they are, may be helpful. During the earlier years of the study of this condition, hardly any controls, appropriate or otherwise, were obtained, and this was little improved over time. Without the critical appraisal enabled by well-chosen control material, a spurious or overblown relation would

Table 6.4 Effect of Insulin Treatment on Perinatal Mortality (PNM) in Gestational Diabetic (GD) Pregnancy

Years of Study[a]	Treatment		p
	Routine Care or Diet[b]	Insulin ± Diet	
1960–1969	15/306 (4.90)	11/293 (3.75)	> .05
1970–1979	11/674 (1.63)	10/381 (2.62)	> .05
1980–late 1990s	4/770 (0.52)	8/510 (1.57)	> .05

[a] Citations (first author only). 1960–1969: O'Sullivan 1966; 1970–1979: O'Sullivan 1974, Stallone 1974, Opperman 1975, Gyves 1977, Pedersen 1977, Adashi 1979, Coetzee 1979, Hadden 1979, O'Shaughnessy 1979; 1980–late 1990s: Lavin 1983, Cousins 1984, Muylder 1984, Olofsson 1984, Persson 1984, Weiss 1986, Leikin 1987, Thompson 1990.
[b] PNM/GD (% PNM).

go unchallenged. This is especially so because of the close correlation among most of the confounding variables associated with perinatal mortality. It is especially regrettable that this question was not raised during the very years when the considerable mortality frequency prevailed, which may have yielded helpful clues.

Fortunately, among the reports of diabetes with onset during pregnancy made in the last 40 years or so that considered perinatal mortality, a handful were identified that included control (ie, nondiabetic) subjects of some sort. They show that the frequency of perinatal mortality in the group supposedly at risk was not greater than in the controls (Table 6.4). If these studies are representative it may be argued that gestational diabetes never significantly augmented the background level of perinatal mortality and that concern with this purported outcome was largely misdirected.

A case might still be made for this untoward outcome if, as Ales and Santini (1989) remarked, insulin could be shown to have had a rescuing effect, which again would have been most conspicuous in the earlier years. But this door, too, was shut by the evidence that there was no difference in perinatal mortality between insulin-treated and untreated gestationally diabetic pregnancies (see Table 6.4).

GESTATIONAL DIABETES AND CONGENITAL MALFORMATIONS

The results of a survey of diabetic births in Copenhagen in 1926–1965 noted that 3 of 62 gestationally diabetic women (called class A) had congenitally malformed infants (Mølsted-Pedersen et al. 1964). The abnormalities unfortunately were not named, nor were they mentioned in a detailed list of malformations in infants of pregestationally diabetic mothers, also included in the survey, which the present author obtained soon after the article was published.

Lack of such details and of various others complicated the task of analyzing the association of congenital malformations and maternal diabetes. The most troublesome impediment to analysis was the practice of many authors of merely stating the number malformed, omitting the clear or complete naming of the conditions possessed by offspring. Thus, it was impossible to know whether inadmissible or debatable items were included. The latter consist of conditions of little or no medical concern and those whose known or probable etiology absolve them of being due to or associated with maternal diabetes, in distinction to abnormalities the consensus considers as medically serious, those known as "major congenital malformations." The full consideration of major malformations appears in Chapter 8.

A total of 83 articles from 1964–1994 yields information regarding the occurrence of congenital malformations in gestational diabetes. The information was recently summarized (Kalter 1998). The full data are obtainable from the author. The nine reports in the 1960s noted a total of 11.4% named and unnamed malformations, an apparently greater frequency than the approximately 2–3% of major congenital malformations usually found in well-examined newborn children (Kalter and Warkany 1983). This frequency was brought into line with the background level, when only those abnormalities were admitted whose status as major malformations could be assured by being named. The malformations in perinatal mortalities, presenting no such uncertainties, yielded a frequency not significantly different from that in overall perinatal mortalities in this decade (Kalter 1991).

In later years, up to the time of this writing, the frequencies of major congenital malformations continued at about the background level. Thus, the recorded data of over 30 years of nearly 7000 gestational diabetic pregnancies clearly revealed that this form of diabetes is not teratogenic. Indeed, if these frequencies are unusual in any way it is that they are on the low side, which probably indicates that the offspring were as a rule not well examined (Kalter 1998). The exceptions were the generally more closely examined perinatal mortalities, whose malformation frequencies were about 20–30%, closely matching those found in contemporary overall perinatal mortalities (Kalter 1991), again supporting the non-association with the maternal illness.

GESTATIONAL DIABETES IN LOCAL GROUPS

The Pima Indians

In certain ethnic and racial groups the prevalence of impaired glucose tolerance or gestational diabetes greatly exceeds the usual range of 1–5% found in most populations. In these groups the level of noninsulin-dependent diabetes also often exceeds the usual one. The best known and best studied of such groups are the Pima Indians of the Gila River Indian Community in southern Arizona, who have the highest known prevalence of noninsulin-dependent diabetes in the world (Knowler et al. 1978).

The first striking feature of this "biologically unusual" people (Hadden 1986) is that, contrary to the unimodal, fairly symmetrical frequency distribution of glucose tolerance levels widely prevalent elsewhere, in these American Indians the distribution is distinctly bimodal, the right-hand curve consisting of values for age groups 35 years and above (Rushforth et al. 1971). The disease nevertheless often has a relatively early onset (Knowler et al. 1978), with the consequence that abnormalities of glucose tolerance often occur in women even during early childbearing years and hence in many pregnant women (Comess et al. 1969). Because of this extraordinary feature and because some of the effects of the condition upon pregnancy outcome present some unusual aspects, the findings in the Pima Indians will be examined in some detail.

Up to the present there has only been limited examination of these consequences (Comess et al. 1969, Bennett et al. 1978, Pettitt et al. 1980, 1985). In the earliest study, made in 1965–1967, all 237 nonpregnant parous Pima women aged 25–44 years were glucose tolerance–tested, and on the basis of the results were divided into three groups: nondiabetic (<140 mg/dL plasma glucose), indeterminate (140–159 mg/dL), and diabetic (≥160 mg/dL). To the last group were added 10 previously well-documented diabetic women of this age. The indeterminates unfortunately were not further considered. The 1207 prior pregnancies of the diabetic and nondiabetic women exceeding 20 weeks of gestation whose medical records were available were examined. Children of the diabetics born before the date of diagnosis of the diabetes were considered offspring of prediabetic pregnancies and those born afterward, offspring of diabetic pregnancies (Comess et al. 1969).

Strangely, perinatal mortality, a subject uppermost in the minds of investigators of gestational diabetes during these years, was barely alluded to. Aside from the remark that the births included stillbirths and that some of them occurred in the diabetic pregnancies, this subject was not further mentioned. Only in the second report, which appeared 10 years later, were a few more details forthcoming, and then only in the discussion following the conclusion of this paper (Bennett et al. 1978). There, it was divulged that in 1960–1965 the perinatal mortality rate was 25% in the diabetic pregnancies and that it had decreased to 7% in 1970–1975. The possible causes and meaning of this great decrease were left unconsidered, except for a statement that implied that no difference in management of the pregnancies of the diabetic women had been instituted that could account for the improved picture. What the rate was in nondiabetics in these two spans of years was not stated. A study was made in which pregnant women were glucose tolerance–tested, mostly in the third trimester (Pettitt et al. 1985). In these cases, the perinatal mortality rate in women with a blood glucose levels of 140 mg/dL was 2.6%. All in all it appears that so far as perinatal mortality is concerned, the Pima Indians did not present a picture outside the usual.

The focus of the earlier two reports, to which the mortality question was obviously subordinated, was an inquiry into congenital malformations. The original findings with respect to this subject had it that the malformation frequency in the offspring of the diabetic pregnancies was about eight times that in offspring of nondiabetic and prediabetic ones, although the further accumulated results presented in the second report modified this to about three times. Nevertheless, this result appeared to indicate that the form of diabetes prevalent in this small population was teratogenic.

My analyses of these data modified this conclusion. A striking fact concerned the relation of the malformation frequency to maternal age at diabetes onset. Of the 13 abnormal children born to the diabetic women, 9 were among the 42 whose mothers were in the younger onset age group, 15–24 years, whereas the other 4 were among the 72 children of the older onset group, a statistically significant difference ($P<.025$). Complementing this, 10 of the abnormal children occurred in the 46 births of the insulin-treated women, and the remaining 3 in the 68 receiving oral glycemic drugs or no treatment, also a significant difference ($P<.01$). Thus, it is clear that the congenital malformations occurred almost exclusively in the children of a "small subpopulation" of diabetic women whose disease had an early onset and in whom it was severe enough to require insulin administration; a severity also evidenced by the fact that in many of them vascular complications developed during their childbearing years (Comess et al. 1969). Thus, although childhood diabetes was apparently rare in these people (Bennett et al. 1979), what was probably a very precocious and severe form of insulin-dependent type 2 diabetes was not, and this, it seems, had the same harmful effects on pregnancy outcome as had been reported for pregestational diabetes in other populations.

That, however, is not the end of the tale. Most of the detailed results of this investigation were reported in the initial publication. It was learned from them that the nondiabetic, prediabetic, and diabetic women together had 53 malformed children, and that over half of their 63 different malformations had been discovered postneonatally. But no information was given about how many of the children of each of these three groups had been diagnosed as malformed before leaving the hospital and how many after the neonatal period. These are crucial facts, as has been emphasized repeatedly.

In order to compare and judge malformation frequencies, in addition to the obviously vital requirement that a definition of the term be widely accepted, there is a further necessity. This is that the malformations be the ones discovered in the first days of life, when children are still in hospital, and that the malformations that appear or are discovered in later infancy and childhood be discounted for this purpose. The reasons for this are outlined in Chapter 10.

Therefore, because the malformations discovered in the newborn period were not identified and because the congenital nature of some of the abnormalities is uncertain, doubt must linger that the diabetic pregnancies contained an excess frequency of congenital malformations.

Finally, attention must be directed to a misinterpreted malformation. One child of a diabetic pregnancy was diagnosed as having a "pattern of anomalies consistent with the sacrococcygeal syndrome reported to be associated with diabetic pregnancies" (Bennett et al. 1978). Yet the table in this article listing the anomalies mentioned no vertebral malformation. What was mentioned were malformed femora, which apparently were equated with sacral dysplasia—in doing which the authors may be forgiven, since they were merely following the lead of a contemporary publication (Passarge and Lenz 1966), which made the same mistake, as a recent analysis made evident (Kalter 1993) and as will be further explored in Chapter 14.

Other Groups

Several other noncaucasian ethnic and racial groups were discovered to have a bimodal blood glucose concentration (Rosenthal et al. 1985, Dowse et al. 1994), and some also had a high frequency of diabetes during pregnancy (Sicree et al. 1986, Doery et al. 1989, Benjamin et al. 1993, Murphy et al. 1993)). Retrospective surveys of some of these groups revealed increased stillbirth rates (Balkau et al. 1985, Sicree et al. 1986), with their attendant difficulties of interpretation, whereas no untoward or equivocal pregnancy outcome was reported in other groups with high levels of noninsulin-dependent diabetes during pregnancy (Forsbach et al. 1988, Contreras-Soto et al. 1991, Hollingsworth et al. 1991).

The pregnancy outcomes in the diabetic women in these populations, in whom the disease may reflect the premature appearance of a severe expression of type 2 diabetes, is of much interest. Even the relatively sparse information available gives the impression that, as in gestational diabetes generally, there was an excess of stillbirths and neonatal deaths in the past, though this would be difficult to prove, but with no indication that an excess exists at present (eg, Contreras-Soto et al. 1991).

CARBOHYDRATE METABOLISM AND PREGNANCY OUTCOME

The previous sections of this chapter were concerned with the risk of adverse outcomes in gestationally diabetic pregnancy. This will now be turned around and consideration given to the occurrence of impaired carbohydrate metabolism in pregnancies that had such outcomes. Since these metabolic disturbances during pregnancy were considered harbingers of the development of overt diabetes, the discussion can be taken as being related to the similar one devoted to prediabetes.

It was commonly found, in the days when the original formulation of the concept of prediabetes had currency, that excess perinatal deaths occurred in the earlier pregnancies of women who in their current ones were judged to be gestationally diabetic. But the salient fact was ignored that in many cases one of the criteria by which the women were selected for glucose tolerance testing was that they had unexplained stillbirths.

In the latter days of this concept, while it was in its death throes and even after its demise, several publications reported an increased frequency of abnormal glucose tolerance in women whose past pregnancies had ended with offspring death. Some had even occurred many years previously, and the glucose testing had usually been done long afterward (eg, Long and Freeman 1969, Salzberger and Liban 1975, Sutherland and Fisher 1982). Other authors reported the same pattern for women delivering congenitally malformed children (Navarrete et al. 1967, López-Quijada and Carrion 1974, Goldman 1976). Wisdom made its appearance only years later when it was realized that "retrospective analyses of data collected in this way with the object of identifying any association between gestational diabetes and reproductive failure is a temptation to be resisted" (Farmer and Russell 1984), except perhaps when combined with matched controls (Maresh et al. 1989).

It was also sometimes noted that congenital malformations were more common in offspring of women with elevated blood glucose levels (Farmer et al. 1988). This was not restricted to the "diabetic" end of the distribution, which implied that abnormal blood glucose was a common factor in the etiology of malformations generally. Other studies of this type, however, yielded no such outcome (Weiner 1988, Little et al. 1990, Berkus and Langer 1993); nor did studies of unselected nondiabetic pregnant women, made to examine the usefulness and practicality of universal glucose tolerance testing, find perinatal mortality or congenital malformation frequency to be associated with blood glucose level (Abell and Beischer 1975, Jacobson and Cousins 1989).

7

CLASSIFICATION OF DIABETES IN PREGNANCY

We now turn to the form of diabetes in pregnancy that was and continues to be the main concern of the patient and physician, insulin-dependent diabetes of pregestational origin. In addition to general classifications of diabetes, promulgated from 20 years ago to the present (National Diabetes Data Group 1979, Wareham and O'Rahilly 1998), others were especially devised for diabetes in pregnancy (White 1949, 1965, 1974, 1978, Pedersen and Mølsted-Pedersen 1965, Brudenell 1975). Their main purpose was to attempt to predict fetal hazard, particularly mortality, which being foretold would alert caretakers to institute special management procedures. Others, though less stressed, were to afford understanding of the connection between the maternal disease and fetal risk and to allow geographic and temporal comparisons of patient samples, treatment regimens, pregnancy outcomes, and so on.

One scheme, used at one time in parts of Great Britain, outlined a simple system: gestational diabetes and established diabetes, that is, diabetes already present before pregnancy either with few or no complications or serious complications. What greater purpose this classification was intended to serve, in the way of predicting outcome or facilitating management, was not mentioned (Brudenell 1975).

Another system sought to make individualized prognoses of fetal outcome by identifying possible danger signs appearing during pregnancy. It attempted to predict and thus it was hoped to avert adverse outcomes of pregnancy in diabetes by recognizing what were rather clumsily named "prognostically bad signs occurring during pregnancy," or PBSP, such as pyelitis, acidosis, and toxemia, as well as "neglecting" women (Pedersen and Mølsted-Pedersen 1965, Pedersen 1977). Its appropriateness was supported by the three- to fourfold larger perinatal mortality rate in the infants of women with such signs than without them. There was an even greater correlation when the PBSP and the White systems were combined. The two were therefore seen as supplementing each other—the one relying on features preceding pregnancy and the other on those occurring during pregnancy. A major inadequacy of the PBSP system was that it did not provide a graded estimate of risk, all the signs seeming to be about equal in indicating deleteriousness (Pedersen and Mølsted-Pedersen 1965). Perhaps for this reason, aside from some Danish and other centers, and that not for too long, the PBSP did not find favor.

By far the most widely used classification was that dividing diabetes existing before pregnancy into classes of increasing seriousness, according to several criteria (White 1949).

THE WHITE CLASSIFICATION SYSTEM

By 1949, when White introduced her scheme for evaluating maternal and especially fetal risk factors in diabetic pregnancy, study of the causes of the persistently high perinatal mortality rate in these pregnancies—little changed over the 27 years since the discovery of insulin—had yielded little understanding of its basis and only vague insight into its prevention. Noting that age of onset of the disease, its duration, and the presence of certain pathological maternal characteristics were often correlated with fetal death, she integrated these features into a classification of seriousness of the disease—a brave exercise in giving some order to a disjointed struggle to deal with a major problem.

Strangely though, the first application White put the system to was not in gauging its relation to fetal death, but as an indication of the doses of sex hormones to use therapeutically (see p. 31). This oddity was partly remedied not long after, when she and colleagues noted a suggestive continuous decline in perinatal survival with advancing White class (White et al. 1953).

Problems With the White System

Disagreement with the White classification was soon voiced. Pedersen (1954a) found that fetal mortality increased with duration of diabetes, but not with age at onset or with severity of vascular complications and recommended modifying the White proposal to take these inconsistencies into consideration. It was this dissatisfaction, no doubt, which prompted him to formulate his own system, mentioned above (Pedersen and Mlsted-Pedersen 1965). Oakley (1953) also differed with the White plan, but even more so, since he found that neither age nor duration was associated with fetal mortality.

A more fundamental question asked what constituted "severity" of diabetes; that is, what were the correlates that best represented and were most applicable to the fetal mortality quandary: historical factors and extent of maternal vascular damage or clinical indicators, represented primarily by insulin dose requirements and difficulty of maintaining control? Each of these views had its vigorous supporters (Jones 1956, Dampeer 1958). Pedersen (1952), advocating the clinical approach, recommended that "alterations in the daily dose of insulin [be] used as a measure of alterations in the severity of diabetes." Jones (1953), finding a poor correlation between the historical and clinical indications, felt that the White grading was an inefficient predictor of fetal loss, but later, although concluding that insulin requirement and fetal loss were related, found that the former seemed less important than the historical features and vascular progression of the disease in rating its severity (Jones 1956). Although it was thought cumbersome and needed modification to make its use in obstetrical units feasible, the White system was felt to be a major advance and soon had "virtual semiofficial recognition" (Anon 1954, Jones 1956).

The White System—Prepregnancy-Based

Since White worked in a long-established clinic largely devoted to the care of juvenile diabetics from the time the disease had its onset, she could assess the condition from an early age (White et al. 1952, 1971). Thus, and because she felt it was "best done" at that time (White et al. 1953), her system of clinically grading the severity of diabetes was "based upon the pre-pregnancy state..." (White 1949). The pregestational basis of her system made for at least two problems: the difficulty of applying the criteria to patients usually not seen until they were already pregnant and the tendency of investigators in later years to confuse the mildest degree of diabetes of pregestational onset and the usually mild diabetes of intragestational onset.

OUTLINE OF THE WHITE SYSTEM

The system of grading diabetes severity devised by White (1949) over 50 years ago has stood the test of time well. It consists of steps of increasing degrees of severity, denoted by the letters A to R, according to age at onset, disease duration and severity, and extent of certain vascular and other complications. In time the system underwent several expansions and modifications, outlined in the following pages. Insulin is always required in the more serious of the classes, but usually not in the mildest.

Class A

The mildest degree of the disease, called class A, consists of a slightly elevated blood glucose concentration, as detected by glucose tolerance testing, but with fasting concentrations that are normal or near normal and a diabetic state that is asymptomatic. No criteria with respect to age at onset and disease duration apply to this class. Normalization of the glucose level is usually achievable by dietary means alone. The "condition" may in fact largely represent the upper end of the normal range of glucose tolerance in the population (Victor 1974, National Diabetes Data Group 1979). One puzzling thing, already alluded to, which to my knowledge has never been explained, is why and how a nonpregnant person with a possibly borderline, asymptomatic state would routinely come to the attention of medical personnel in a diabetes clinic.

Of all the White classes, this has been the most confused and confusing, since views of it and its definition have shifted and altered over the years. The essential problem, it seems to me, is whether mild glucose intolerance in a nonpregnant individual is to be equated with a similar state in a pregnant one.

The recognition of the existence of mild degrees of glucose intolerance prompted new thinking about a number of things. It helped to displace the concept of prediabetes by substituting for it the idea that there existed a covert or latent situation that the stress of pregnancy could uncover. It followed, if this were true, that all women should be examined to detect this latent state, a prelude to the later advocacy of universal glucose tolerance testing of pregnant women. It also led to the later confusion between pregestational class A diabetes and the gestational form; exemplified by Peel and Oakley's (1949) statement that "pregnancy in most cases increases the severity of an existing diabetes or, when latent, brings it to light." Others soon echoed these ideas (Kinch 1958).

Examining the effects on pregnancy outcome in true class A diabetics was made more difficult as the strict definition initially given by White (1949) was increasingly less often adhered to and class A women became ever more commingled with gestational diabetics. However, data that allowed examination of their consequences separately showed that neither of these mild degrees of glucose intolerance had discernible effects on spontaneous abortion or perinatal mortality (Kalter 1987).

Class A Subcategories

It was noticed early that a small proportion of pregnant class A diabetic women had a fasting hyperglycemia that called for insulin administration. This required the creation of separate categories for women of this sort and those satisfactorily managed by dietary means alone. The major rationale for these subdivisions was the possibility that they may carry different prognoses. So far as offspring are concerned this has not been substantiated. A last word. The White classification is not ironclad. Occasionally the classification of a patient may change, either from pregnancy to pregnancy or during a pregnancy. For example, class A becomes B if otherwise uncontrollable abnormal blood glucose levels occur and necessitate insulin or oral hypoglycemic drug administration.

Insulin-Dependent Diabetic Pregnancy

It must be acknowledged that while insulin has been a lifesaver for diabetic individuals, this great medical achievement had innumerable unintended consequences, as the historians put it. For young diabetics the paradox was well phrased years ago, when it was said that "the problem of diabetic pregnancy was created by the introduction of the insulin treatment" (Andersson 1950), and "the advent of insulin has given rise to a new problem. The juvenile diabetic who has been helped to survive, mature, and marry and reproduce faces the problem of premature vascular sclerotic changes" (Reis et al. 1950).

These vascular effects formed part of the basis of White's classification, together with insulin need and age and duration considerations. Diabetic women who required insulin were placed in classes B and beyond. The age at onset of the diabetes in these advancing classes was progressively less and the duration of the disease greater, and they presented increasingly more severe complications of the disease.

As a testimony to the by-then conventional use of insulin, and a refreshing reminder of a bygone more innocent age, we recall the comfort Tolstoi (1949) gave his patients when he emphasized that "insulin *cannot* be taken by mouth but that it is not 'dope,' even though it must be given by 'needle.'"

In class B there was adult onset (≥20 years), a duration of <10 years, and clinical absence of vascular disease; in C and D, respectively, a juvenile (10–19 years) and childhood (<10 years) onset, a duration of 10–19 and ≥20 years, and no or minimal evidence of vascular complication; and classes beyond D (mostly F, H, and R) no age and duration criteria, but serious, often advanced stages of renal, coronary, and retinal pathology. (For other details and implications of the classes see, eg, Kitzmiller et al. 1982, and Hare 1989, 1994).

This scheme has gone through several modifications and expansions (White 1965, 1978). Classes C and D were subdivided, the first according to age at onset and disease duration and the second according to type of disease complication. In addition, further classes were added to accommodate newer problems. Not all of the newer classes were generally used, and one of the older ones was discarded (Hare and White 1980). Furthermore, as perinatal mortality greatly diminished, this salient distinction among classes B, C, and D almost disappeared, and it is questionable whether their formal definitions are still apposite (Kitzmiller et al. 1981). The revised classification, as it stands presently, was described by Hare (1989, 1994).

Variations in Distribution of White Classes

Has the distribution of the White classes varied geographically and temporally along with changes in demography and prevalence of insulin-dependent diabetes? For the present monograph, examining such variations had as its main purpose determining the effects such changes may have had on rates of perinatal mortality and congenital malformation. These questions will be addressed below.

Table 7.1 Temporal and Geographical Variation (%) in Distribution of White Classification of Type 1 Diabetes in Pregnancy

Era	B	C	D	> D	Pregnancies[a]	Mean[b]
				America		
1940s + 1950s	42.2	29.7	21.1	6.9	4404	1.93
1960s	32.6	26.1	34.1	7.0	1893	2.16
1970s	52.4	26.5	15.9	5.2	2566	1.74
1980s to mid 1990s	41.2	30.0	17.2	11.5	2586	1.99
				Europe		
1940s + 1950s	43.7	31.1	16.8	3.3	1117	1.79
1960s	37.6	25.9	28.6	7.9	4814	2.07
1970s	32.3	34.0	26.8	6.8	3205	2.08
1980s to mid 1990s	32.0	29.3	29.2	9.4	4242	2.16

[a] Number of classified as class B and beyond.
[b] The mean severity was obtained by assigning the number 1 to class B, 2 to class C, 3 to class D, and 4 to classes beyond D.

Aside from examining such topics, the inquiry immediately revealed a conspicuous change. This was a shift, which was manifested very early, that occurred in distribution of the classes at the lowest end of the system, as class A was rapidly invaded, and it may be said corrupted, by its confusion with the concept of gestational diabetes, as was already discussed. The upshot of this was that the proportion of cases classified as A mounted (see Table 6.1) as the concept took hold and the practice among obstetricians grew of routinely testing pregnant women for carbohydrate intolerance (Beard and Oakley 1976). Note from the table that this fashion caught on in America sooner and reached greater heights than in Europe, perhaps because of European conservatism or lack of enthusiasm about this latest American innovation.

In the same way, parts of Europe, particularly Great Britain, at first resisted adopting the White classification as a whole. To discover whether variations occurred in the distribution of the remaining White classes it was necessary to negate the distorting effect of class A by omitting it from consideration. The results of an exercise using these data (Table 7.1), if interpretation be dared, seem to point to a continual increase in Europe in average severity of diabetes in pregnancy and in America a "plateauing" of severity. Can the former possibility be related even remotely to the widely reported growing prevalence of childhood diabetes in Europe (Levy-Marchal and Czernichow 1992)?

8

CONGENITAL MALFORMATIONS—WHAT, WHEN, WHERE?

It is truly remarkable that so few babies are born malformed. Considering the many misdirected paths that may be lying ahead for the creature at the start of its course, encoded in the gametes whose union will commence its being, and the many extrinsic perils that can bombard it from the instant of conception, one can only marvel that prenatal development so seldom goes awry. But morphological abnormalities of development—malformations—do happen, and these happenings have loomed ever larger as over time many medical problems of the newborn have been reduced in number and seriousness. It is to this topic we turn, asking what are malformations, what causes them, how often do they happen.

WHAT ARE CONGENITAL MALFORMATIONS?

Malformations can occur at any time in the life of an individual, in childhood or later, as a result, for example, of trauma or infection. The concern here is with a specific type, those that are present at birth, congenital malformations. Various terms have often been used interchangeably for such abnormalities (Taffel 1978): congenital abnormality, congenital defect, congenital anomaly, birth defect. Since there is no good reason for this multiplicity except elegant variation, only congenital malformation will be used here. Incidentally, the term "birth defect" is a misnomer, easily misconstrued and leading to misunderstanding, since it can imply that it refers to damage caused by and originating at birth. Its use at present, to be laid at the feet of popularizers, is to be discouraged. It will be shunned here.

Congenital Means Present at Birth

Defining congenital malformation presents two difficulties. The immediate one deals with the meaning of "congenital" and its connotations. *The Shorter Oxford*

English Dictionary on Historical Principles states that the word, which made its first appearance in English in 1796, means "existing from birth or born with." There is a conflict in this, since one part, but not the other, seems to exclude existence before birth. *The Funk and Wagnalls Standard College Dictionary*, making one of these explicit, says that the word means "existing prior to or at birth..." But it adds to its definition, as does *The American Heritage Dictionary of the English Language*, "but not hereditary," thereby resurrecting a usage that had almost expired. The present scientific meaning of congenital simply is "present at birth" and connotes nothing of etiology.

This obviously signifies that such conditions arise prior to birth, but does not exclude that, while present at birth, they may be covert and not detected or expressed till sometime afterward. For the primary purposes of this work, however, attention will dwell almost exclusively on conditions evident and ascertained in the first days of life, because most malformations, especially the medically serious ones, are found in the neonatal period and because the great majority of reports that have been made of congenital malformations in offspring generally, as in those of diabetic pregnancies, were concerned with neonatal infants. The subsidiary consideration of the postneonatal appearance or discovery of malformations will be the subject of a later section in Chapter 10.

Malformations Are Abnormalities of Structure

Defining "malformation" is the greater challenge. Broad definitions, such as "abnormalities attributable to faulty development" (McKeown and Record 1960), or "structural defects present at birth" (Warkany 1971), leave their key terms unsettled. Although abnormalities from the submicroscopic to the glaringly gross, strictly speaking would be admitted by the term "structural," in practice such semantic quibbles make for no difficulty, because the conditions predominantly considered in clinical and epidemiological teratology are those that are discovered almost entirely by the unassisted eye or with the aid of standard clinical instruments. Such are the conditions relevant to the subject discussed here, and abnormalities included by the studies discussed below that did not conform to this limitation—molecular, cellular, metabolic, endocrine, functional, and so on—were discounted to the extent possible.

The term "faulty development" can also be reasonably dealt with, by limiting malformations to those resulting from disturbances of development of parts having to do with the laying down, early in prenatal life, of basic embryonic structures and the formation of organ systems. This excludes conditions such as tumors, nevi, angiomata, and others.

Also excluded were two other varieties of abnormality. The first, because in themselves they are of little or no medical significance, are relatively common conditions such as minor defects, trivial blemishes, tissue abnormalities, anatomical variants, and abnormal biochemical and other functional states; and the second, because they have a known or probable etiology, exempting them from being attributed to maternal diabetes, such as defects of chromosomal, genic, and possibly exogenous or complex origin, such as trisomies, chondrodystrophy, cretinism, dwarfism, deafness, mental retardation.

Major and Minor Malformations and Other Variants

Many different sorts of aberrant or unusual physical characteristics have their origin during prenatal life. Note that in this sentence the word "abnormal" to designate deviant was studiously avoided. "Abnormal" and "abnormality" indicate something beyond or different from normal and are easily told apart from it. But saying what is normal is itself not easily pinned down, because the word, presenting a philosophical dilemma, can mean so many things descriptive—regular, standard, usual, ordinary, symmetrical, healthy, common, typical, natural, average, expected, and so on.

The difficulties that grappling with this conundrum can lead to were inadvertently alluded to by a writer who held that "truly discontinuous phenomena in nature are excessively rare, particularly in biology" (Murphy 1966). He may have meant by this that in science the concept of abnormal is pointless, since the location along a continuous distribution at which the normal is departed from is indeterminable.

On the contrary, in a critical phase of existence, embryonic life, discontinuities may be common; but only revealed when developmental processes fail to overleap quantitative thresholds and give rise to outcomes that differ qualitatively from what would have eventuated otherwise (Fraser 1976). These are not outcomes that deviate in shape, dimension, relation, or any other manifestation of degree, or do not lie at the extremity of arrangements of finely shaded, progressively diverging appearances, but are species without link to what they are marked off from. Such phenomena, regardless of how the word is defined, it cannot be denied are abnormal.

However, not all of what are called developmental abnormalities have the same medical import. Thus what abnormal means for the purposes of this work calls for some distinctions to be made between those with different consequences for viability, health, and well-being. The distinction most often made in this regard is that between what are called serious or major congenital malformations and minor or inconsequential defects, aberrations, variants, and so on. There are good, pragmatic reasons for this separation. The former are those that cause or are associated with embryonic or perinatal death, require surgical or medical care soon after birth, or are gravely physically handicapping. Understandably, therefore, they have gained much attention from the medical and biological world, as well as the lay public. And because of this they have long and widely been registered and thus form a body of record against which comparison and analysis is to be made (Warkany and Kalter 1961, Kalter and Warkany 1983).

Major congenital malformations, ironically, are among the most frequently occurring of developmental abnormalities and include numerous types of malformations of the central nervous, cardiovascular, orofacial, gastrointestinal, urogenital, skeletal systems, and so on. Considering that many of these malformations were usually lethal or impaired reproduction in the days of premodern medicine, what this means as far as evolution is concerned would be an interesting topic for discussion.

Many types of developmental aberrations also occur that consist of lesser departures from the typical or affect parts that are not vital to the body economy.

These, minor congenital malformations, as they are called, usually entail no or only trivial medical or cosmetic difficulty. The instance of Ann Boleyn may be mentioned here, one in which such a defect—in her case, the presence of "a rudimentary sixth finger on her left hand" (Mattingly 1941, p. 246)—did not interfere, at first at any rate, with her attractiveness.

A huge quandary here is defining what is a minor abnormality, since, depending on the inclusiveness of the term (and there is little consensus here) and the assiduity of the search for them, the number of such conditions an individual may be discovered to possess can vary from few to many, and the frequency of the newborn population so affected can likewise vary greatly. Examples of this predicament follow.

In an early foray into this uncharted field, unselected newborn infants were examined for 26 different "minor anomalies" and one or more, mostly of the ear and hand, discovered in 14.7%; in addition 14.3% had 1 or more of 14 "normal phenotypic variants," again mostly affecting the ear (eg, folding over of the upper helix) and face (hemangiomas) (Marden et al. 1964). In another, an expanded search, children not exposed in utero to certain drugs were examined for the presence of 104 unnamed physical features, called minor malformations, and 42.9% found to have one or more of them (Holmes et al. 1985). Other studies similarly found that some large percentage of infants have such minor physical features, in the absence of associated major congenital malformations (Méhes 1983, 1988, Merlob et al. 1985, Leppig et al. 1987).

Acknowledging the perplexity presented by this *embarras des richesses*, students of these phenomena attempted to put them into perspective by arbitrarily dividing them into those occurring in less and greater than some percentage of infants (eg, 4%) and calling only the less common ones defects (Smith 1971), on the reasonable assumption that very common ones could not be "abnormal." Because there has been no agreement about what features are relevant and meaningful, such categorical measures can hardly hold promise of diagnostic or other usefulness (especially since most of them are doubtlessly physical or morphometric variants and seldom have the least medical significance). Evaluating their heuristic significance thus is impeded by the absence of agreement as to which of the isolated "nonvariants" is to be accepted as minor defect and which not (Pinsky 1985, Leppig et al. 1987, Merlob 1994).

Thank God, these controversial matters are of little concern here, where it is necessary simply to know that there are generally two varieties of congenital abnormalities: first, the major congenital malformations, those that historical judgment and practice have made into the canon; and second, minor malformations and trivial physical variants, which have been rejected for this role. The task in this work will be to examine the data that have accumulated during the past five to six decades for the purpose of judging the widely held belief that congenital malformations, for the most part those of the major variety, occur excessively in children of diabetic women. Minor malformations will not be ignored, however; questions regarding them in diabetic pregnancy will be aired on pp. 109 et seq.

CAUSES AND FREQUENCY

The subject of the etiology of congenital malformations is of obviously vital importance here, being integral to examining the association of such conditions to diabetic pregnancy. It has been pursued by countless investigators from many avenues over the decades into modern times, ever since humankind first observed what were and remain bewildering events and pondered their meaning (Ballantyne 1894, Warkany 1977).

From numerous surveys during the past 60 years, the consensus emerged that approximately 3% of well-examined newborn infants are affected by major congenital malformations (eg, Malpas 1937, McIntosh et al. 1954, Böök and Fraccaro 1956, Leck et al. 1968, Saxén 1983, Regemorter et al. 1984). To this figure is added a similar proportion with medically relevant but less harmful anomalies not usually detected for months and years after birth (McIntosh et al. 1954, McKeown and Record 1960, Ekelund et al. 1970, Klemetti 1978). If the search for abnormalities is widened by relaxing the definition or extended by different kinds of follow-up, the result may be such as was found in one study, in which the frequency ranged from 2.1% to 7.4% (Mellin 1963). But it is only malformations discovered in the neonatal period that in the main will be dealt with here, since with relatively few exceptions offspring of diabetic pregnancies have been examined for congenital malformations only at this time.

As to the causes of major congenital malformations, to make a long story short, little is known with certainty at the present time. Though clearly of heterogeneous causation, the numerous and diverse catalogue of abnormalities they comprise has yielded some rough order and a classification (Warkany 1971). It consists of five broad categories: single major mutant genes; chromosomal aberrations; interactions between hereditary susceptibilities and usually undefined nongenetic factors; discrete environmental factors; and all others—those still with no unambiguously identified cause. Of these categories, a well-constructed calculation assigned about 7.5% of major malformations to a monogenic basis; 6% to association with chromosomal aberrations, 5% to identified discrete environmental causes; 20%, on the basis of various lines of evidence, to the combined action of genetic and environmental components—the so-called multifactorial and ecogenetic defects—and the remainder, over 60%, still unknown (Kalter and Warkany 1983). These categories will be recalled in Chapter 10 where the association of diabetic pregnancy with congenital malformations will be discussed, since those occurring in the infants of diabetic women that are of known genic, chromosomal, or nondiabetic environmental origin must be discounted when assessing the association.

While hardly satisfactory, this knowledge must be considered a vast leap beyond some of what was accepted by medical people in the past, for example, that "maternal impressions" could be responsible for deforming infants in utero (Gould and Pyle 1898, p. 81). A humorous, but perhaps semiserious example of this belief occurs in Chapter 75 of Melville's *Moby Dick,* where a "harelipped" whale is reported with a "fissure...about a foot across," whose mother "...during an important interval was sailing down the Peruvian coast, when earthquakes caused the beach to gape." The author at least was rationally deterministic in timing the catastrophic event to an embryologically susceptible interval.

The reported frequencies of all and of individual congenital malformations have often been very different from one another. This is not surprising, since in addition to variations of definition their frequency depends on numerous factors—demographic, environmental, temporal, geographic, surveillance practice and efficiency, observer skill and experience, birth registration and hospital record completeness and accuracy, and so on (Kennedy 1967, Klingberg and Papier 1979, Janerich and Polednak 1983, Leck 1984, 1993, Khoury, 1989). But studies that have been aware of such difficulties and applied uniform criteria and ascertainment procedures have, as already stated, usually found the background rate of major congenital malformations to be about 3%, a figure that has not greatly varied in the last 60 years of such studies (Warkany and Kalter 1961, Kalter and Warkany 1983).

PRENATAL AND PERINATAL DEATH AND MALFORMATION

As estimated from examining unselected spontaneous abortuses, human embryos and fetuses have an overall frequency of anatomical abnormalities that, though admittedly difficult to establish, is perhaps six to seven times greater than the approximately 3% of congenital malformations present in newborn children (Sentrakul and Potter 1966, Poland et al. 1981, Shepard et al. 1988, 1989). Thus, although the causal relation between these anatomical abnormalities and prenatal death is unclear (Rushton 1985), the greatly reduced malformation frequency present at birth is due to the powerful effect of spontaneous abortion in selectively eliminating many malformed embryos and fetuses (Warkany 1978, Shiota 1993).

The frequency of congenital malformations in stillbirths and early neonatal deaths is also considerably larger than the overall 3% occurring in newborn infants, although again a causative relation between malformations and perinatal death is often not apparent. Also different from the overall newborn malformation frequency, which seems not to have shifted since its earlier determinations, is the fact that in perinatal mortalities it has increased steadily over the years, as the mortality rate has decreased.

An example that vividly demonstrates this inverse relation is the contrast between surveys made in Vienna in 1934–1953 and 1981–1983, which showed that as the perinatal mortality rates fell the malformation frequency in the mortalities increased from 5.6% in the earlier period to 23.4% in the later (Fink 1955, Huber and Reinold 1985). This inverse relation was well supported by a recent comprehensive review of 50 years of hospital-based reports (Table 8.1, Kalter 1991).

This trend has been arrested and perhaps reversed in some localities by the practice first introduced 15–20 years ago of terminating pregnancies in which a lethal abnormality was recognized prenatally (Powell-Griner and Woolbright 1990). In one area, for example, nearly half the decline in the perinatal mortality rate in a 9-year period was due to this practice; consequently the frequency of perinatal death due to congenital malformations declined from 23% at the beginning to 14% at the end of the period (Northern Regional Survey Steering Group 1992).

Table 8.1 Inverse Relation Between the Perinatal Mortality Rate and the Frequency of Congenital Malformations (CM) in Stillbirths and Early Neonatal Deaths (END)*

Decade	SB		END	
	% Death	% CM	% Death	% CM
		America		
1940s	14.9	12.0	12.7	16.4
1950s	12.0	10.4	11.9	17.7
1960s	12.3	9.4	11.0	15.9
1970s	6.2	14.7	8.4	43.6
1980s	4.9	11.8	3.6	31.4
		Europe		
1940s	20.5	5.4	22.2	6.5
1950s	15.3	12.3	18.4	15.4
1960s	14.5	11.5	14.1	16.8
1970s	8.1	13.4	6.5	21.4
1980s	5.9	18.3	2.2	36.3

* Taken from Tables 1 and 2 in Kalter 1991.

Table 8.1 shows that stillbirth and neonatal death have behaved differently in malformation frequency, having increased over time far less or not at all in the former than the latter. Since 50 years ago the frequency was similar in both, this divergence points at least partly to differential success in overcoming the causes or concomitants of death in these two phases of existence. Certain facts point to reasons for this: sharp distinctions between the predominant types of malformations occurring in them, in stillbirths 75–85% being of the central nervous system (mostly failure of neural tube closure), whereas in neonatal deaths the most common types are cardiovascular defects, types carrying very different prognoses for viability and well-being (Kalter 1991). How these facts impinge on the topic of the association of congenital malformations and diabetic pregnancy will be pursued in Chapter 10.

9

CASE REPORTS OF MATERNAL DIABETES AND MALFORMATIONS

The clinical impression that maternal diabetes is associated with an increased occurrence of congenital malformations has a long history. As far back as 1933, Skipper considered that there was an "unusual tendency for the children of diabetics to show congenital abnormalities," though the evidence—various disparate abnormalities reported in several publications—was too scanty "to allow definite conclusions to be drawn." Attention given to the subject during the ensuing 60 or more years largely turned to surveys of series of hospital-based births of diabetic women, but scattered publication of individual instances of diabetic women having malformed children continued as well. These isolated occurrences included many types or complexes of malformations, but four predominated: caudal dysplasia (also known by various other names), caudal regression/sirenomelia, femoral dysplasia, and holoprosencephaly. Case reports of the association of these malformations with diabetic pregnancy are the subject of this chapter.

A PROPOSED SPECIFIC DIABETIC EMBRYOPATHY

Numerous surveys of diabetic pregnancies have chiefly indicated that malformations in the offspring of diabetic women, as in the population in general, formed no particular pattern, but consisted of a cross-section of numerous types of defects. This was and frequently continues to be the prevailing opinion (Driscoll 1965, Neave 1967, 1984, Pedersen 1977, Holmes 1992).

Opposed to this is the opinion that the offspring of diabetic women as well as possessing an increased frequency of a nonspecific assortment of malformations also have even more excessively a particular syndrome of malformations, a specific diabetic embryopathy, a term coined by Lenz and Passarge (1965). A similar term, embryopathia diabetica, introduced some years earlier (Mayer 1952), merely encompassed the long-recognized newborn features macrosomia, organomegaly, etc, although it was later broadened to include congenital malformations generally (Mayer 1964) even as it continued to be used in the original sense (Majewski et al. 1979).

As used by Lenz and colleagues, however, the term had a specific connotation. It held that maternal diabetes caused directed defects: particular abnormalities of the lower limbs, a view based on anomalies in several children of diabetic women (Lenz and Maier 1964, Lenz and Passarge 1965) and supported, it was believed, by limb and lumbar defects in older children of diabetic mothers noted by orthopedic surgeons (Blumel et al. 1959). It appeared from these initial cases that the postulated diabetic embryopathy consisted primarily of defects of the leg above the knee.

This perspective changed when it was appreciated that sacral defects were present in orthopedic cases about as frequently as femoral ones. The name of the syndrome was therefore changed from the earlier suggested "caudal regression" to "caudal dysplasia," and redefined as malformations of the lower extremities, most commonly hypoplasia of the femur, absence of the sacrum and coccyx, or both (Passarge and Lenz 1966). A further modification seemed to exclude femoral defects, and the entity was finally described as composed of lower vertebral abnormalities alone (Lenz and Kučera 1967).

The previous apparently misplaced emphasis on the femur may have stemmed from the deceptive appearance of the legs of individuals with sacral defects. In many of these instances, especially of more extreme examples, the legs are held in what is called the frog-leg position, being rigidly flexed at the hips and hyperextended at the knees. Despite the consequent bizarre appearance of the upper leg, the femur is seldom shortened. The lower legs also usually appear abnormal, but this is due not to their position but to hypoplasia or absence of muscles supplied by the affected spinal nerves, causing atrophy of the calves and giving them a withered look.

In essence then the final depiction of the malformations considered to be typically associated with maternal diabetes were those, especially absence, of the lower vertebral elements and seldom of the femur. What was apparently meant to be a precise term designating a circumscribed anomaly-picture was soon loosened, however, and the concept weakened by addition to it of a heterogeneous spectrum of defects of the caudal axis and others (eg, Kaplan 1979, Ullrich 1979, Welch and Aterman 1984).

Frequency of the Proposed Embryopathy

It was estimated—guestimated perhaps, since the basis for the calculation was not stated—that this anomaly-picture occurred in "possibly about 1%" of the infants of diabetic women and, according to the pooled data of several publications, that 16% [sic] (10/72) of all individuals with the picture were born to diabetic women (Passarge and Lenz 1966). These figures have been uncritically repeated in numerous publications since that time (eg, Jones 1988, p. 575, Buyse 1990, p. 297).

The first figure, however, was soon revised in accordance with the analysis the authors made of reports of 48 series of diabetic pregnancies that extended over the previous 30 years, which yielded nine instances of "caudal regression" in 7101 births, that is, a frequency of 1.3 per 1000 children of diabetic women (Lenz and Kučera 1967, Kučera 1971a). (These nine instances will be scrutinized on p. 134.) This frequency was 227 times that of the condition reported in all births in Czechoslovakia in 1961–1963 (Kučera and Lenz 1967), but only 4.5 times that in a multicountry control series (Kučera 1971a).

In addition to the many reasons noted by Kučera (1971a) himself to be skeptical of the validity of many of the series he cited, there is one he did not mention, namely the frequent misconception of what comprises caudal regression or caudal dysplasia. Many of these erroneous ideas stemmed from the writings of Duhamel (1961), discussed on p. 87. To give but two examples, anal atresia and other abnormalities (but not lower vertebral ones) have often been labeled caudal regression (Miller 1972, Kubryk et al. 1981, Boutte et al. 1985, Lage et al. 1987, Petit et al. 1987, Shanberg and Rosenberg 1989); even more ludicrously, miscellaneous skeletal abnormalities in a stillbirth and an abortus were called the caudal regression syndrome for no more reason it seems than that they were the products of diabetic women (Perrot et al. 1987).

The "16%" estimate of affected individuals born to diabetic women is also open to criticism. It was based on the information concerning 72 cases of congenital sacral abnormalities reported in three articles and a personal communication from the author of one of them (Blumel et al. 1959, Russell and Aitken 1963, Stern et al. 1965). Fifty of the cases had been reported by Blumel et al. (1959), but only eight were their own orthopedic patients, the others being learned of through a postal survey—poorly replied to—mainly of orthopedic surgeons.

It is important in considering the frequency of these sacral abnormalities to know that most persons with them have first been reported by neurosurgeons, urologists, radiologists, and orthopedic surgeons, and seen at ages beyond infancy, since these conditions are seldom diagnosed at birth (Pang and Hoffman 1980, Borrelli et al. 1985, Pang 1993, Van Dyke et al. 1995). For example, of the 56 persons whose ages were noted in the three papers cited in the previous paragraph, only two were neonates (Stern et al. 1965), the ages of the others when diagnosed or examined ranging from 2 to 41 years. Obviously, this means that only the most severe examples of sacral abnormalities are recognized at birth, most instances in the general population of newborns being overlooked. Hence, comparison of the prevalence of such defects in these individuals with that in the generally well-examined infants of diabetic women is hardly credible.

Case Reports of the Proposed Association

Because the association of maternal diabetes and a specific malformation complex was first proposed in the mid-1960s, the present overview was confined to reports made following this time. In addition, since components of the complex are shared by various other entities—of known and unknown etiology (McKusick 1992, vol. 2, pp. 1028–1030)—to lessen the possible heterogeneity of the material and the analytical imponderabilities thus engendered, the condition considered was limited to sacral absence.

A search of the postmid-1960s literature identified 37 reports of 41 children with sacral absence born to 40 women with diabetes. Many also had other vertebral and a wide variety of nonskeletal malformations (Kalter 1993; the citations can be obtained from the author). Twenty-six of the 40 children whose ages were stated were diagnosed under 1 year of age, probably indicating that they were more severely affected than the majority of individuals with this abnormality. This surmise was supported by about 78% of them having total absence of at least the sacral elements of the vertebral column (in contrast with the far smaller percentage in the examples reported in surveys of older patients noted on p. 87). In part also, the early diagnosis may have been prompted by the growing awareness of the condition, which is attested by the increasing volume of such reports: of the 37 articles six were published in 1968–1969, nine in the 1970s, and 22 from 1980 to the time of writing this chapter. Finally, at least 27 of the 40 mothers of the children were insulin-dependent diabetics; the status of most of the others was uncertain or not relevant.

Such case reports, even when valid, while possibly adding some details to the picture of the complex,[11] do little to strengthen the connection between it and the disease, characterized as they are by their wholly biased ascertainment. The limitations of case reports for establishing etiology were well outlined by Leck (1993).

With respect to the frequency of the proposed association, the number of such occurrences reported during the past 30 years is a minute fraction of those expected according to the estimate of 1.3 per 1000 diabetic women (Kučera and Lenz 1967). In the US alone, with approximately 113 million births from 1965 through 1995, and a frequency of insulin-dependent diabetic pregnancy of about 5 per 1000 (Chung and Myrianthopoulos 1975b, Mills and Withiam 1986), over 700 such children should have been born to diabetic women in this period. If far fewer have been medically reported, it may in part be due to editorial reluctance to publish negative or non-newsworthy items, to estimates of their frequency being exaggerated, or to both.

Retrospective Surveys of Caudal Dysplasia

The validity of the purported association of maternal diabetes and caudal dysplasia may be tested by determining the strength of the association in individuals brought to medical attention because of these abnormalities. In a case-control study, this would be attempted retrospectively by comparing the frequency of exposure to the imputed cause of affected persons with that in persons not so affected. Since no such comparisons have been made, one must attempt to judge the question by information that is available, namely, from that in reports of individuals with the complex.

To my knowledge 25 reports of two or more instances of this abnormality complex were reported from 1965 to this writing, which dealt mainly with the orthopedic and urologic problems of 335 patients that stemmed from their vertebral defects. One hundred-sixteen patients not randomly ascertained, but selected because of one feature or another, are not further considered here.

---

11 For example, the cases make it clear that if maternal diabetes and sacral abnormalities are associated, the association is predominantly with *symmetrical* absence of sacral vertebral elements (with or without absence of more rostral vertebrae.)

Most of the remaining patients were far older at examination or diagnosis than the isolated cases previously noted, not surprisingly since the majority of the reports were made by orthopedists, urologists, and radiologists. From this it follows that their defects should be less extensive as well, which was the case, since 44% of the patients for whom the relevant information was supplied had complete sacral or lumbosacral absence, compared with 78% of the infants. In addition, about 14% had only unilateral absence of sacral elements, that is, hemisacrum, compared with perhaps as few as 3% in the younger cases noted above.

About 14% of the patients for whom such information was presented had diabetic mothers, but for most it was not made clear whether the diabetes antedated the index pregnancy, the only form of the disease considered teratogenic (Chung and Myrianthopoulos 1975b, Pedersen 1977, Mills 1982). It must also be recalled that after 1965 the suggested association of maternal diabetes and caudal abnormalities became widely known and accepted as fact. This cannot be discounted as a biasing factor in directing attention to this possible, and sometimes misunderstood, association, as when, for example, gestational diabetes, so-called prediabetes, noninsulin-dependent diabetes, or even a family history of diabetes was sometimes thought apropos (Banta and Nichols 1969, Sarnat et al. 1976, Mariani et al. 1979, Pang and Hoffman 1980). These data do not support the belief that caudal dysplasia and pregestational diabetes are significantly associated.

THE CAUDAL REGRESSION SYNDROME

It is instructive to consider the origin of the term "syndrome of caudal regression" and its evolution as it took on additional layers of meaning when it came to be applied to the proposed diabetic embryopathy. Two issues are intertwined here, which must be separated and clarified. The first concerns the original concept: that there exists a complex of progressively more severe interrelated congenital malformations, the syndrome of caudal regression (Duhamel 1959, 1961); and second that one of the features of this syndrome, lower vertebral absence, is increased in frequency in diabetic pregnancy.

Duhamel postulated the complex to consist of a graded series of malformations—limb, urogenital, anorectal, and lumbosacral—of increasing severity, extending from defects of the anal region at the mildest end to symmelia (or sirenomelia) at the most extreme. The scheme was based on (a) clinical observations of the frequent association of such malformations in nonsymmelic individuals and (b) experiments with chicken embryos that apparently supported the idea that the comprehensive syndrome stemmed from variably localized defects in the formation of the caudal region (Wolff 1948, pp. 165–170).

It was Duhamel's theory (which, incidentally, was formulated without reference to maternal diabetes) that formed the basis of Passarge and Lenz's (1966) suggestion that "minor malformations of the caudal region of the body [as seen in their cases]...were related to symmelia and sireniform monsters in a teratogenic spectrum which may include anorectal and urogenital anomalies," and hence that their cases possibly were examples of the caudal regression complex enunciated by Duhamel.

The suggestion that symmelia is sacral regression carried to its utmost degree (Passarge and Lenz 1966), since then widely accepted (eg, Källén and Winberg 1974, Kaplan 1979, Källén et al. 1992) and even equated with it (eg, Schwartz et al. 1982), coupled with the supposition that sacral defects are associated with diabetic pregnancy, if taken to its logical conclusion, leads to the inference that symmelia too must be associated with maternal diabetes. This idea will be explored right after the symmelia complex itself is considered.

The Symmelia Syndrome

The existence of a "sirenoid" complex has been accepted for many years with little reservation. For example, O'Rahilly and Müller (1989) wrote that "in less extreme forms, the caudal regression syndrome consists of sacral agenesis or merely imperforate anus." In their discussion of the developmental mechanisms of median anomalies these authors seconded an older theoretical scheme (Feller and Sternberg 1931), which ascribed the features of this complex to the extent of a median defect in the caudal region of the early embryo, narrower and shallower defects being associated mostly with vertebral abnormalities and broader and deeper ones with symmelia, and so on.

In an extended critique of this theory (only briefly summarized here) Gruenwald (1947) noted several difficulties with it. First, in Wolff's (1948) experiments with chicken embryos the initiating cause of the radiation-induced symmelia was localized destruction of prospective axial organs, which is not the mechanism initially proposed for the origin of human symmelia (Kampmeier 1927), nor is it of any of the mechanisms since proposed (David and Fein 1974, Chappard et al. 1983, Stevenson et al. 1986). Second, the theory requires (a) that the defects be determined in early stages (according to O'Rahilly and Müller 1989, by stage 11, ie, about 24 days postovulatory) and (b) that their extent and respective locations be unchanging in time—in other words that the parts concerned must develop independently of one another. But such implied mosaicism, that is, development without correlation of parts, is contrary to what is known about the interdependence of tissues and organ primordia in the early embryo (Hamburger 1988).

For these reasons it is doubtful that the several components of the symmelia complex can be due to variability in the extent of the putative initial caudal fault and hence that any one or more of them by themselves represent intermediate degrees of the so-called symmelic syndrome.

Are Symmelia and Maternal Diabetes Associated?

In support of the claimed connection between caudal dysplasia and maternal diabetes and the almost axiomatic contention that lower vertebral abnormalities and symmelia are lesser and extreme forms respectively of one and the same syndrome of caudal regression, it was proposed that symmelia is also associated with maternal diabetes (Passarge and Lenz 1966). On the basis of the following facts, this proposition cannot be accepted.

A search of post-1965 sources yielded 75 reports and personal communications of 157 symmelic fetuses and infants (including a concordant twin and a sib pair—references obtainable from the author). In 116 of the 119 accounts of pregnancies in which information regarding maternal health or the course of pregnancy was noted, it was made clear or highly probable that none of the mothers had pregestational insulin-dependent diabetes. In the three others, one mother had gestational and two had type 2 diabetes (Stocker and Heifetz 1987, Martin et al. 1990, Gürakan et al. 1996). Looking further back, of 28 symmelics reported in 1927–1964 (Stocker and Heifetz 1987) apparently only one had a known diabetic mother, who, however was not clearly insulin-dependent, and another a mother who had received insulin shock therapy for emotional illness.

Considering only the more recent 119 cases with known maternal health condition and using the mean of several estimates of the prevalence of symmelia of 1.37 per 100,000 (Butler and Bonham 1963, Stevenson et al. 1966, Leck et al. 1968, Källén and Winberg 1974), the cases represent approximately 8.5 million births. Taking 5 per 1000 once again as the approximate frequency of pregestational diabetic pregnancy, among this number of total births over 42,000 occurred to diabetic women of this type. The apparent rarity of reports of symmelia in these diabetic births seems to indicate that its relation to diabetes is indeed minuscule or nonexistent. Their nonrelatedness is further indicated by the dissimilarity of the supposed pathogeneses of the two conditions (Jones 1988) as well as by various morphological considerations (Colwell et al. 1991).

Finally, in the innumerable articles published since the 1920s read by this author concerned with thousands of pregnancies of diabetic women, five instances of symmelia were reported, in three hospital-based and two population-based series (Gellis and Hsia 1959, Kučera 1971a, Steel et al. 1982, Vadheim 1983, Becerra et al. 1990), not all for certain occurring in offspring of indisputably pregestational insulin-dependent diabetic women.

FEMORAL DYSPLASIA AND MATERNAL DIABETES

Following the initial claim of the existence of a specific diabetic embryopathy (Lenz and Maier 1964), a large miscellany of isolated instances of congenital malformations and anomalies was alleged to be associated with maternal diabetes. Some of these defects, discussed here and later in the text, have been reported often enough to merit special attention.

In the light of hindsight it is ironic that the deformities of the very first infants that were considered to form a "special spectrum" (Lenz and Maier 1964, Passarge 1965) were not those that later came to represent the typical diabetic embryopathy. As previously noted, the first cases reported had femoral abnormalities, not the sacral ones that later came to be regarded the hallmark of the anomaly-picture.

It is probable that Passarge's (1965) case was actually an example of a separate entity, one that has also been alleged to occur nonrandomly in infants of diabetic women. This infant, in addition to short femurs, had a pronounced cleft palate, micrognathia, and glossoptosis, that is, the Pierre Robin syndrome (a photograph of this infant appears on p. 999 in Warkany's 1971 vade mecum), and hence is included among the cases with facial abnormalities considered in the following section.

With respect to the femoral defect itself—known especially to orthopedists as proximal femoral focal deficiency (Ring 1961)—from 1965 to the time of this writing, depending on definition, perhaps 18 alleged instances of the condition have been reported (references obtainable from the author). As with caudal dysplasia, these cases were ascertained in various ways. They too will be discussed further below.

Facial and Femoral Abnormalities

In another early report, a child, originally presented by Lenz and Maier (1964), with femoral and other long-bone abnormalities was incidentally also noted to have "a remarkably long upper lip [and] a cleft palate...." (Kučera et al. 1965). A photograph included in the article clearly showed that the child had an "odd-appearing" face, but this was not specifically alluded to. Some time later she and her features were recalled by Daental et al. (1975), and together with further instances of this combination of femoral defects and unusual facial features (long philtrum, thin upper lip, short nose with a broad tip, and so on) were offered as representing a newly recognized entity, named the femoral hypoplasia-unusual facies syndrome. Up to the present writing, 42 instances or purported instances of this syndrome have been reported (references obtainable from the author). All were single cases of infants or young children, apparently ascertained through their malformations, by pediatricians and clinical geneticists. What makes this and the femoral dysplasia syndromes relevant here is the presence of diabetes in the mothers of some of the cases. This aspect will be considered on p. 91. First, the two syndromes will be compared.

Are These Different Syndromes?

There is uncertainty about the distinctiveness of the femoral dysplasia and femoral hypoplasia-unusual facies syndromes. Many of their facial and other features overlap, so that if they do constitute different entities it is difficult to know what demarks them. This criterion should perhaps be the so-called unusual facial features present in the latter syndrome. These, however, consist of two very different sets of anomalies: one, a collection of morphometric features that in toto labels a face "unusual," and the other a set of "conventional" malformations—cleft palate and micrognathia. Both sets present problems: the first because they may be open to arbitrary judgment and because of their possible transience, and the second because they are frequently found in both syndromes.

There has been much uncertainty and difference of opinion over the diagnosis of the syndromes. Daentl et al. (1975), in the original delineation of the femoral hypoplasia-unusual facies syndrome, found that three facial features were unequivocally shared by all their cases. But this standard was not accepted by others (eg, Johnson et al. 1983), and many dissenting opinions have been expressed.

Thus, Eastman and Escobar (1978) felt that two of Daentl et al.'s own cases may not have had the unusual facies syndrome; Lord and Beighton (1981) questioned whether this syndrome has a separate identity; and Graviss et al. (1980) and Maisels and Stilwell (1980) doubted that such an entity existed and on the contrary asserted that the supposed unusual facial features were typical of the Pierre Robin syndrome.

The conventional orofacial malformations sometimes found in the syndromes have also been a source of disagreement. It has been maintained that the abnormalities in the Pierre Robin syndrome constitute a distinct entity, even when associated with femoral dysplasia (Walden et al. 1971, Holthusen 1972, Graviss et al. 1980, Maisels and Stilwell 1980), whereas they have also been held merely to be additional components of the femoral hypoplasia-unusual facies syndrome (Hurst and Johnson 1980, Burck et al. 1981, Pitt et al. 1982, Johnson et al. 1983). In any case, it appears that cleft palate, per se, as a feature distinguishing the two syndromes can be of no use, since in the instances that have been reported the present author has discovered no statistically significant difference between them in its frequency (7/19 versus 23/39, $P > .05$).

It appears suitable therefore to consider these two supposedly distinct entities as one in getting to the nub of the question—their imputed association with maternal diabetes. Together, they amounted to 58 isolated cases of femoral dysplasia with or without facial anomalies. Eighteen had diabetic mothers: 12 insulin-dependent (11 pregestational, one of uncertain onset time), two noninsulin-dependent, three gestational, and one described merely as "diabetic." Thirty of the cases had cleft palate, but the conjunction of this defect and maternal insulin-dependent diabetes was not statistically significant (6/12 versus 24/46, $P > .05$). Ultimately, however, the question of the relation of the femoral defect to diabetes is clouded by the problem of possibly biased ascertainment. Some help may be offered by the apparent absence of diabetes in the mothers of 186 patients with the femoral defect, usually without the facial abnormalities, in three orthopedic surveys of affected individuals (Hamanishi 1980, Koman et al. 1982, Kalamchi et al. 1985).

OTHER MALFORMATIONS AND MATERNAL DIABETES

As mentioned, a diverse and heterogeneous assortment of congenital abnormalities, singly or multiply, mostly not associated with vertebral defects, has been reported since 1965 in infants of diabetic women. It is unnecessary to describe and discuss or even name them all, since most are without merit. Two, however, will get further attention, since reports of their occurrence in offspring of diabetic women led to a directed search for and subsequent discovery of them in other children of such women. This is exemplified first by the alleged association with diabetic pregnancy of the transient functional intestinal obstruction, neonatal small left colon syndrome, an initial report of which (Davis et al. 1974) led to the discovery of further such coincidences (Davis et al. 1975, Berdon et al. 1977), a route of recognition that vitiates its confirmatory role.

Holoprosencephaly

In a similar sequence the finding of holoprosencephaly in two infants of diabetic women (Barr and Burdi 1978) led to surveys at three unnamed medical centers, which over the course of 4 years uncovered five further occurrences of one or another of the various forms of this malformation in an unspecified number of infants of such women. In one of the total of seven cases, the karyotype was not determined; this is relevant since chromosome abnormalities occur frequently in individuals with this defect (Cohen 1989). Another of the cases did not have a brain morphology typical of the condition and two others were without facial features typical of it, the latter two with various abnormalities unrelated to the supposed diagnoses. Such variability is perhaps expected.

The preliminary report also "stimulated recognition" of the association of holoprosencephaly with maternal diabetes and led to personal communications to the authors of nine other such occurrences in 8 years. As said above, the usefulness of data obtained in this manner for substantiating causative relationships is to be mistrusted. Finally, three such occurrences (including two of the seven noted above) identified through retrospective surveys of 189 diabetic deliveries at two medical centers were said to suggest a frequency of at least 1% for this condition in the infants of diabetic women.

As Barr et al. (1983) carefully pointed out, the evidence for this suggestion was derived solely from tertiary-level referral hospitals and is open to the various biases residing in information obtained from this source. Therefore, the authors' tacit assumption that their estimate of the condition's frequency in diabetic pregnancy is far greater than that in the general population presents problems from the start. Several variables affecting the prevalence of the condition at birth (Cohen 1989) further cloud this proposal.

Findings in a genetic and an abortion study may be noted. In 30 families of 32 patients with holoprosencephaly, two mothers were found to be juvenile diabetics (Roach et al. 1975). Both of their children had less severe forms of the condition. Chromosome examinations were not made, but neither case was considered of karyopathic origin. In the second study, the mothers of 150 induced abortuses with holoprosencephaly were found to have diseases of all sorts no more commonly than did matched controls (Matsunaga and Shiota 1977).

Population surveys of holoprosencephaly suddenly became popular in the mid-1990s, and five made in separate areas were published within a short period (Martínez-Frias et al. 1994, Croen et al. 1996, Rasmussen et al. 1996, Whiteford and Tolmie 1996, Olsen et al. 1997). Reported were 381 occurrences with frequencies of 0.5–1.2 per 10,000 live- and stillbirths, with a mean of 0.75 per 10,000. Six of the mothers of the 316 cases for whom this information was given had insulin-dependent diabetes, but whether of pregestational origin was not stated. On the face of it this is a frequency of 19 per 1000, much larger than the usual overall population level. To provide firm evidence of the association with maternal diabetes, further details would have been required. Since holoprosencephaly has a very heterogeneous etiology, a considerable fraction of instances (one-third to one-half) having a chromosomal basis or forming part of monogenic or other known syndromes, or furthermore possibly resulting from numerous nongenetic risk factors (eg, see Croen et al. 1996), information about the maternal condition of cases with and without identified etiology would have been useful. Without such information and also without at least some matched control group, inferences regarding the association of holoprosencephaly and maternal diabetes derived from such studies can have but little credibility.

Cyclopia

It is appropriate to round out the discussion of this malformation by noting, as alluded, that the condition known as holoprosencephaly is in fact a general term for a series of progressively more severe median abnormalities of the face and fore- and midbrain (DeMyer et al. 1964). As the term cyclocephaly originally proposed by Saint-Hilaire (1832–1837 vol. 2, pp. 423–424) better intimates, this graded series of defects culminates in cyclopia, which displays a single or partially divided median eye in one orbit and a large anterior cerebral cavity (Kalter 1968, p. 240).

This leads ultimately to this question: If cyclopia is the extreme expression of holoprosencephaly, as symmelia is said to be that of the caudal regression syndrome, and if holoprosencephaly, as claimed, is associated with maternal diabetes, it follows that cyclopia should also be so associated. Population surveys of the condition might be helpful with this question. Cyclopia, like symmelia, is rare. An overview of more than 10 million births in various countries since 1965 revealed perhaps 121 instances of cyclopia for an estimate of about 1.2 per 100,000 (Källén et al. 1992). Later, more precise estimates reported a total of 28 cases in slightly over 4 million births, giving a mean frequency of 0.69 per 100,000 live- and stillbirths (Croen et al. 1996, Rasmussen et al. 1996, Whiteford and Tolmie 1996, Olsen et al. 1997). The condition of the mothers of these cases unfortunately was not stated. The earlier survey (Källén et al. 1992) found that in four of the occurrences maternal diabetes was recorded, but absence of information about the specific maternal disease makes this number unhelpful. Skepticism is supported by the rarity of cyclopia in diabetic pregnancies in hospital-based reports; only four were discovered in articles published from the 1920s to the present: one in births at the King's College Hospital in London during 1951–1960 (Seligman 1963), one in 1950–1984 in the maternity hospitals of Dublin (Drury 1966), and two from India, whose mothers, said to be diabetic, turned out to be a gestational and a noninsulin-dependent diabetic, respectively (Soni et al. 1989).

CONCLUSION

In evaluating the alleged association of malformations and diabetes, especially as made by case reports, it is obviously pertinent to recall that both congenital malformations and diabetes are common human afflictions. The relatively great frequency of the former has been mentioned often above (Kalter and Warkany 1983). Diabetes is no less pervasive (Harris et al. 1987). Considering these facts, as well as the largely biased nature of the conduct of the majority of the case studies outlined in the previous text, it must be concluded, being extravagantly generous, that the evidence at most but barely suggests a causal relation between maternal diabetes and the various congenital malformations the condition has been alleged to be associated with.

Finally, it must be said that an association of specific congenital malformation patterns with maternal diabetes, as surely must be recognized intuitively, cannot be established by isolated reports of their concurrence. It is only by careful analysis of well-described surveys of unselected diabetic pregnancies, supported by meticulously planned and executed epidemiological efforts, that definitive conclusions regarding claims that they are causally related may perhaps be arrived at.[12]

12 A version of this chapter appeared in *Clinical Genetics* vol. 43, pp. 174–179, 1993.

10

MATERNAL DIABETES AND CONGENITAL MALFORMATIONS

INTRODUCTION

The waning of perinatal mortality brought congenital malformations to the foreground as the most pressing enigma of diabetic pregnancy. Since 1930, and especially from the 1940s, a large number of hospital-based publications appeared, which detailed the outcome of pregnancy in insulin-dependent diabetic women. What they recorded about congenital malformations in the offspring of these pregnancies, perishing and surviving, will be dealt with in this chapter.

This and subsequent chapters address various questions about these abnormalities: whether their overall frequency is greater in the children of diabetic women than in those of nondiabetic women; whether certain malformations or combinations of them are disproportionately increased in diabetic pregnancy; and whether the possibly increased frequency can be prevented by strict metabolic management of diabetes started before or very early in pregnancy.

Early Difficulties

Different points of view about these matters arose early and have persisted, essentially because the evidence regarding the ultimate matter of the frequency of congenital malformations in the offspring of diabetic women has been flawed, fragmentary, and ambiguous. Inadequacies of much of the data, especially of earlier years, and faulty appreciation of concepts regarding congenital malformations, it can now be seen, made resolution of these questions hardly possible. What the several difficulties were will be briefly noted here, and dealt with later in this chapter.

In addition, it is now known that whether diabetes antedates pregnancy or is gestational is relevant to the problem, since only the former state has been found to be associated with an increased frequency of malformations. But this was not well understood at an earlier time, and women with both types of diabetes were included in many studies without distinction and the outcomes of their pregnancies usually not reported separately. This practice is understandable, however, since the foremost problem of that day, the exceedingly high perinatal mortality rate, was shared by both types of diabetes, but still it has hindered examining the relation of malformations to offspring death and to the maternal disease generally.

It is fundamental that determining whether a given situation causes or is associated with congenital malformations must be preceded by widely accepted agreement about what is a congenital malformation. The herculean task of defining and agreeing upon definition has been wrestled with by professionals whose interests lay in this area. It is the long disregard of the need for definitional standards by clinicians caring for diabetic women and by others that has made for the confused state of the data which, at first blush, all but defied attempts to determine whether diabetes causes congenital malformations.

But it was not any of the innumerable elements outlined in great detail elsewhere in this work that has principally underlain the confused observations and inconclusive interpretations about this question. That role has been played by the disorder of the abnormalities that have been recorded: rarely was the admissibility of the reported hodgepodge of abnormalities questioned, because their association with the maternal disease was a priori unquestioningly accepted. Only of just less moment was the seldom recognition of the impact that numerous ingredients have upon the diagnosis of malformations: infant age at examination, means of diagnosis, inclusion or omission of perinatal deaths, autopsy rate and the thoroughness of the postmortem examination, interests and experience of the investigators, accuracy and completeness of records, representativeness of the pregnant women, and so on. And seldom has it been realized that in evaluating the studies of this subject such factors must enter the judgment.

The Prevailing Opinion

Without questioning how it was arrived at, the prevailing opinion, beginning at least 40 years ago, has been that the frequency of congenital malformations is increased, perhaps threefold or even more, in the offspring of insulin-dependent pregestationally diabetic women (eg, Hagbard 1956, Gellis and Hsia 1959), and despite some isolated demurrals and skepticism (eg, Miller 1956, Farquhar 1959, Rubin and Murphy 1958, Warkany and Kalter 1961, Simpson 1978) that consensus has continued until today (eg, Neave 1984, Mills and Withiam 1986, Reece and Hobbins 1986, Greene 1989, Cousins 1991b, Landon and Gabbe 1995, Coustan 1998).

Nevertheless, doubts linger about the proposition. To try to resolve this problem, the malformation and other data will be subjected to critical scrutiny for the purpose of determining their basis and credibility. The inquiry will largely hinge on hospital-based reports of the outcome of diabetic pregnancies, but will also consider public health and epidemiological records that may be pertinent.

The daunting challenge to such an undertaking lies in rectifying the various incommensurabilities contained in these publications, especially regarding ascertainment, definition, and diagnosis of congenital malformations. It is but little consolation to discover that the struggle of reading and making sense of the records of the past is not rare. Morison's (1971, p. vii) exasperation at the struggle led to these words: "All honest efforts to throw light on historical darkness...have my enthusiastic support. But it has fallen to my lot...to read some of the most tiresome historical literature in existence. Young men seeking academic promotion, old men seeking publicity, neither one nor the other knowing the subject in depth...write worthless articles, and the so-called learned journals are altogether too hospitable to these effusions." Morison was well over 80 years old when he wrote and felt free to express himself as he pleased. As candid also was an editor of the *British Medical Journal* when he said "...much of what is published in peer reviewed journals is of very low quality" (Smith 1994).

Diagnostic Problems

Sources of These Problems

Many of the difficulties of judgment and comparison that one has had to deal with were contained even in more recent studies, but some older ones were perhaps more vexing. The nature and sources of many of these problems were stated by Warkany (1971): "There exist many publications that contend that the incidence [of congenital malformations in the offspring of diabetic mothers] is definitely increased, but some of the statements rely on impressions that are not adequately controlled and suffer from lack of clear definition of the term 'congenital malformations.' Some include stillbirths and necropsies; others deal with surviving children. Some conclusions are based on single examinations, others on repeated examinations. It is also probable that infants of diabetic mothers often are more thoroughly examined than the controls. ...The continued discussion of teratogenic effects of maternal diabetes illustrates the difficulties of ascertaining maternal factors in the etiology of congenital malformations" (pp. 124–125).

Some writers were aware of the workings of these and like factors even further back. Farquhar (1959), perhaps thinking in part of findings such as White's noted in the next section, explained the wide variation in malformation frequency reported in diabetic pregnancy in the decades before he wrote as follows: some authors, he said, "include every trivial abnormality found on clinical examination, whereas others used technical aids to diagnosis or recorded only lethal malformations discovered at autopsy. Some have mentioned only those anomalies which are obvious in the first week whereas others have followed their cases and have added those malformations which were discovered later." Most vexing, as Miller (1956) bewailed, was the fact that "few reports bother to list the kinds of anomalies encountered." It is in this vexation that the present author has felt himself most at one with Miller.

Clearly, studies that failed to enumerate malformations, or included trivial departures from normality, or commingled findings in newborn and older children, and so on, could be of no help in the quest for answers to the question whether the frequency of malformations in offspring of diabetic pregnancy was greater than in the general population, when the latter was derived from serious, conspicuous malformations detected in the neonatal period. It is these inadequacies and other discordances between the numerous publications whose pages have yielded the data on which this work are based that the present author has attempted to reconcile and analyze.

Examples of These Problems

Flagrant examples may be mentioned of studies that attempted to gauge the effects of maternal diabetes on prenatal development without taking into consideration the need for agreement on procedure and endpoint. Almost ludicrous was a statement of White's (1952). Summing up her experiences with congenital malformations in the Joslin Clinic in Boston, she said that "congenital anomalies…have occurred in 80% of the infants of our diabetic mothers…and include defects of the skull and heart, cysts of the kidney, ovary, pancreas, mouth; angioma, syndactylism, claw hand, club foot, web toes, congenital hip, dwarfism, feeblemindedness, and Mongolian idiocy." Questioned as to how these facts had been arrived at (Rubin and Murphy 1958), she replied, "Many of the abnormalities had been revealed by subsequent visits of these children, during x-ray examinations, etc. Every deviation from normal has been counted…and included are such slight abnormalities as a nevus, shovel rib, ear nodules and many other things…. The figure was based on a pilot study…conducted not only on the newborn, but on children of diabetic mothers up to age twenty." In Europe, too, such confusing practices could be found. Koller (1953), for example, not only reported "serious" malformations found at birth, but also included conditions dubiously labeled malformations as well as those found at follow-up examination of older children. Even in more recent years egregious examples of the looseness of the definition of congenital malformation may often be found in the diabetes literature, which give an idea of what a reviewer has had to contend with (Neufeld 1987).

Because some types of malformations may be less apparent during the neonatal than at later periods, serial examination of children at various postneonatal ages will increase the yield. However, when only older children are examined, as was sometimes the case (see the following text), the results are biased by the presence of abnormalities that become obvious only at later ages and also by absence of malformations fatal at younger ones. Although such extended coverage may be important for complete detection of abnormalities, and is valuable for other purposes, in studies made to determine the possible prenatal consequences of a discrete influence like maternal diabetes, it is mandatory to set a clear limit to the age of children to be examined. Clearly it is most logistically feasible and satisfactory that this be the neonatal period. However, when older children are included, the findings of each period must be presented separately. It should not be surprising, then, that when no uniformity of ages examined is adhered to and furthermore merely the total frequency of malformations found, without naming them, is reported, the already variable outcomes of a potentially prenatally harmful situation are magnified and difficulties of comparison and interpretation made further problematic.

The first of these sources of discrepancy between studies was recognized by Hagbard (1956, 1958), when he presented the results of observations made during the first week of life separately from those at later ages. This care was vitiated, however, by his failure to list the malformations discovered, for which his reporting of the overall frequencies was little compensation, since only a listing can enable the reviewer to analyze the acceptability of the defects found. The same fault was committed by Stevenson (1956), who, it may be said, compensated a bit for this omission by making the astute observation that "an interesting feature of many of these cases is the high incidence of abnormalities of the limbs," anticipating some assertions of the next decade, discussed above; and also by asking rhetorically why "if a metabolic disturbance does play a part in human development it should be limited to this particular time," that is, of limb bud development. In essence by this remark, he recognized that defective prenatal development occurs early in gestation, as did others of that generation, for example, Corner (cited by Miller 1956) and Hagbard (1956), who stated "We are concerned mainly with the first trimester of pregnancy, as most deformities develop during the first 7 to 8 weeks of embryonic life...." Thus, the stunning revelation by Mills et al. (1979) that malformations in infants of diabetic women occur early in gestation had been foretold at least 25 years previously. Nevertheless, to some this revelation seemed "almost revolutionary" and again a "veritable revolution in biological thought" (Opitz 1994, discussion in Holmes 1994).

Jones (1952) was an innovator in being among the first, if not the first, to report minor congenital malformations (which to him corresponded to those that were "correctable") separately from those that were severe or incompatible with life. But again, unfortunately, he did not name any defect and hence prevented insight into his method of classification.

How to Deal With These Problems

In order to reach the primary goal of comparing and analyzing malformation frequency in diabetic pregnancy, the present writer was presented with the necessity (1) of shearing away all reported abnormalities that did not conform to the usage of the term major malformation used here (as explained later), and (2) of being certain that the malformations were found only in the neonatal period. It was not always possible to be sure of both, because—presenting a total impediment to satisfactory analysis—a listing of the specific kinds of malformations encountered was not invariably provided, a problem recently a bit less prevalent than when Miller (1956) lamented over it, but not overcome yet; and some reports (fortunately not too many) did not identify the age of the infants in whom some of the malformations reported were diagnosed. A final point, ending this litany of complaints, is to note the rarity over the years of control subjects, matched or not, obligatory for valid judgment of the findings in the offspring of diabetic women.

The major concern of this work requires, once again, that congenital malformations as used here be defined. Because they comprise the basis of universal comparison, the primary emphasis is on those, called major malformations, present at birth that cause or are associated with perinatal death, need surgical intervention for continued life, or are a dire threat to health and well-being. Excluded are malformations with a known or probable cytogenetic, genic, or environmental etiology. Other aspects of this problem are not ignored. Minor malformations, as they have come to be called, are discussed on p. 109 et seq. Developmental abnormalities discovered upon examining children during postneonatal months will be considered in Chapter 13 and elsewhere.

MALFORMATIONS IN DIABETIC PREGNANCY

Early Observations

Pre-insulin Era

It is illuminating to read the earliest reports of the outcomes of diabetic pregnancies that carry a mention of a malformed child, often a dead child, and see the difficulties of interpretation they often embodied, beginning with the first one, by Lecorché (1885), often cited as substantiating the conviction that diabetes is teratogenic. Lecorché noted two children with hydrocephalus in five cases, one dead late in the neonatal period, and the fate of the other uncertain at 10 months of age. The diabetes in the mother of one of the children was said to have disappeared during pregnancy. Since hydrocephalus has a heterogeneous etiology and frequently arises postnatally as a result of infection or trauma (Russell 1949), the nature of the occurrences is unclear, and the return to normal during pregnancy in one of the mothers (? which one) casts doubt on the correctness of the diagnosis. There seems not to have been another report of a malformation in a child of a diabetic pregnancy during the pre-insulin years till the birth of a girl in 1922. Although described as healthy at birth, she died at 13 days of age with a congenital heart defect. Her mother died 9 months later in a diabetic coma (Rosenberg 1924).

During the first two decades of the insulin era such occurrences were apparently rare, despite the increased prevalence of diabetic pregnancy. In all, seven children with malformations from mothers with diabetes were reported (Gray and Feemster 1926, Nevinny and Schretter 1930, Peckham 1931, Skipper 1933, Hurwitz and Irving 1937, Allen 1939), but the maternal circumstances of many of them were such that today they would not be ascribed to the maternal disease.

Early Joslin Clinic Observations

Other such findings came from a long-existing Boston diabetes center, the Baker Clinic (afterward the Joslin Clinic). Earlier ones are detailed here; those of studies in later years are given on p. 112 et seq. The first report presented data beginning with the early days of the clinic, 1898–1935, from 166 pregnancies of the pre-insulin and insulin eras collectively (White 1935). In seven of the cases, children were found to be abnormal, which the author felt bore out her contention that "congenital defects occur frequently" in these cases. The conditions of two of the children, however, are hardly to be attributed to the maternal disease—one, a "Mongolian idiot," a state now known to be due to a chromosomal abnormality (Lejeune et al. 1959), and the other, an achondroplasia, not further described, but conditions so named are known today to be largely gene-caused. The others were microcephaly, gastrointestinal atresia, two instances of congenital heart defect, and a "monster." Omitting the first two defects gives a frequency of 3.0%, corresponding to the figure usually reported for the overall population (Kalter and Warkany 1983).

A parenthesis is called for. One abnormality (unspecified) occurred in one of the seven stillbirths, and White (1935) attempted to put this frequency (1/7) into perspective by comparing it with that of congenital defects (5/306) in a control of sorts—stillbirths in consecutive births in approximately the same years reported by Dippel (1934). Apart from not knowing which defect occurred in the diabetic stillbirth—which confuses the comparison—the data chosen for the comparison, obtained from the records of a Baltimore hospital of women probably different racially and otherwise from the Boston patients were obviously not well suited for the task. This is underscored by the strangely low frequency of congenital defects in the "control" series, probably due to the preponderance of deaths from infectious diseases, especially syphilis. Even a contemporary death certificate study (a notoriously unreliable source) in Philadelphia discovered a higher rate of malformed stillbirths (Murphy 1939). But more to the point are American hospital-based perinatal mortality studies made before 1959, a review of which found that 12.0% of 3540 stillbirths and 16.4% of 1696 first-week deaths were malformed (Kalter 1991). Thus, White's (1935) finding of one abnormal in seven stillbirths was not unusual.

Three other earlier publications from this clinic (White et al. 1939, White and Hunt 1943, White 1949) presented the results of successively supplemented pregnancy numbers, whose data, however, are not consistent and so must be evaluated individually. The first, concerning patients seen in 1936–1939, reported 3 children with congenital malformations in 35 deliveries—congenital heart defects, hand and foot abnormalities, and isolated bilateral dislocation of the hip.

The last defect requires some comment. First, to call it congenital (present at birth), although that is the conventional designation, is incorrect, since usually only the slight anomalies that predispose to dislocation exist prior to birth, whereas the defect itself is probably precipitated by later trauma. Next, it is a relatively common defect (a fact known since its recognition by Dupuytren almost 150 years ago), but nevertheless presents diagnostic difficulties. Third, it frequently has an appreciable genetic component. Last, it very often undergoes spontaneous restitution (Hass 1951, Barlow 1962, Warkany 1971, p. 992 et seq., Anon. 1992, Rosendahl et al. 1992). For all these reasons, bilateral hip anomalies will not be included in the toll of congenital malformations under consideration here as associated with maternal diabetes.

The next in the series, overlapping the preceding, encompassed the years 1936–1945 and concerned 125 infants of whom—discounting the three noted above—17 were said to have congenital anomalies (White and Hunt 1943). Among these were numerous conditions whose being endowed with the appellation "malformation" can be disputed: pancreatic rests, short tendon, ovarian cysts, angioma, cysts of the mouth, varices of the heart. Others of known etiology (Mongolian idiocy and cretinism) or heterogeneous states of unclear origin (dwarfism and mental retardation) it is difficult to hold the maternal disease responsible for. Those qualifying as congenital malformations were an encephalocele in a child who died after the "second week" and, perhaps, two instances of skull defects not further specified, which were combined with kidney cysts.

The last of these publications (White 1949), bringing the record up to 1949, reported congenital anomalies in 6 of 439 deliveries—bilateral renal agenesis, anencephaly, "hemorrhagic disease," and the remainder unnamed. In a follow-up of the survivors, there was said to be a "high incidence of [unspecified] congenital defects most of which have been slight in character…."

The few findings just outlined—suspect and heterogeneous—can be of little use in grappling with the question of whether congenital malformations were of any but perhaps the slightest significance so far as the excessive perinatal mortality rate was concerned or understandably whether malformations were present excessively in diabetic pregnancy generally. More definitive information started to appear in the 1940s when congenital malformation data began to be more regularly and more informatively presented, especially for perinatal mortalities separately. The latter, as previously noted, were in fact the only reliable indication of congenital malformation frequency for diabetic births of that time, since investigators, being chiefly concerned with explaining the deaths, paid great attention to them, and on the contrary seldom mentioned the survivors with regard to malformations at all.

MALFORMATIONS IN PERINATAL MORTALITY

Introduction

Analysis of the association between congenital malformations and diabetic pregnancy must recognize a pair of most consequential facts. First, perinatal mortality rate and malformation frequency are inversely related; thus, as the former has decreased over time in diabetic pregnancy, the latter has continually increased. (This relation was discussed extensively elsewhere on p. 82 et seq.) Second, the malformation frequency in offspring generally has not increased, but has remained essentially unchanged over time (Warkany and Kalter 1961, Kalter and Warkany 1983, Kalter 1991). Therefore, because this change has taken place in the former but not the latter, perinatally dying and surviving offspring cannot be considered together but must be looked at separately.

It is also necessary to note that the frequency of congenital malformations is much greater in perinatal deaths than in surviving infants. Most past practitioners were unaware of or ignored this; hence they seldom presented data regarding surviving and nonsurviving offspring individually. Such mixing of heterogeneous data obstructed valid examination of the relation of congenital malformations to diabetic pregnancy.

Comparability is not always achieved even when observation is limited to malformations in mortalities because: first, stillbirths—a significant component of perinatal mortality—may often not be well examinable because of maceration, that is, autolysis following in utero retention (Keeling 1987); second, many grave malformations are not inevitably lethal, especially as their prognosis has improved with medical advancement; and last the relative frequency of malformations in perinatal mortalities has increased over time as the overall rate of such deaths has decreased (Kalter 1991), making judgment against current vital statistic and other material even more necessary. This was true even in the early years, as when Hagbard (1961) found the proportion of fetal deaths with malformations to have increased from 9% in 1948–1951 to 20% in 1956–1960, as a result of decline in other causes of death.

Studying malformations in perinatal mortalities has certain advantages: it provides fuller information, since dead infants are usually closely examined and autopsied; and since most malformations in perinatal mortalities are major ones, questions about major versus minor and other unsettled matters do not intrude. Some authors, especially earlier ones, actually confined the reporting of malformations to those found in the mortalities, almost certainly because one of their main focuses was uncovering the causes of the great perinatal mortality rate in diabetic pregnancy. In some instances (eg, Clayton 1956, Gellis and Hsia 1959) the only congenital malformations mentioned were those found in mortalities.

Six early publications of this sort cited by Miller (1956) reported malformation frequencies of 0–5.7%. Reid (in a private communication to Miller 1956, p. 152) reported that 2.4% of the infants of diabetic women had lethal malformations compared with 0.75% in nondiabetics in the same hospital (a rare instance of such a comparison, even in later years). Incidentally, this figure of 2.4% was found in the Joslin Clinic population, the same institution in which the overall frequency of 80% was noted by White (1952).

Malformations, however, were not high in many earlier author's list of conditions believed to underlie the persistently excessive perinatal mortality rate in diabetic pregnancy (Henley 1947, Pease et al. 1951). But even so their possible part in contributing to these deaths were matters of some dispute. For example, Ronsheim (1933) held that deaths of "monstrosities" were part of the large number of mortalities, while Skipper (1933) equivocated, considering that though there seemed to be an "unusual tendency" for diabetics to have congenitally abnormal children, the facts were too scanty "to allow a definite conclusion to be drawn."

These mixed opinions continued into the next generation, as the following quotations illustrate. "The evidence does not suggest that congenital defects are responsible for the greatly increased mortality rate" (Henley 1947). "...[N]ot a single deformity was found" (Hall and Tillman 1951). "Congenital malformations... account for a very small proportion of neonatal deaths" (Pease et al. 1951). "There was no significant increase of associated congenital anomalies..." (Given et al. 1951). "Congenital malformations do not play a large part in fetal loss; their role is largely confined to late neonatal death" (Bachman 1952). "The evidence for the increased incidence of congenital abnormalities in infants of diabetic mothers is still unsatisfactory.... In none of these cases could the abnormality be considered to play any part in the death of the infant" (Cardell 1953). "Congenital anomaly was not responsible for an important segment of the fetal loss" (Jones 1958). Others, though they left no memorable quotations, found no malformations in the perinatal deaths occurring in their series, many of which were probably autopsied (Brandstrup and Okkels 1938, Herrick and Tillman 1938, Potter and Adair 1938, Mengert and Laughlin 1939, Hall and Tillman 1951).

Countering a growing conviction that maternal diabetes was associated with increased malformation risk, Hall and Tillman (1951) found not a single deformity in 104 babies of diabetic women. Unfortunately, what was considered to be a

Table 10.1 Frequency of Congenital Malformations in Perinatal Mortalities in Diabetic and Overall Pregnancies Since the Early Insulin Era

Era	Europe			America		
	No. of Studies	SB[a] (%)	ND[b] (%)	No. of Studies	SB (%)	ND (%)
Diabetic Pregnancy[c]						
1930s + 1940s	9	4/38 (10.5)	6/44 (13.6)	24	4/75 (5.3)	35/218 (16.1)
1950s + 1960s	41	31/229 (13.5)	96/464 (20.9)	23	9/118 (7.6)	44/199 (22.1)
1979 to mid 1990s	28	13/70 (18.6)	45/94 (47.9)	22	19/94 (20.2)	23/72 (36.9)
General Population[d]						
1940s		73/1352 (5.4)	79/1215 (6.5)		423/3540 (12.0)	278/1696 (16.4)
1950s + 1960s		999/8381 (11.9)	1525/9323 (16.4)		456/4640 (9.8)	501/3046 (16.4)
1970s + 1980s		410/2870 (14.3)	579/2373 (24.4)		505/3982 (12.7)	282/877 (32.2)

[a] Stillbirth (specifically designated)/total births.
[b] Neonatal death (specifically designated > 97% early neonatal death, that is, occurring in the first postnatal week)/total births.
[c] A very small number of not clearly identified gestational diabetic pregnancies were unavoidably included.
[d] Taken from Kalter 1991.

malformation was not indicated, nor whether autopsies were attempted on the 19 perinatal mortalities, most of which were stillbirths, many macerated. Another inadequacy was not separately reporting the fetal and neonatal mortality and morbidity outcomes of insulin-dependent and noninsulin-dependent patients. Most telling also are the words of Palmer and Barnes (1945): "Although congenital defects were greater than normal in the group of living children they were not common, and none of major nature occurred except in one instance, in which the child was proven deaf and dumb."

These negative impressions were supported by the several findings of malformation frequencies in perinatal mortalities that did not differ from those in perinatal deaths in general (Kalter 1991). Such impressions, however, may have been due to the large perinatal mortality rate then current in diabetic pregnancy, which would have obscured any increased malformation rate that was present. If this were the case, the mortality rate falling in later years would have allowed any such increase to be revealed.

Stillbirth versus Neonatal Death

During the years when the perinatal mortality rate in diabetic pregnancy was extraordinarily high the search for its cause was intense. The presence of congenital malformations was frequently noted, and a small number of authors, perhaps more sophisticated, presented such findings in stillbirths and neonatal mortalities separately.

Whatever their motive, it enabled the disclosure of an important fact: that malformations occurred far less frequently in stillbirths than in neonatal deaths. Two reasons for this may be conjectured. In the earliest years especially, only or mostly nonmacerated stillbirths may have been examined—assuming maceration was disproportionately associated with malformation; and as well as having an intrinsic basis, hinted at as the overall mortality rate abated, by the generally slower and smaller increase in the congenital malformation frequency in the former than the latter (Table10-1).

Table 10-1 shows that, for the latter reason and perhaps others as well, in diabetic stillbirths the frequency increased little in the earliest decades surveyed, despite the substantial overall decrease in the perinatal mortality rate itself during this period, and that in more recent years the increases were only modest. On the contrary, the frequency in the neonatal deaths increased continuously over the entire span in a fashion closely inversely related to the death rate (see Tables 4.1, 10.1). These patterns reflect differences in the types of malformations predominating in stillbirth and neonatal death and perhaps the variable success in correcting them: those of the central nervous and cardiovascular systems, respectively (Table 10.2), resembling in this respect overall perinatal mortalities (Kalter 1991).

Diabetic versus Nondiabetic Mortality

The question remains whether the malformation frequency in deaths from diabetic pregnancies, many of which were autopsied and thus presumably closely

Table 10.2 Types of Congenital Malformations in Stillbirths and Neonatal Deaths in Diabetic Pregnancies in America and European Countries[a]

Area	CNS	CV	GI	GU	MS	Total
			Stillbirths			
America	47.8[b]	43.5	–	4.3	4.3	49/455 (10.8)
Europe	72.2	5.6	–	–	22.2	68/561 (12.1)
			Neonatal Deaths[c]			
America	24.6	49.1	5.3	10.5	10.5	128/581 (22.0)
Europe	17.8	58.3	6.0	7.1	10.7	188/713 (26.4)

CNS, central nervous system; CV, cardiovascular system; GI, gastrointestinal; GU, genitourinary; MS, musculoskeletal.

[a] Limited to articles describing stillbirths and neonatal deaths separately, and to specifically named malformations.

[b] Percentage of all malformed (omitting miscellaneous anomalies).

[c] Overwhelmingly early neonatal deaths.

Table 10.3 Autopsy Studies of Perinatal Mortalities in Diabetic Pregnancy

			Malformed (n)	
Reference	Years	Autopsies (n)	Index	Control
Helwig 1940	1931–37	9	1	1/9
Miller 1946	1928–48	32[a]	7	
Hurwitz and Higano 1952	1932–50	32	4	
Kloos 1952	1945–51	5	1	
Warren and LeCompte 1952	1937–49	50	9	
Cardell 1953	1947–52	24	6	20/99
Thosteson 1953	–	14	3	
Given and Tolstoi 1957	1949–55	28	6	
Dekaban 1959	–	16	3	0/5
Driscoll et al. 1960	1940–56	95	19	
Komrower and Langley 1961	1951–60	35	7	
Mølsted-Pedersen et al. 1964	1926–63	82	16	
Hubbell et al. 1965	1959–64	39	10	
Seligman 1963	1951–60	31	8	
Naeye 1978	1959–65	26[b]	4	
Farquhar 1969b	1948–66	65	6	
Persson et al. 1979	1959–66	74	21	
Beláustegui et al. 1980	1970–76	27	5	2/19
Nielson and Nielsen 1993	1976–90	11	1	
Soler et al. 1976	1950–74	94	25	
Ballard et al. 1984	1956–78	26	3	
Totals		815	165 (20.2%)	23/132 (17.4%)
	1928–56	344	69 (20.0%)	
	1951–78	471	96 (20.4%)	

[a] Another 24 autopsies not further described.

[b] Nineteen others macerated.

examined, was greater than in those of pregnancies from nondiabetic women. The data are summarized in Table 10.3. Since control material was almost never collected, for comparison it was necessary to resort to data from hospital-based general population births for approximately the same stretch of time, taken from a recent compilation (Kalter 1991).

The data for the earliest decades show that the impression of the clinicians of old—that malformations in diabetic pregnancies, as reflected by those in mortalities were not increased—was correct. And for the most part the results for recent years have continued to show no credible increase. Only in European neonatal deaths, on the basis of very sparse numbers, may an increase have occurred. Confirming this will be ever more difficult, since perinatal mortalities have so decreased that they are seldom ever mentioned in articles these days.

Thus, resorting to perinatal mortalities, even with more accurate account of major congenital malformations, yielded an almost uniformly negative answer to the question whether there is a significant elevation in the level of congenital malformations in the children of diabetic women. Have pathology studies of perinatal mortalities from diabetic women confirmed this?

Pathology Studies

Since there was almost complete agreement that malformations played little if any part in the high diabetic perinatal mortality rate in older decades, other explanations were sought for them. Pathology studies later joined clinical efforts, and though they revealed several unusual features they had no more real success than the latter, perhaps justifying the skepticism of Baird et al. (1954), who said that the numerous autopsies "showed no consistent pathologic change in any organ that could provide convincing explanation of death." Early studies often found fetal pancreatic islet cells to be hypertrophic and hyperplastic (Helwig 1940, Miller and Wilson 1943), which was thought to be the basis of the frequent transient neonatal hypoglycemia. However, it was contended that these features were not directed related (Miller and Ross 1940).

The heart was also noted to be markedly enlarged (Hurwitz and Irving 1937, Miller and Wilson 1943) in association with neonatal macrosomia, but disproportionately so, relative to increase in size of other organs (Naeye 1965). The enlargement proved to be transitory, serial x-ray examination showing progressive return of the heart to normality, achieved by 2 months of age or less (Miller and Wilson 1943, Given et al. 1950).

Since that time it was learned that cardiomegaly and cardiomyopathies occur very frequently in infants of diabetic women (Wolfe and Way 1977), and in the last 25 years or so have received a good deal of attention. Advanced techniques identified the basis of fetal heart overgrowth as a transient hypertrophic subaortic stenosis (Gutgesell et al. 1976), and later more fundamentally as interventricular septal hypertrophy (Gutgesell et al. 1980), an exaggeration of the normally disproportionately thick fetal septum (Weber et al. 1991, Veille et al. 1992). Although the septal hypertrophy was found to be related to the third-trimester maternal glycosylated hemoglobin level and that good control of the maternal diabetes reduced its incidence (Cooper et al. 1992), such management did not always ensure its prevention (Rizzo et al. 1991, Weber et al. 1991), much as was true of macrosomia itself (Knight et al. 1983, McCance and Hadden 1989).

Two further points bear attention: first, the septal hypertrophy occurred equally in fetuses of women with several forms of diabetes: insulin-dependent, type 2, gestational, and class A (Cooper et al. 1992, Veille et al. 1992, Gandhi et al. 1995), indicating it to be a late gestational phenomenon and unrelated to any possible consequence of the maternal condition during early gestation; second, septal hypertrophy was sometimes associated with septal defects (Cooper et al. 1992).

Considering the gravity in former years of the problem of diabetic perinatal mortality, it is remarkable that so few autopsy studies looking into its basis appear to have been conducted. A mere handful of reports, stretching from 1940 to the 1990s, makes up the record (see Table 10.3). That they added little to understanding the problem hardly mitigates the surprise. But even in what they might have been expected to accomplish—furnish an enlarged and more detailed picture of the morphological state of the dead children than clinical observations could do—they were a disappointment. Approximately the same malformation frequency was noted in the autopsied material as in clinical studies of perinatal mortalities, and as the latter had also shown, the difference from the admittedly sparse controls was not statistically significant.

One extraordinary matter that Table10-3 reveals should be pointed out: the malformation frequency in autopsied diabetic mortalities did not increase with time, remaining steady over the years at about 20%, contrary to its steady temporal increase in all perinatal mortalities. This fact may indicate that autopsies were not done on an unselected sample of mortalities from diabetic births; as Farquhar (1965) commented, "the pathologist's population is not a fair sample of that seen at birth by the clinician."

The variety of malformations found was limited, predominantly cardiovascular and urogenital; the one unusual one, a symmelia (Driscoll et al. 1960, originally reported by Gellis and Hsia 1959), obviously did not depend on autopsy for its revelation. Within organs, however, a wide spectrum of heart defects was found, a remarkable variety according to Rowland et al. (1973), which were tabulated by Rowe et al. (1981, p. 677).

Only in a minority of the autopsy studies were stillbirths and neonatal deaths reported separately, and in these the proportion of the former was unrealistically small; part of the reason for this no doubt being that many stillbirths were autolyzed and thus poorly examinable, but also probably because neonatal deaths were the uppermost challenge.

A different slant came out of autopsies of nearly 3000 mortalities conducted by Mason Barr (personal communication, 1993). He noted a significantly increased frequency of several malformations in specimens from pregestational diabetic women compared with those from nondiabetic women, including central nervous system and genitourinary, but not cardiovascular and skeletal malformations. The individual number of stillbirths and neonatal deaths was not stated, however, making it difficult to understand the findings. A large proportion of the specimens had been sent to him, presumably unselected for maternal diabetes; but this was made questionable by the greater than usual percentage of cases with pregestational diabetes and frequency of malformations—1.7 and 59.1%, respectively.

Table 10.4 Frequency of Major Congenital Malformations[a] in Surviving Offspring[b] of Pregestational Diabetic Women

Era	Europe		America	
	Studies (n)	Survivors[c]	Studies (n)	Survivors[c]
1930–49	6	6/279 (2.2)	13	9/629 (1.4)
1950–69	21	39/1682 (2.3)	8	15/731 (2.0)
1970 to mid 1990s	26	46/1473 (3.1)	21	29/1084 (2.7)

The data this table is based on are found in the Appendix.
[a] Omitting minor malformations, those of known or probably known etiology, and those otherwise inadmissible or not named (see Appendix).
[b] Liveborn offspring exclusive of neonatal deaths.
[c] Malformed/total (%).

MALFORMATIONS IN SURVIVING INFANTS

The final subject to discuss is the frequency of malformations in surviving infants, that is, liveborn offspring not dying neonatally. The sources from which this information was gathered, in distinction to the specialized clinics caring for pregnant diabetic women (discussed in Chapter 11), were hospitals large and small, located in cities and communities of every size, extracted from over 100 publications. They are not individually cited here, but are named in the Appendix. Articles reporting survivors and perinatal mortalities collectively were excluded since their reports were contaminated by data from the latter, in which though its contribution decreased with time its malformation frequency increased (see Table 10.1).

The 100 or so articles that yielded the facts contained in the Appendix and summarized in Table 10.4, form a relatively small proportion of the literature dealt with in this work in its entirety. These are the comparative few that explicitly reported the occurrence of major malformations in surviving offspring, as previously defined, or from which this fact could be extracted.

The findings show, first, as is true generally, that the frequency of malformations in surviving infants of diabetic women has remained fairly constant over the last 60–70 years, and, second, that it was comparable to that noted in hospital-based reports of overall populations of surviving infants (see Table 10.4). Although the comparison was hindered by only a handful of articles being found in which such information was given or could be ferreted out and because the comparison required judgment as to which of the sometimes indiscriminate inclusion of defects was relevant, the overwhelmingly likely conclusion again is that the frequency of congenital malformations was not increased in diabetic pregnancy.

MINOR CONGENITAL MALFORMATIONS

Differences of opinion about the definition, prevalence, and significance of minor congenital malformations and morphological variants have continued for years. Some of these matters were touched on in previous pages. The reader interested in fuller details is directed to articles and books especially concerned with these topics (eg, Méhes 1983, Pinsky 1985, Merlob 1994). Matters of these sorts impinge on consideration of whether such conditions occur more often in the children of diabetic than of nondiabetic women.

Aside from their intrinsic interest or importance, of great implication here is another role minor malformations have been assigned—that of indicators or monitors of major prenatal maldevelopment. This function was bolstered by the finding that unselected children with major defects had more minor ones than normal children (Ekelund et al. 1970, Leppig et al. 1987) and that children exposed in utero to known teratogenic anticonvulsant drugs had more minor defects than those not so exposed (Janz 1982, Koch et al. 1992). Thus, according to these ideas, if insulin-dependent pregestational diabetes is teratogenic, infants of diabetic women should have a greater frequency of such lesser defects than occurs generally (Pinsky 1985).

A primary obstacle to determining whether this inference is true has been the wide practice of congenital malformations occurring in diabetic births being reported without differentiating between those that are conventionally designated as major and those not so considered. In the previous section in which the overall frequency of congenital malformations in diabetic pregnancy was dealt with, in the instances in which the abnormalities were actually named to the best of my ability, minor and other questionable ones were excluded. One rare example of an author drawing this distinction was Pengelly's (1961) noting that patent ductus arteriosus "...can hardly be regarded as an abnormality...." Far more common, for example, was Connor's (1967) practice of considering a minor deviation, in this instance a vestigial thyroglossal duct, an acceptable malformation and including it with the others found. Of course, only because he listed the abnormalities was it possible to discover this. In the following analysis, to avoid argument, only reports will be considered in which the data for major and minor malformations were presented separately.

Twenty-seven articles, published in the last 40 years, were identified in which this was done. But only nine of this handful included a further vital ingredient, a control group, especially important for contemplating the frequency of minor defects because, compared with the fairly good agreement about what is a major congenital malformation, there is near chaos regarding what is reckoned a minor one. Hence only the inclusion of a comparably examined control with equally defined entities can permit a convincing judgment.

The 27 articles themselves vividly typified the discord by taking conditions as falling into this category that varied from narrowly delimited to widely inclusive. As a result, the frequency of whatever was called a minor defect, or any of its congeners, ranged in them from 1.3% to 91.0%! The distribution of the percentages, however, was very skewed, with 19 of the 27 finding levels of less than 10% for a mean of 3.3%. The defects scored in these instances were probably the most obvious ones, those that might be adjudged "major minor."

But only the articles that included controls can contribute to the inquiry here; they are listed in Table 10.5. In only one of them did the diabetic group have a statistically significantly larger frequency of minor conditions than the control. In that one, the defects scored—144 "minor physical features"—were not individually named, and whether the cases and controls differed in type as well as in fre-

Table 10.5 Frequency of Minor Congenital Malformations in Studies Containing a Control Group

Reference	Diabetic Group	Control Group	P
Mølsted-Pedersen et al. 1964	11/853 (1.3)	12/1212 (1.0)	> .05
Chung and Myrianthopoulos 1975b	49/499 (9.8)	3523/47408 (7.4)	> .05
Day and Insley 1976	6/117 (5.1)	8/205 (3.9)	> .05
Simpson et al. 1983	23/106 (21.7)	12/41 (29.3)	> .05
Holmes et al. 1987	95/165 (57.6)	2993/6977 (42.9)	< .001
Hanson et al. 1990	11/491 (2.2)	3/206 (1.6)	> .05
Rosenn et al. 1991	12/110 (10.9)	10/55 (18.0)	> .05
Hod et al. 1992	24/117 (20.5)	74/380 (19.5)	> .05
Van Allen et al. 1994	121/133 (91.0)	73/81 (90.0)	> .05

[a] Number of malformed/total (%).

quency was not noted and could not be determined. A larger proportion of infants of diabetic women with a major malformation (some considered thus are debatable) were also reported to have minor ones, but the difference was not statistically significant.

In sum, in the preponderance of studies no increased level of minor defects occurred in the offspring of diabetic women. So far as the theoretical inference noted above is concerned, with respect to insulin-dependent diabetes this result may mean that minor defects do not "serve as reliable measures of intrauterine teratogenicity" (Pinsky 1985), but it was not explained why this might be the case for this category of environmental insult and not others. Or, it might mean, of course, that insulin-dependent diabetes is not teratogenic.

11

STUDIES BY DIABETES CENTERS

It will be helpful to trace the course taken by the most active of the medical centers in the US and Europe studying the problems of diabetic pregnancies in order to examine the difficulties of interpretation and analysis entailed in their efforts.

DIABETES CLINICS

The Joslin Clinic

Probably the first center for the study and care of diabetic individuals, which is still active today, was the Joslin Diabetes Center in Boston (originally named the Baker and then the Joslin Clinic). By 1915, after 17 years, Dr. Elliott P. Joslin had treated about 650 severely affected female patients, only 10 of whom had become pregnant. This infertility problem greatly improved with the introduction of insulin, and by the 1950s over 1000 viable diabetic pregnancies had been followed in the clinic. By 1978, this number had reached 2307 (White 1978).

In an early summary of the outcome of 125 consecutive completed diabetic pregnancies in 1936–1942, 115 of which occurred in women whose disease predated the index pregnancy, 20 infants were reported with "congenital anomalies" (White and Hunt 1943). This high frequency, as already noted, was clearly the result of including conditions ineligible here, such as "cretinism, feeble mindedness, and Mongolian idiocy." The total incidence of anomalies was further augmented later to 80% of infants of diabetic mothers (White 1952), a figure that obviously included every conceivable defective state found at various ages of childhood, as White herself confirmed in the interview with Rubin and Murphy (1958) noted in a previous chapter.

In the publication introducing her convenient scheme for grading obstetrical diabetic patients according to the prepregnancy state of the disease, White (1949) reported 439 viable pregnancies personally observed during the preceding 15 years. Because the clinic was a referral center, it is not surprising that the great majority (95%) had the insulin-requiring severe grades of diabetes. In this report only the congenital defects found in the 78 perinatal mortalities (17.8% of those born) were reported, 2.9% in the 34 stillbirths, and 16.0% in the 44 neonatal deaths. The percent in the former was significantly less than was present in overall perinatal mortalities in the United States at that time (Kalter 1991), indicating perhaps that the search for defects in the stillbirths had not been thorough or entirely possible.

The next report from the clinic that is relevant here was forthcoming 10 years later (Gellis and Hsia 1959), but again was not entirely satisfactory for the analysis of the problem, since it mentioned only the congenital malformations associated with the neonatal deaths, 12.5% of 104 such occurrences, which was somewhat less than the rate for neonatal deaths in the overall population of the day (Kalter 1991). The deaths were autopsied and the malformations listed (Driscoll et al. 1960).

Following this account came one that provided some general data, but still had various gaps. It dealt with 504 pregnancies lasting more than 22 weeks of diabetic patients of the clinic who delivered at the Boston Lying-in Hospital in 1959–1964, almost all of whom were insulin-dependent (Hubbell et al. 1965). A control group of sorts was included, which consisted of consecutively delivered premature infants, that is, of 2500 g birth weight or less, born in the same hospital to nondiabetic women in 1962–1964. Both groups were part of the Collaborative Perinatal Study of the National Institute of Neurological Diseases and Stroke (as it was then named) and thus probably conformed to its protocols for examining newborns, stillborns, and so on (Niswander and Gordon 1972). But these matters were not discussed, and this and the failure to list the malformations found made it impossible to judge the assertion that "significant" malformations were found in 13.5% and 6.5% of the test and control groups and were the primary cause of neonatal death of 25.6% and 7.1%, respectively.

The most ambitious investigation undertaken up to that time (and perhaps even to the present) to look into the possible teratogenic effects of maternal diabetes was made by Neave (1967), mentioned here because almost half of the subjects of the study were Joslin Clinic patients. A full discussion of this important paper is reserved, however, for Chapter 12.

A small, somewhat different step in the story came next with Holmes et al.'s (1976) prospective survey of neural tube defects in 18,155 live- and stillborn infants born in 1972–1975 in the Boston Lying-in Hospital. Of these births, 283 were to "diabetic" women, a prevalence of 15.6 per 1000, far higher than that usually found (Kalter and Warkany 1983), probably partly the result of many being Joslin Clinic referral patients, but possibly also due to other forms of diabetes having been included. One infant, it seems, had a neural tube defect (0.35%) compared with 0.14% in the presumably nondiabetic remainder–hardly of significance, especially in light of the various unanswered matters regarding this investigation.

Carrying the Joslin Clinic series forward was the report of Kitzmiller et al. (1978) of a review of 175 diabetic pregnancies in 1975–1976. No control group was mentioned. Twenty-one of the pregnancies aborted spontaneously, and seven were electively aborted, three because of ultrasonic diagnosis of anencephaly upon routine scanning. Malformations were found in 13 of 150 pregnancies (8.7%), including the three abnormal induced abortuses. But since the condition of the other four was not mentioned, it is misleading to include any of the seven in this sum. Omitting them gives a frequency of 6.8% (10/147). Two of the malformations were persistent ductus arteriosus, not ordinarily considered a serious abnormality because it frequently closes soon after birth; whether that happened in these cases was not stated. The authors failed to mention that no major malformations occurred in the infants of the 16 gestationally diabetic women; the malformation frequency in the pregestational diabetics (omitting anencephalics and ductus) was therefore 5.3% (7/131). Overlooked as possibly contributing to the high frequency of anencephaly—3 in 159 (ie, minus the offspring of the gestational diabetics) or 18.9 per 1000—is the fact that Boston has a considerable population of Irish ancestry, an ethnic group with a history of one of the highest newborn prevalences of neural tube defects in the world, in that city (Naggan and MacMahon 1967) as in Ireland (Coffey 1974). In this connection it is to be noted that the clinic patients were predominantly white. Whether the increased anencephaly and overall malformation frequencies were related to the possible biased ascertainment of the diabetic patients might have been resolved by including a suitable control group.

Later studies from the clinic had as their purpose determining whether elevated levels of glycosylated hemoglobin in early diabetic pregnancy were associated with an increased frequency of congenital malformation or spontaneous abortion (Miller et al. 1981, Greene et al. 1989) and sonographic diagnosis of malformations in diabetic pregnancy (Greene and Benacerraf 1991). These questions are addressed elsewhere in this work.

London Studies

Another venerable center for the study of diabetes is the King's College Hospital in London. But with the exception of an early publication, not until recently have its reports been of much help in answering the questions of concern here. The early report (Peel and Oakley 1949) surveyed 142 diabetic pregnancies occurring in 1942–1949 and found nine (6.3%) instances of "more serious" malformations. How many and which of these abnormalities may have occurred in the considerable perinatal mortalities (25.5%) were not stated. The 6.3% was compared with the 0.94% found in 4829 nondiabetic pregnancies in the same hospital during these years, and though it was implied that little trust could be placed in the latter figure it was felt that an increase could not be doubted. More recent exaggerated risk estimates based on such unrealistic background frequencies are noted on pp. 137, 151, 153.

The next article from this center expressed a different opinion. It reported 201 pregnancies of 176 patients with preexistent diabetes in a series consecutive to the one just noted (Clayton 1956). Although the perinatal mortality rate continued to be high, a "disastrous" 27%, the possible role of congenital malformations in contributing to it was minimized, because it was felt that "such abnormalities are seldom gross enough to cause intrauterine death, and the malformed foetus is usually born alive." As can be realized in hindsight, Clayton was partly right, since the larger the perinatal mortality rate, in diabetic as in nondiabetic pregnancy, the smaller generally is the proportion due to congenital malformations. The only malformations mentioned at all were those in five neonatal deaths (with the cogent remark that their pattern varied greatly). It may be that this changed opinion was brought about by Cardell's (1953) pathology study from this hospital in which congenital anomalies were not significantly more frequent in autopsied specimens from diabetic than nondiabetic pregnancies. The work from this center continued not to be helpful with a report stating that in 1958–1963 just four instances of significant (though unnamed) fetal abnormalities in 31 perinatal deaths occurred (Oakley (1965).

The next communications were brief, but brevity was their least inadequacy, since they reported results of examinations only of older children using a definition of anomaly that was unacceptably broad (Watson 1968, 1970). These will be discussed further in Chapter 16.

Equally unhelpful was the report noting that in 1968–1972 seven infants from diabetic pregnancies were born with severe congenital abnormalities, since the total number of such births during this period was not clearly stated (Essex et al. 1973). The report evaluating the significance of elevated glycosylated hemoglobin in diabetic pregnancy in King's College Hospital (Leslie et al. 1978) will be discussed in Chapter 15.

The most recent full account from this center, overlapping that of Essex et al. (1973), reported 294 consecutive diabetic pregnancies including 34 gestational in 1968–1976, but the two groups were not presented separately (Gamsu 1978). Most of the article was not devoted to congenital abnormalities. All together, 20 infants (6.8%) were said to have severe congenital abnormalities, and a list of sorts was given. Seven were among the 13 neonatal deaths, but what defects they had was not stated. Minor abnormalities occurred in 19 infants, but whether they were isolated or associated with the severe ones was not stated.

Brief mention of congenital malformations (Essex 1976, 1979) noted that they were the most common single cause of perinatal death in diabetic pregnancy in the hospital and that their overall 7% frequency in 230 such deliveries in 1971–1977 contrasted with the 2.5% found in a control group reported by Watson (1973) in an unpublished thesis, a comparison not to be taken seriously.

Edinburgh Studies

The first report from the Simpson Memorial Maternity Pavilion in Edinburgh mentioning malformations in diabetic pregnancy recorded only one such occurrence, an anencephalic, in 16 perinatal deaths seen in 1950–1953 (Rolland 1954). A decade of studies followed, beginning with a general article whose predominant interest was the later development of children born to women "known to have diabetes mellitus" (Farquhar 1959); thus, the physical abnormalities reported were those largely inferred to have been present at birth. In the initial report, such conditions were found in 10 of 93 children when reexamined at older ages. This seemingly large frequency nevertheless furnished no contrast with the state of the children of 93 matched nondiabetic women, 13 of whom had abnormalities, especially since one of the index children had Down syndrome and two others "mental defect."

The upshot of the analysis of an enlarged series of babies of diabetic women born in 1948–1959 continued to be negative (Farquhar 1965). Those that died perinatally and a like number of randomly selected perinatal deaths of nondiabetic women were autopsied and compared and found to have similar frequencies of congenital malformations. The surviving children were examined at several postnatal ages; the findings will be discussed in Chapter 15.

Farquhar's final report (1969b) was of a further enlargement of the series. The entire sample consisted of 329 children born in 1948–1966 to diabetic women, 89% of whom were insulin-dependent. Only 5 of the 69 perinatal deaths had malformations, none of which were cardiovascular ones, as determined by the pediatric pathologists conducting the autopsies "with care," in whose opinion heart defects would not have escaped detection, even in the 28 macerated fetuses. These 5 plus the 10 malformations found in survivors, many examined at ages up to 18 years, which were likely to have been seen or diagnosed neonatally, gave a malformation frequency of 4.6%. The author concluded, based on the control data in his 1965 paper, that though "no difference in incidence was found, the nature of the defects in the diabetic group were more serious," an opinion commented on elsewhere in this work (see pp. 138, 141).

He also recognized and called attention to the important fact that the geographical variations that occur in the frequency of certain congenital malformations in the general population may be reflected in the outcome of diabetic pregnancies, which despite their exaggerated presence maintain the regional variations. Thus, in Farquhar's collection the frequency of anencephaly was 4/329 or 12.2 per 1000 total births, whereas the population frequencies in Scotland in the years 1939–1958 and 1956–1966 were 2.6 and 2.8 per 1000, respectively (Record 1961, Elwood and Mackenzie 1971). This accords with the relation in Copenhagen between the albeit much lower anencephaly frequency in diabetic pregnancy of 4.7 per 1000 (Mølsted-Pedersen et al. 1964) and that in overall pregnancies in that city in 1959–1961 of 1.6 per 1000 (Villumsen 1970). Increased occurrence of this malformation was not always the case however, as will be seen below. An account of neural tube defects in diabetic pregnancy will be given in Chapter 14, dealing with specific malformations.

Since the focus of Farquhar's articles was the follow-up of the children to various older ages, the entire body of these results will be fully discussed in Chapter 15, as will later studies from the Edinburgh center that dealt mainly with the ameliorative effects on fetal maldevelopment of metabolic control of maternal diabetes begun very early in pregnancy or even before conception. (Steel et al. 1982, 1984a,b, 1989, 1990).

Birmingham Studies

A letter to Lancet was the first publication from the Maternity Hospital in Birmingham to deal with this subject (Dunn 1964). This, a brief note lacking various details, reported the births of 69 offspring to women with "frank" diabetes in 1960–1961. Only one malformation was found, in one of the 12 perinatal mortalities, and the outcome was matched against the malformation frequency in offspring and perinatal deaths of nondiabetic women born in the hospital during this period, 3.3% and 22.2%, respectively. This negative result was apparently contradicted by the finding of 5.8% major (but unnamed) congenital malformations in 306 infants of diabetic mothers in the same hospital in 1950–1964 (Malins 1968), but neglected was Dunn's practice of attempting to put the findings into perspective by comparison with a control.

A subsequent article rectified this omission. It reported outcomes of 205 babies born in 1969–1974, 57% the offspring of insulin-dependent pregestational diabetics (Day and Insley 1976). Malformations causing death, needing surgical correction, or likely to lead to deformity or handicap were classed as major; all others were called minor except for those posing insignificant problems, such as skin flaps and small nevi. Overall major malformation frequencies of 12.2% and 5.8% were found in the diabetic and control groups, respectively. But the only statistically significantly increased frequency occurred in the offspring of the insulin-dependent women (9.4% versus 2.6%), 7 of the 11 defects being fatal. The minor malformations, which were not named, were relatively few and not elevated in the diabetic pregnancies.

The list of the malformations in the insulin-dependent group included some whose admissibility as a serious abnormality is disputable: a microcephaly, which, as will be discussed on p. 123, is often not easy to diagnose; and two occurrences of patent ductus arteriosus, whose inclusion may be questioned since children only up to the age of 10 days were examined and anatomical closure of the ductus, which is frequent, may not occur until 2–3 weeks following birth (Taeusch et al. 1991). Omitting these conditions yields a malformation frequency that is not a statistically significant increase.

Another report from this hospital made the same year surveyed a much longer period (Soler et al. 1976). What accounted for the dual publication by two different sets of authors, one from the Neonatal Department, the other from the Diabetic Clinic, was not explained. The report concerned 701 "viable" infants (which was current obstetric jargon for being at least 28 weeks of gestation) born in 1950–1974 to 585 diabetic women of classes B to F, that is, insulin-dependent, and 116 of class A, that is, not requiring insulin. The congenital malformation frequency for the entire period was 8.1% (6.3% major and 1.8% minor, according to the listing of the malformations).

The class A women had two malformed offspring, neither a perinatal mortality. Since the malformation frequency in this type of diabetes is probably not increased, it is fair to omit them, giving a total frequency of major malformations in the insulin-dependent pregnancies of 7.2%. But this figure includes 90 perinatal deaths, which should be considered separately, for the reasons already adduced. Omitting the deaths, which had a major malformation frequency of 26.3%, leaves 3.6% of the survivors malformed, not very different from that in the general population.

Since the Soler et al. (1976) and Day and Insley (1976) studies originated from the same hospital and the series they reported overlapped in time, it is not surprising that there was a duplication in the malformations recorded by them, but because of the ways they were listed it was impossible to establish exactly which were repeated. The former also included two instances of patent ductus arteriosus and an isolated microcephalus among the major malformations. Others also probably misclassified were meconium ileus (apparently unaccompanied by other symptoms), congenital heart block, a condition frequently without obvious evidence of cardiac maldevelopment and, furthermore, compatible with a long and active life (Warkany 1971, p. 583), and Hirschsprung's disease, frequent familial occurrence of which suggests possible genetic determination. Discounting these still further reduces the significance of the malformation findings.

A further report, adding 100 consecutive diabetic pregnancies in 1974–1977, noted a similarly suspicious frequency, of about 9.0%, major malformations (Soler et al. 1978). A noteworthy item in the two publications by Soler and colleagues is that among the abnormal children they reported were two cases of the Ellis-van Creveld syndrome, a relatively uncommon condition, one born before 1974 and one after. As Warkany (1971, p. 793) noted, repeated observation of the condition in siblings and the high rate of consanguinity in parents of such cases strongly suggest its recessive inheritance. Soler et al. (1978) seem not to have recognized this possibility and thus did not mention whether the two children were related. A report summarizing some results of the Birmingham studies (Wright 1984) noted that malformations in fatalities were 4.5% of all diabetic births in 1974–1979, approximating that found in earlier years, a statistic less useful than the proportion malformed of all the perinatal mortalities would have been.

Belfast Studies

Like that of the studies just described, the main and practically only concern of the earliest study of the pregnancies of diabetic women in the Royal Maternity Hospital in Belfast was their high perinatal mortality rate, its causes and prevention (Stevenson 1956). Thus, it is not surprising that the only reference to malformations was the casual observation, devoid of any details, that 6.1% of the 114 viable offspring born in 1940–1955 had a "foetal abnormality"; nor that no controls were obtained, since there was no doubt that the perinatal mortality rate was high and needed none to verify it.

The next study examined whether progress had been made in dealing with this primary problem and concerned 109 offspring of mostly pregestational diabetic women delivering in 1956–1963 (Harley and Montgomery 1965). These patients and the previously reported ones were almost all referred from the diabetes clinic of the Royal Victoria Hospital, which the maternity hospital was affiliated with. The frequency of diabetic pregnancies in this period was about 6.6 per 1000 deliveries, which is somewhat greater than the prevalence of frank diabetes in random samples of women of reproductive age often found elsewhere at about the same time; thus, the sample of women attending the hospital may not have been entirely representative of the general population of diabetic women in Northern Ireland, as was undoubtedly true of many referral centers (eg, White 1949). Major congenital malformations were found in 4.7% (5/105) of liveborn infants, in two of the nine neonatal deaths and three others (the condition of the four stillborns was not specifically noted). The absence of controls made this figure tentative, but obviously the level of malformations was not impressive. Again, however, the interest of the study was focused on the most glaring problem, the persistent high perinatal mortality picture.

By the next report, the situation had changed. The mortality rate had greatly decreased, and attention turned to the increasing importance of a residual cause of death, prenatal maldevelopment, so much so that it was titled "Congenital malformations in infants of diabetic mothers" (Glasgow et al. 1979). In the years 1963–1978, there had been 184 pregnancies of diabetic women lasting 28 weeks or more, most of whom were treated with insulin. Congenital malformations, defined as structural abnormalities present at birth and recognizable with the naked eye, by x-ray examination, or at necropsy, were divided into more severe ones, that is, causing death or affecting a major organ system and resulting in serious incapacity, and less severe ones, which were not explicitly defined. The oldest offspring age examined was not stated.

There were 19 malformed offspring with 24 abnormalities. Only the latter were listed (another occasional hindrance to analysis), but it was possible to deduce that 10 offspring had major malformations (those of the more severe variety) and 9 had minor ones or regarded as questionable. The major congenital malformation frequency was thus 5.4%, with cardiovascular defects predominating. Two anencephalics occurred, giving a rate of 10.8 per 1000, apparently somewhat larger than the prevalence in the general Belfast population in that era, of about 4.0 per 1000 (Elwood 1975). But clouding this likelihood were the great regional variations within the city in the frequency of this defect and the high frequencies in women with abnormal reproductive history (Elwood and Elwood 1984). Others reporting from this center felt that the high rate of this defect in their patients probably reflected the high rate in Northern Ireland as a whole (Glasgow et al. 1979). A further publication from this center (Traub et al. 1983) muddied things because it surveyed diabetic births in years that overlapped those studied by Glasgow et al., and it is difficult to determine whether the observations noted were additional or duplicating.

A still later paper, reporting diabetic births in 1979–1983, remedied this shortcoming, but enlarged the purview to add numerous other Northern Ireland obstetrical units, introducing other imponderables (Traub et al. 1987). Altogether, there were 221 pregnancies of insulin-dependent diabetic women, 121 of whom were patients of the Belfast center or referred during pregnancy to it. Fifteen infants had major congenital malformations, but only those in four prenatally diagnosed and therapeutically aborted were named, and four unnamed minor malformations. Omitting the 17 spontaneous abortions gave a major malformation rate of 7.4%.

Two facts threw doubt on this outcome. The prevalence of pregnancies in diabetic women of reproductive age was only 1.6 per 1000 total deliveries in the country, far less than is usual (contrary to the previously mentioned Irish finding), despite a diligent attempt to trace all such patients, and supporting suspicion that data from centers with large referral clientele may sometimes or in some ways be unrepresentative, the perinatal mortality rate of the women referred during pregnancy to the Belfast hospital was nearly six times that of the diabetic patients cared for throughout pregnancy in that facility. The malformation frequency for the series was compared with that in the overall population, a procedure that hardly satisfied the need for a well-matched control, especially since the most glaring residual problem, the overall diabetic perinatal mortality rate, was approaching the background level.

The latest report from this facility, a brief summary, again omitted naming the malformations (Hadden et al. 1988). About 11% major congenital malformations was reported in offspring of insulin-dependent diabetic women born in 1979–1986, but only the two anencephalies in induced abortions were specifically named, aside from the cryptic remark that "half were potentially fatal." And yet the writers complained that another author's report was "incomplete."

Dublin Studies

The paper introducing the long-ongoing overview of the outcome of diabetic pregnancies in Dublin, being the first Graves Lecture to the Royal College of Physicians in Ireland, began with the obligatory comprehensive historical review of the subject (Drury 1961). Emanating from the National Maternity and the Combe Lying-in Hospitals, one of its main topics was offspring mortality, which was appreciable: 14.3% of the offspring of the 178 pregnancies seen in about 1950–1960, most already advanced in pregnancy when referred. But congenital malformations as one of the causes of the latter was not overlooked. Consistent, however, with findings from other centers during these years, malformations were found in relatively few of the perinatal mortalities, as might have been expected of a time when the mortality rate was high and most deaths were not of developmental origin. But 9 of the 12 stillbirths were macerated, and whether they were examinable was not mentioned. Altogether only five malformations were noted, three major ones in the deaths, and two of a minor variety—a talipes and a hypospadias. (Incidentally, the latter was also mentioned, as occurring in an adult, in an earlier work from a Dublin author [Joyce 1922, reprinted 1986, p. 402].)

A fuller account next considered 269 offspring of diabetic women born in 1950–1965, 14 (5.2%) of whom were malformed, 4 in the 26 perinatal mortalities, a cyclops being additional to the 3 just noted (Drury 1966). An agreeable surprise—the abnormalities were enumerated—and thus it was possible to learn that five of them were inadmissible or questionable: a "Mongol," a laryngomalacia, two talipes, and a hypospadias. Ninety-eight percent of the women were said to be insulin-dependent, although 9.5% were class A, a form not usually needing insulin. Again, many of the 16 stillbirths were probably not examinable. Nevertheless, in balancing these facts it does not seem that an increased frequency of malformations occurred, but absence of a control left the question up in the air.

Publications over the next 10–15 years brought the record up to date (Dundan et al. 1974, Drury et al. 1977), until the last of them detailed the findings in 687 infants of consecutive diabetic pregnancies from early 1951 to mid-1979 (Drury 1979). Disappointingly, only the frequency of malformations found in the 58 perinatal mortalities (20.7%) occurring during these 28 years was mentioned, and aside from two malformed stillbirths in 1975–1979, one anencephaly, the other iniencephaly, no other abnormality was specified.

An earlier paper, recording the outcome in 558 offspring from 1951–1976, gave a full account of the malformations (Drury et al. 1977). In this sample, 36 infants were malformed, including 11 instances of defects that are inadmissible, of the sorts enumerated above, leaving 25 with major malformations (4.5%). Whether this was a real increase above the background rate, the continued absence of a comparison group makes difficult to judge.

One incidental bit of evidence may be helpful. Since the ordinarily rare malformation iniencephaly may be more frequent in areas where anencephaly is more common (Paterson 1944), the two instances of neural tube defects mentioned above may be considered together. These were apparently the only ones found over the entire 28-year period of 1951–1979 in the 687 viable offspring, giving a rate of 2.9 per 1000 in a population whose prevalence of anencephaly was among the highest yet recorded, averaging 4.3 per 1000 for the years 1953–1973 (Coffey 1974). A later summary brought the total of such defects to four, one iniencephaly and three anencephalies, in 941 viable infants, a rate of 4.2 per 1000 (Drury 1986), matching the population level and thus different from the apparent increases in this malformation found elsewhere, mentioned earlier on p. 116.

One last word. In the Banting Lecture given before his death, Drury (1989) stated that 5.6% major malformations had occurred in 1066 viable infants of diabetic women in 1951–1987. Drawing on evidence presented in earlier papers, the 60 cases on which this frequency was based clearly included some significant number of minor abnormalities. For example, Drury et al. (1983) remarked that nearly 40% of the malformations noted were minor ones, and an even larger proportion of minor defects was detailed by Sheridan-Pereira et al. (1983).

Copenhagen Studies

Any early doubt that diabetes was teratogenic largely evaporated upon the presentation of the findings of an investigation by Mølsted-Pedersen et al. (1964). They examined the records of 853 infants weighing 1000 g or more born to diabetic women in the two maternity wards of the Rigshospitalet in Copenhagen, Denmark, in 1926–1963, 80% of them after 1946. Taken into account as malformations were structural abnormalities present at birth or diagnosed before the 10th day of age and recognizable by the naked eye, with the exception of the "most negligible abnormalities." The malformations included major—fatal or seriously handicapping—as well as minor ones, not further defined, but apparently different from "negligible" defects. Also included were autopsied perinatal deaths in one of the maternity wards between 1954 and the end of the study period.

The infants were compared with a control of sorts: newborn children born consecutively in both of the maternity wards during a 6-month period in 1959–1960 and examined by pediatricians in a separate study. Its primary objective was to investigate the possible teratogenicity of antihistaminic preparations, but strangely the report gave no information regarding malformations or their frequency (Zachau-Christiansen and Villumsen 1962).

The bottom line, as the current parlance has it, was that malformations were found in 6.4% of the infants of diabetic women and 2.1% of the control group, and in 19.5% of the diabetic perinatal mortalities and 6.6% of the control ones, thus indicating that infants of diabetic women had about a threefold increased risk of being congenitally malformed.

Since this study was a pivotal one in the unfolding history of the belief that maternal diabetes and congenital maldevelopment are associated, a close look will be taken at it from a number of points of view—first concerning another aspect of controls. It is axiomatic in animal research and should be so in clinical investigation that not only must the control match the study group in all ways known to be relevant, but it must be contemporaneous as well, to obviate the changes in conditions and diagnostic procedures that the passage of time can bring.

Neither injunction was observed in this study. Even if only the majority of the diabetic births be considered, they stretched over almost 17 years, and the control births only during 6 months toward the end of the study period. Social conditions and the state of medical practice were no doubt quite different, especially at the end of World War II, from what they were 12–13 years later, differences that may have made an imprint on care during pregnancy and parturition. In this regard, and possibly of even greater moment in a study of this sort, is the well-documented fact that the frequency of particular congenital malformations may vary cyclically over time. Examples of such shifts of importance here were noted during the years in question, for example, in a number of Czechoslovakian maternity hospitals (Kučera 1971b).

These facts in themselves could impair the validity of the control material, but there is further cause for doubt. The diabetic and control mothers were in hospital for a variety of severe complications and thus were not representative of the diabetic nor of the general population as a whole, since, as noted (Villumsen and Zachau-Christiansen 1963), these maternity wards received women who were expected to have a pathological delivery, were unmarried, or were admitted during difficult delivery. Another factor throwing doubt on the randomness of the control women is the large number (who were excluded) of diabetics among them, in frequency 15.8 per 1000, about three times that reported in unselected series of insulin-dependent pregestational diabetic pregnancies (Chung and Myrianthopoulos 1975b, Kalter and Warkany 1983).

Infants of less than 1000 g were excluded from both groups, but whether premature and growth-retarded offspring formed similar proportions of the two was not stated, a point of possible relevance, because Danish illegitimate infants, as often elsewhere, had a increased rate of low birth weight (Matthiessen et al. 1967), and the frequency of malformations can differ in different weight groups (Goldenberg et al. 1983, Berry et al. 1987, Kalter 1991).

A further matter, perinatal mortality rate was not usefully detailed. In neither group was the overall death rate noted, which made for additional difficulties of comparison, since the rate in Denmark changed appreciably over the years surveyed (Matthiessen et al. 1967).

Finally, the important question lingers of whether the control infants were as thoroughly and competently examined for congenital malformations as those of the diabetic women probably were. An insight into this question was provided by a report that studied all the children born in the two Copenhagen maternity wards during 1959–1961 (Villumsen and Zachau-Christiansen 1963), some of whom presumably made up the control group for the Mølsted-Pedersen et al. (1964) survey. This report, also focusing on the putative teratogenic effect of antihistaminics, omitted many details that might have supported its validity as a control.

Concerning the outcome phenomena, there were 55 malformed infants, 44 with major malformations and 11 with minor ones. Since, however, the authors considered that the "classification of congenital malformations according to severity is largely subjective," their apparently personal scheme was unclear since the malformations were not listed in the publication.

Fortunately, such a list, which included the designations of major and minor, was made available and a copy was obtained at the time. Inspecting the list proved instructive. Four of the major defects, for one reason or another, were inadmissible: Pseudohermaphroditism, male or female, can have a varied etiology (Warkany 1971, p. 1107 et seq.), and without details its status could not be judged.

Clubfoot is a fairly common malformation occurring more often in males than in females and having a strong familial tendency (Wang et al. 1988). Strangely, the latter was listed as a major malformation in one infant and a minor one in another, even though in the latter it was accompanied by a short femur. Microcephaly, first, is not always easy to diagnose in newborns, and, second, when occurring in the absence of other abnormalities, as was true in this instance, is frequently attributable to recessive inheritance. Last, Down syndrome, having a chromosomal origin, which in those years was already established (Lejeune et al. 1959), could not be due to maternal diabetes. This was definitively clarified much later, when an investigation from this same center found that insulin-dependent diabetes did not increase the risk of chromosomal abnormalities (Henriques et al. (1991). Excluding the four inadmissible abnormalities and the 11 minor ones left 40 congenitally malformed infants in 853 births, or 4.7%.

An important omission should be pointed out: 18 (17 in the supplied list) of the malformed offspring died perinatally of their presumably lethal malformations. But the number of all perinatal mortalities was not specified, without knowledge of which the frequency of malformations in survivors cannot be determined. A partial clue to this figure can be derived from the information given for the 82 diabetic births that died and were necropsied in the last nine and three quarter years of the study, of whom 16 had malformations. Subtracting these deaths from the total born gives a malformation frequency in the survivors of 3.1%, possibly an overestimation, but not a large one. It can be concluded that an increased malformation frequency did not emerge from this study.

Incidentally, seven of the cases cited by Kučera et al. (1965) in support of the theory that maternal diabetes was associated with a specific diabetic embryopathy (see Chapter 12) were among the infants reported by Mølsted-Pedersen et al. (1964). But the detailed list revealed that only one of them had a sacral abnormality.

Important studies continued from this active Copenhagen center. An astute observation was made that the frequency of malformations in perinatal mortalities increased as improved maternal and neonatal care caused the overall rate to decrease (Mølsted-Pedersen 1967, Pedersen et al. 1974); the significance of this temporal variation in the overall malformation frequency was apparently not appreciated, however. Malformation occurrence was reported spottily and uninformatively during the 1970s, only total frequency being given without specifying the defects found; this was true of the control as well, precluding close analysis (eg, Pedersen 1975). Overall frequencies of major and minor ones were stated separately (Pedersen 1977, p. 192, Damm and Mølsted-Pedersen 1989), which was helpful. Autopsied infants from diabetic mothers, as reported previously (Mølsted-Pedersen et al. 1964), continued to have a higher malformation frequency than controls, with cardiovascular and central nervous system abnormalities predominating.

During the mid-1970s, a change was made in the manner of diagnosing congenital malformations: to the previous definition of malformations—structural abnormalities present at birth or recognized by external examination—was added those detected by x-ray study, upon clinically indicated need (Pedersen 1975); then came a further addition: "Some malformations were diagnosed only postmortem" (Pedersen 1977); both arrangements rather vague. What difference these alterations may have made to the outcome was not considered.

Seeming to shift his earlier view that certain malformations (particularly short femur) were characteristic in offspring of diabetic women (Pedersen 1977, p. 105), Pedersen later stated that "the correlation between maternal diabetes and congenital malformations in the progeny is of an unspecific nature" and that the apparently increased frequency of certain malformations in such children was due to an "increase in incidence and severity of the usual types of malformations" (Pedersen 1977, p. 194), a statement that is nothing if not ambiguous.

By the mid-1970s, the Copenhagen series included four cases of "total caudal regression" (Pedersen 1977, p. 194), a term supposedly meaning sacral absence, which constituted a 600-fold increase over the general population rate (Kučera 1971). As noted, the above-mentioned list of malformations included only one sacral abnormality, although Kučera et al. (1965) considered that there were seven such cases in this material. What accounted for these discrepancies? Were they partly caused by change of definition of the entity in midstream? Or, was it as well, as the pathologist Benirschke (1987) suggested, that the term "embraces…a host of malformations that are very dissimilar," or as a team of epidemiologists put it, that its prevalence "depends on which forms are included…" (Källén et al. 1992).

Many later papers from this center were mainly concerned with prenatal evaluation of fetal growth and development in diabetic pregnancy and other matters; they will be discussed in Chapter 16. Others summarized findings in series during different time periods. One study, comparing diabetic pregnancies cared for in 1966–1977 at the two hospitals in Copenhagen with those outside the area, introduced further changes in the definition of malformations and further increased the difficulties of analysis (Pedersen and Mølsted-Pedersen 1978). A distinction was made between major malformations and a subset of these, "severe" ones, the latter causing death or necessitating major surgery in the first 6 months of life. The total malformation rate was 8.2%, but, since none of the conditions was named, scrutiny was again precluded. The mention in a contemporaneous paper (Pedersen 1979) of five occurrences of "caudal regression" did nothing to lessen the difficulty. A publication appearing 10 years later (Damm and Mølsted-Pedersen 1989) presented data for a series of patients considerably overlapping the one just mentioned, yet only one case of sacral absence was reported in this larger group of infants.

Finnish Studies

The study of diabetes in pregnancy has a long history in Finland, perhaps engendered by its relatively high prevalence of type 1 diabetes (Tuomilehto et al. 1991). All of the several hospitals in Helsinki that have been engaged in this work will be considered. The first such report to mention congenital malformations, from the First Women's Clinic of the University of Helsinki, of births in 1949–1955, noted two abnormal infants in 81, one with "frog position of the limbs," often a sign of caudal dysgenesis. Congenital malformations were not mentioned among the causes of the neonatal deaths, but most of the many stillbirths were probably macerated and not autopsied (Jokipii 1955).

Abnormalities were noted in 7 of 162 infants in 1951–1960 in the Central University Hospital, 3 in the 16 neonatal deaths. At least two of the remaining four defects were minor or negligible. The condition of the 30 stillbirths was not mentioned. Several of the usual difficulties were present: the diabetic women were a selected group, having "complications" of pregnancy, referred from all parts of the country; over 20% of them had gestational diabetes; the stillbirth rate was high, and most were macerated and not examined. The cases reported by Jokipii partly overlapped this group of women (Österlund and Rantakallio 1964).

Congenital abnormalities occurred in 12 of 123 births in 1961–1966 in the Institute of Midwifery. Six were in 47 children of class A mothers, one a Down syndrome; the others minor defects. The others, from insulin-dependent pregnancies, were all called major, including a "defect of sacrum," but were not further described (Tiisala et al. 1967).

A later report, from the Department of Obstetrics and Gynecology of the University Central Hospital, compared the outcome of pregnancies in 1970–1971 in which the diabetic management was the conventional one of the day with those in 1975–1977 given intensive metabolic control. In the first period, malformations occurred in 4 of 54 infants, and in the later period in 4 of the 136 born. Whether the apparent improvement was thought to be connected to the difference in management was not said (Teramo et al. 1979).

Consecutive to the last study was one of glycosylated hemoglobin in pregnancies of insulin-dependent diabetic women in 1978–1982. Congenital abnormalities were found in 17 of 146 offspring, including 3 malformed induced abortuses diagnosed by ultrasound, 10 or 11 of which were major. These included 2 with caudal regression syndrome (one in an abortus, called "typical" [Ylinen et al. 1981a], raising the questions of what that meant, and whether the second was not typical). The infants were obviously well examined: neonatologists saw them at least three times before discharge from the hospital, and if a congenital defect was "suspected further diagnostic studies were carried out when necessary." The patients were referred, but the reason was not stated. Controls were not mentioned (Ylinen et al. 1984).

Other American Studies

Strangely, aside from the Joslin Clinic in Boston, very few American clinics and hospitals have carried on long-term programs devoted to charting progress in the study and care of pregnant diabetic women, and most of these few entered the field fairly late.

Iowa City

An exception were the studies from the University of Iowa Hospital at Iowa City, the first report from which appeared very early in this unfolding saga. It described the pregnancies in 1926–1938 of 33 insulin-requiring diabetic women and their outcomes. The seemingly high incidence of diabetes noted of 3.6 per 1000 hospital pregnancies was attributed to the patients' being a selected group.

No congenital anomalies were seen, but not all the perinatal mortalities were autopsied (Mengert and Laughlin 1939).

Thirty-one years passed before the appearance of the next paper from this institution. In the intervening period, 334 viable offspring were born to diabetic women, a large number of whom apparently were referred, and nearly one-third were class A. Congenital defects, undesignated except for the comment that "No particular defect predominated," affected 3.9% (Delaney and Ptacek 1970).

The most recent report from this hospital, so far as can be determined, was primarily concerned with evaluating the postnatal development of 80 children of diabetic women, about 76% of whom were insulin-dependent. Twenty of the children had abnormalities, mostly trivial or minor, supposedly found in the neonatal period, but several were probably diagnosed only postneonatally. The definition and means of detecting abnormalities were not spelled out. One abnormality, an L5-S1 fusion—thought possibly to represent a partial expression of the caudal regression syndrome—was no doubt found by x-ray examination. But what prompted that procedure and at what age it was done were not stated. Because of such considerations, the frequency of major malformations in these children could not be calculated. Little, in fact, was certain other than that four of the nine neonatal deaths had major defects (Stehbens et al. 1977).

Los Angeles

Reports of studies from the Los Angeles Women's Hospital, begun only in the mid-1970s, throughout had the shortcoming of naming only the malformations occurring in some of the mortalities, with the possible exception of one case of sacral absence (Gabbe et al. 1977, 1978, Artal et al. 1983, Golde et al. 1984). This plus absence of control observations made any contribution to understanding the entire question by these studies impossible.

Cincinnati

A series of studies made at the University of Cincinnati Medical Center extended into the 1990s. The reports began with a comparison of the effects of two treatment protocols instituted consecutively in 1956–1978 on pregnancies of insulin-dependent women. Nineteen of the 176 infants were found with congenital abnormalities, but the admissibility of perhaps seven was dubious for different reasons: for example, one was chromosomally aberrant and one had what was called a "persistent ductus arteriosus," although the children were examined for abnormalities in the first 3 days of life only (Ballard et al. 1984).

Focusing on another of the abnormalities is instructive, the three labeled "caudal dysplasia." The authors in this instance did the reviewer the kindness of indicating the basis of this designation and thus revealed that only one had sacral absence, another merely lower-limb defects, and the third sacral vertebral abnormalities—a concrete example of the lumping of heterogeneous conditions under a single misleading rubric, as warned against by Benirschke (1987) and Källén et al. (1992).

There was a puzzling difference between the earlier and later treatment periods. In the years before 1970, when the management consisted of the customary practice of the time, only one abnormality was noted in 69 offspring, the ductus arteriosus already mentioned, whereas in the years after 1970, when "a more rigorous approach to diabetic control was undertaken," about 10% of the 107 offspring had major malformations. Could this indicate that in the later period there was also a more rigorous approach to detection of malformations?

Interim studies from this ongoing program covering different succeeding periods also had conflicting results. The first reported a polydactyly (Lavin et al. 1983), a defect, though not further characterized, is a fairly common and usually negligible one in blacks (eg, Altemus and Ferguson 1965), a group comprising a large proportion of the diabetic patients of this center (Neave 1967). A lengthier series was next reported: 205 infants of recruited insulin-dependent diabetic women prospectively collected in 1978–1986, 13 of whom had major malformations, predominantly cardiovascular. Caudal dysplasia was seen three times, but apparently did not include sacral absence, the supposed hallmark of the diabetic embryopathy. Routine ultrasonography was done in the second trimester and thereafter to detect malformations. Whether any of those found was discovered in this way was not mentioned (Miodovnik et al. 1987, 1988).

The most recent reports from this center of concern here noted benefits to diabetic patients enrolled in a specialized prepregnancy program, including reduced spontaneous abortion and offspring malformation frequency (Rosenn et al 1991, 1994, Miodovnik et al 1998). These are discussed in Chapter 3.

BIRMINGHAM HOSPITAL STUDY: A DETAILED LOOK

In my opinion, the long-ongoing programs conducted by diabetes centers such as those just previously described bear the major responsibility for the mistaken belief that diabetic pregnancy poses an increased risk of defective babies. For the purpose of closely examining this allegation, as a paradigm the outcome of pregnancies of diabetic women studied in the diabetes clinic of the Birmingham Maternity Hospital is scrutinized.

The most detailed of the reports from this clinic noted that 8.1% of the 701 offspring born in 1950–1974 had congenital malformations (Soler et al. 1976a). Two of the malformed children can be excluded, having been delivered by the 116 women with an abnormal glucose tolerance test (mistakenly equated, incidentally, with class A diabetes), leaving 9.4% of the remainder abnormal. How did this excessive frequency come about?

The information imparted indicated that the mothers of these children were not a random sample of the diabetic women in the Birmingham of the day, at least not during about the last 15 years of the study, when the hospital became known as a referral center for more severely affected diabetic women. It was during these years that a significantly higher frequency of malformed children and especially of children with lethal malformations occurred than in the earlier period. This, at a time (as the authors commented) when the frequency of malformations in infants of normal pregnant women in Birmingham did not alter.

Several maternal features and disease severity were considered as possibly involved in the increase. Disease duration and maternal age at time of pregnancy were not implicated, confirming many previous studies. There was, however, an undoubtedly greater malformation frequency in children of mothers with disease onset at ages less than 20 years and a progressive increase in advancing White class, although my analysis showed the latter not to entail a significant trend.

Thus, at least in the later period the diabetic women delivering at this facility were a selected and atypical group, their less seriously affected, and perhaps older, diabetic peers giving birth at local hospitals or at home, a quite common practice at the time. Whether the elevated frequency of malformations was associated with some aspect of seriousness of the illnesses of the referred group, or with some other features that marked them as different from the run of the mill diabetics, or with still other biasing factors is unknown. What seems difficult to deny is that the increase in the later years was directly or indirectly influenced by the biased ascertainment of the patients.

Other factors distorting the findings may be related to the qualifications and attitudes of the physicians examining the children. Attesting to the thinking of Takeuchi and Benirschke (1961), special attention was paid to them since they were looked after over the years by "a number of pediatricians…with an active interest in the management of the infant of the diabetic mother." Whether the group of examiners remained the same over this period was not stated.

Important considerations also are the diabetic perinatal mortality and autopsy rates, for reasons that the authors themselves pointed out: "…infants of diabetics are likely to have been examined in greater detail; more *post mortem* examinations were carried out amongst infants of diabetics because of their higher perinatal mortality and the rate of recognition of congenital abnormalities at autopsy is higher than in living infants." The perinatal mortality rate during this period was 14.1%, and the autopsy rates were 93% for stillbirths and 98% for neonatal deaths, much greater than the overall 60% in Birmingham in those days (Leck et al. 1968). It is to be noted that although the malformation frequency was greater in the latter period of the study than the earlier, the mortality rates in the two intervals were almost identical. Whether the autopsy rate varied was not reported. The frequency of malformations in the stillbirths was 17.5% and in the neonatal deaths 38.1%, which perhaps for the former and definitely for the latter is greatly beyond the overall level for these years, as seen in Table 8-1. It can be suspected that these increased frequencies were the result of the extraordinarily high autopsy rates and the particular interest of the pathologists, although the latter was not made explicit.

A most crucial matter is the definition of major malformation. Was the "three to four times higher" frequency claimed by the authors due to inclusion of ineligible entities? Fortunately, a complete list of the malformations was provided, including indications of which were fatal and also which in their opinion were major malformations.

All but 2 of the 26 malformed fatalities had acceptable major malformations, the exceptions being one apparently isolated meconium ileus and one Ellis-van Creveld syndrome—the latter most likely an inherited condition. But among the 31 malformed children surviving the neonatal period, only 11 had acceptable major congenital malformations (Table 11.1).Thus, recalling that two of the sur-

Table 11.1 Nonfatal Malformations Considered Major by Soler et al. 1976 (Accepted or Rejected as Such Here)

Accepted as Major (n)	Rejected as Major or Relevant (n)
Atrial septal defect (2)	Patent ductus arteriosus (2)
Tetralogy of Fallot (1)	Congenital heart block (1)
Cerebral diplegia (3)	"No definite diagnosis" (2)
Encephalocele (1)	Microcephaly (2)
Sacral dysgenesis and phocomelia (1)	Spina bifida occulta (1)
Cleft lip and palate (1)	Deformities of the pinna (2)
Abnormal foot, extra digit, abnormal thumb (1)	Hypoplastic thumb (1)
	Deformed hands (1)
Imperforate anus (1)	Accessory finger (2)
	Congenital hip dislocation (1)
	Talipes equinovarus (2)
	Hirschsprung disease (1)
	Multiple hemangiomas (1)
	Preauricular sinus (1)

viving abnormal children had class A mothers, in all the rate was 5.6% (33/585), almost double that of the background.

Remaining uncertainty comes from the last drawback—the absence of a contemporaneously collected group of matched pregnant nondiabetic women whose offspring were as carefully examined for malformations as were those of the diabetic women. Even this step alone would not have been entirely satisfactory, since it would have yielded a smaller proportion of perinatal mortalities than occurred in the diabetic group. A convincing judgment might have been arrived at by a meticulous comparison of the surviving and nonsurviving offspring of the diabetic mothers with equal numbers of surviving and nonsurviving children of normal women during the same span of years.

The authors did recognize that a control was necessary and resorted to a comparison of the findings of a study of births in Birmingham in the 1950s (McKeown and Record 1960). But they acknowledged that because of incommensurabilities this was a poor choice. They recalled that a control had been included in a smaller study of diabetic births made at their hospital (Day and Insley 1976), which had apparently discovered a markedly increased malformation frequency. A simple two-by-two chi-square test of the data for the pregnancies of the pregestational diabetic women and their controls in this latter study, performed by me, refuted this assertion.

The study made an important finding, namely, that the frequency of the conspicuous central nervous system abnormalities, anencephaly and spina bifida, was increased in the diabetic births, reaching together almost 11 per 1000 offspring, whereas in the 1950–1959 births in Birmingham these abnormalities constituted 3.6 per 1000 (Leck et al. 1968). Whether this increase was related to the fact that inhabitants of Great Britain were at extraordinarily high risk for these malformations (Rogers and Weatherall 1976, Elwood and Elwood 1980), which propensity was possibly exacerbated by maternal illness (as postulated, eg, by Hoet 1986), are subjects that will be discussed further in Chapter 14. But it must be recalled that a similar or even greater propensity to neural tube defects existed in Ireland, yet no such increase was discovered in that region.

These four cardinal faults—biased ascertainment of diabetic women, prejudiced examination of their children, inclusion of ineligible malformations, and absence of an appropriate or even of any controls—were committed by study after study of the outcome of pregnancy of diabetic women, especially of the occurrence of congenital malformations, reported by specialized clinics. It would be flogging an expired equine creature to name them, but they are legion.

CRITIQUE

The preceding pages described investigations of the major US and European centers caring for pregnant diabetic women conducted serially over considerable numbers of years. As medical and social progress brought improvement in the perinatal mortality rate to these pregnancies, a continually increasing fraction of offspring deaths still occurring were due to or associated with a most refractory set of phenomena—congenital malformations. And of greater concern, it also seemed that the overall risk of fetal maldevelopment was increased. Much interest then turned to documenting these conditions and later to attempts at reducing their prevalence.

Outlined in this chapter were not only the findings of these centers regarding the spectrum and frequency of malformations, but also the difficulties impeding efforts to establish beyond doubt that the malformations were indeed extraordinary in type or extent. For the analytic reviewer, the virtual absence of any consideration of these many important factors made his task inordinately perilous. It is tedious to repeat, but these vital ingredients must be emphasized. Doubts largely remain about: how the diabetic women cared for at specialized centers were selected or otherwise identified; how representative they were of the entire population of diabetic women of reproductive age in the regions served by these centers; the definition and means of diagnosing the phenomena considered "malformations"; the assiduity and competence of personnel examining dead and surviving infants for malformations; the validity of the composition of control pregnant women and the diligence of the examination of their children for malformations, in the infrequent instances in which controls were recognized as essential at all; and last the many almost uniformly neglected subsidiary relevant elements in the scheme, familial, socioeconomic, demographic, and so on (Little and Carr-Hill 1984).

Perhaps greatest among these—distorting the outlines of the malformation landscape more than the others—was the practice of the specialized centers of falsely typifying the situation by generalizing from individuals who in one way or another were unrepresentative of diabetic women generally. The patients in these clinics were usually a selected group referred, for example, because of their poor previous reproductive history or the unusually severe nature of their illness, and observations made upon them are not to be considered typical without good evidence. As Williams (1930, p. 602) said years ago of maternal and fetal death in diabetes, so it also may be true of other pregnancy outcomes of diabetes, "...such statistics give too gloomy a picture, as they are based mostly upon severe cases, and do not take into account the milder ones which are usually not reported."

Sometimes even what is meant by "selected" or its opposite "random" may be misunderstood. For example, Pedersen (1954b) called his patients "unselected" because they came to the clinic at all stages of pregnancy, but at the same time noted that they were referred by various private and provincial hospitals and general practitioners. Froehlich and Fujikura (1969), on the contrary, thought that since "the Collaborative Study is a prospective one and the mothers randomly selected, the proportion of 'high-risk' cases such as maternal diabetes would be relatively low;" but Mitchell et al. (1971b) reported a prevalence of "diabetes" among these women of 14 per 1000, some three times that usually found of type 1 diabetes, indicating that the Study had defined the condition very broadly.

An explicit admission of the occurrence and perils of nonrandom selectivity was made by Takeuchi and Benirschke (1961) when, in studying autopsied offspring of diabetic mothers, they stated that it was possible their material was "biased because of the higher incidence of maternal diabetes at the Boston Lying-in Hospital due to its affiliation with the Joslin Clinic," and then, calling attention to another biasing element, noted that "a high percentage of autopsies is obtained in this group because of the interest by the physicians taking care of this group of patients."

Ultimately, problems arise because in the aggregate and for many kinds individually, congenital malformations are relatively common. Thus, a comparatively small increase in their frequency, such as has been claimed diabetes causes, because of the numerous biases and variables confounding the picture, makes recognizing such possible augmentation difficult. The relevance of these facts can be shown by the following. If for purposes of analogy one considers pregnancy in diabetes a pandemic, then the problems entailed in determining whether this state is associated with an excessive level of malformations can be compared with the task undertaken in the early 1960s by those trying to identify the cause of the rash of unusual limb malformations that had suddenly appeared in Germany and elsewhere (McBride 1961, Lenz 1961). It proved incredibly complicated to do, and only upon profound epidemiological analysis, greatly facilitated by the fact that among the most frequent malformations induced were phocomelia and amelia, which are conspicuous and ordinarily quite rare, was it nailed down that the culprit was the recently introduced sedative thalidomide (Lenz and Knapp 1962, Sievers 1969, Weicker 1969).

In the case of diabetes, the situation is reversed. The supposed cause is known, the effects have to be proved. Would it help to do this if the frequency of ordinarily rare and conspicuous malformations were increased? Does sacral absence or holoprosencephaly, both said to be increased in diabetic births (Kučera 1971, Barr et al. 1983), fit this bill? Several difficulties attend this proposition.

Sacral absence is apparently seldom diagnosed in newborn infants; a worldwide review of hospital births noted a frequency of 4.8 per million (Kučera 1971). But such a scarcity is not true in older individuals, as was shown by a survey of a relatively small number of American orthopedic surgeons, which had no trouble identifying at least 50 cases of partial or complete absence of the sacrum (Blumel et al. 1959). This discrepancy appears to indicate that the condition mostly goes unrecognized at birth and that the alleged increase in diabetic pregnancies was owing to diligent examination, more severe defectiveness, or both.

Holoprosencephaly, the general term for a set of related conspicuous craniofacial abnormalities, can hardly be overlooked (DeMyer and Zeman 1963). Though etiologically heterogeneous (Roach et al. 1975, Corsello et al. 1990), it is uncommon, with a mean frequency lately determined to be about about 0.75 per 10,000 total births (Martínez-Frias et al. 1994, Croen et al. 1996, Rasmussen et al. 1996, Whiteford and Tolmie 1996, Olsen et al. 1997). There is evidence that many embryos with these severe malformations are spontaneously aborted, since the frequency in induced abortuses in Japan in 1962–1974 was many times greater than that found at term (Matsunaga and Shiota 1977). The condition should thus be overrepresented in abortuses of diabetic pregnancies, but pathology studies of perinatal mortalities described in Chapter 3 supplied no support for this surmise.

12

BROAD-SCALE STUDIES

In addition to the studies considered in Chapter 11, various other approaches have been taken to the study of the outcomes of diabetic pregnancy, including broad-scale, multicenter, and population-based surveys. The latter will be discussed in the next chapter; the others in this one.

Many attempts have been made in the last 40–50 years by sweeping reviews and analyses of information gathered from multiple sources to survey the broad landscape of congenital malformation in diabetic pregnancy. Their purpose was to overcome the limitations imposed by the sparse numbers of diabetic pregnancies any one clinic or hospital could supply, by collectively examining and interpreting the findings of many isolated and smaller reports. The conduct and findings of such efforts will be looked at—first extensive reviews made early and then multicenter studies.

TWO WIDE REVIEWS

The Kučera Analysis

Not long after the publication of the influential report of Mølsted-Pedersen et al. (1964), there appeared a broad review supporting its finding of an increased occurrence of malformations in diabetic pregnancies (Kučera 1971a), which seemed to clinch the argument. It presented an analysis of a compilation of over 7000 births to diabetic women drawn from nearly 50 case series reported from many European countries and the US in about the previous 30 years. Noting that 4.8% of these offspring "showed anomalies," compared with 1.6% in a control series (the article's summary erroneously gave this figure as 0.6%) derived from a World Health Organization (WHO; Stevenson et al. 1966) study and his "own series of anomalous cases," the author cautiously suggested that there was an increased incidence of anomalies in the offspring of diabetic women.

His caution proceeded from the fact that, as the author conceded, the suggestion was based on data that were flawed in many ways, methodological, conceptual, and so on. Certainly, these were important invalidations, but not less so than one consideration not mentioned—the probable noncomparability of the control and the test material. Although, aside from the general geographic origin of the control, none of its characteristics was described, even this alone showed that the control and test groups were hardly alike. Thus, about three times as many controls were German or Czech as were the diabetic group; some controls were Australian and South African, nationalities not present in the diabetic births at all; and many countries represented in the latter were not present in the controls.

Apparently the source of a considerable proportion of the control series was a study sponsored by the WHO, and some clues as to its formulation and characteristics can be gleaned from the report emanating from it (Stevenson et al. 1966). It appears that only the largest hospitals were recruited for the study and that such hospitals, as Stevenson et al. noted, "with so many births each year are inevitably very busy places and understaffed, so that it would have been unrealistic to expect recording of elaborate information about births." Hence, all other dissimilarities apart, Kučera's findings were challenged by the strong and familiar objection that relatively competently and conscientiously examined infants of diabetic women were compared with superficially and casually examined controls.

Another observation of great influence in future years reported in the Kučera publication was that certain malformations occurred in disproportionate excess in the children of the diabetic women, especially "spinal anomalies including the syndrome of caudal regression." What was meant by this nomenclature was not entirely clear, but if "caudal regression" was synonymous with absence of the sacrum, as the introduction in this article held it to be, and the latter was considered a "specific malformation of fetuses of diabetic women," then this malformation as it occurred in the case series, on which the conclusion was built, must be closely looked at.

Kučera reported that there were nine instances of "caudal regression" in these series, two from the US, one from the United Kingdom, two from Germany, one from Bohemia, and three from Denmark. Reading through the original articles alleged to report this defect, I found the following: In none of the US papers cited was sacral absence mentioned; in one a "spinal defect" was recorded (Thosteson 1953) and in another a "sireniform monster" (Driscoll et al 1960; this was a report of a pathology study of malformations in neonatally dying children of diabetic mothers first reported by Gellis and Hsia 1959, discussed in Chapter 10). Although sirens often have sacral abnormalities, the sacrum is seldom missing. Four of the other seven cases were reported to have sacral absence (Farquhar 1959, Herre and Horky 1964, Mølsted-Pedersen et al. 1964, Kučera et al. 1965); another was a siren (personal communication from Mølsted-Pedersen to Kučera et al. 1965), and two others had unspecified vertebral-column abnormalities (see Kučera et al. 1965).

Since sacral absence seldom comes to medical attention in neonates, only a well-examined matched series of nondiabetic births gathered concurrently with a series of diabetic ones could satisfactorily have decided whether the four clear occurrences of the defect in the 7101 infants of diabetic mothers collected by this review was truly an excess frequency. Questions regarding the frequency of this defect in diabetic and nondiabetic pregnancies are discussed in Chapter 14.

The Neave Analysis

The Study Plan

During about the same time the articles by Mølsted et al. (1964) and Kučera (1971a) appeared, a doctoral thesis was submitted to the Harvard School of Public Health on the subject of congenital malformations in the offspring of diabetic women (Neave 1967). Excellent in conception and execution but relatively little known, perhaps because not otherwise published, except for a relatively brief summary appearing 17 years later (Neave 1984), it presented a substantial and meticulously analyzed body of data that made a case for malformations being much increased in diabetic pregnancy.

The data came from the records of deliveries in 10 university-affiliated hospitals in the northeast US and Canada, stretching from Cincinnati to Montreal, and covered greatly different lengths of time from hospital to hospital in the years 1928–1966, but mainly from the 1950s and 1960s. Very different proportions of the deliveries were contributed by the various hospitals, ranging from 2.1% to nearly 47%, the latter by the Boston Lying-in Hospital, and the number of diabetic women delivering, indicating hospital size or referral status, ranged from about 5–35 per year.

The records, abstracted by trained employees, concerned births to women known to have been diabetic before delivery and hence included women not insulin-dependent and not diabetic before conception of the index pregnancy, and both with and without clinical symptoms. Controls consisted of women delivering next at the same hospital matched for age, parity, and race. Excluded were plural births and offspring of less than 1000 g birth weight and less than 28 weeks of gestational age. This was a thorough investigation of historical records, albeit unavoidably containing great heterogeneity.

The Malformations

The infants were observed from birth to the time of discharge, which varied from hospital to hospital, but no doubt at that time in cases without complications was about 1 week to 10 days. Most of the malformations, however, were discovered in the first 2–3 days of life. Perinatal mortalities were included, of which about 65% of the stillbirths and 80% of the neonatal deaths of both index and control cases were autopsied. In all, records of the births of 2592 index and a like number of control infants, borne by 1939 diabetic and 2592 control women, were available. The malformations were coded according to a modification of the framework presented by Edwards et al. (1964); each infant's abnormalities were encoded and listed in the Appendix of the thesis.

In the index group, 339 or 13.1% were congenitally malformed compared with 5.3% of the controls. These large frequencies were arrived at by including some inadmissible and dubious entities. The most frequently observed abnormalities, in fact, were various sorts of gross morphological defects of the placenta and umbilical cord, states that by no stretch of the imagination can be considered malformations of the infant. [Such conditions, incidentally, were not mentioned in reports of a number of pathological studies of the placentas of diabetic pregnancies (Warren and LeCompte 1952, Driscoll 1965, Singer 1984, Labarrere and Faulk 1991)]. This type of defect was recorded in the absence of any serious abnormality of the newborn child in 75 diabetic and 34 control pregnancies. In addition, numerous isolated abnormalities (ie, occurring in the absence of any others) were included that in themselves are usually trivial or have doubtful health implications, such as single umbilical artery, undescended testis, hypospadias, microcephalus, polydactyly, and so on (see Table 12.1 for the entire number).

The rather large number of one of these isolated defects, single umbilical artery, all but one of which were diagnosed at the Boston Lying-in Hospital, was explained by the interest of the pathologists at that facility in this anomaly. That this undue interest created a biased situation was made obvious by the fact that in a pathology study from the same hospital this defect was found only once in 95 autopsies and that without associated abnormalities (Driscoll et al. 1960). The other doubtful defects also suffered from one drawback or another: Isolated microcephalus, as Neave admitted, is not ordinarily a clear-cut deformity and is subject to variations in diagnostic criteria. Hypospadias is a relatively common and usually trivial defect with an important hereditary component (Harris 1990); 75% of cases or even more are mild (the degree of the defect was not indicated in Neave's thesis) and seldom associated with unrelated defects (Calzolari et al. 1986). Undescended testis is even more common than hypospadias, and in most cases the offending organs have descended by 3 months of age (John Radcliffe

Table 12.1 Number of Infants With Isolated Minor and Unaccepted Abnormalities in Diabetic and Control Group[a]

Abnormality	Diabetic Group	Control Group
Placental/other umbilical	75	34
Undescended testis/other genital NFS	20	12
Single umbilical artery	16	3
Hypospadias	11	3
Ear and ear-related	10	3
Microcephalus	9	0
Poly-/syndactyly	8	8
Down syndrome[b]	6	5
Toe/finger/nail NFS	5	4
Simple umbilical hernia	5	3
Mouth/eye/face/nose NFS	5	3
Talipes	4	6
Hair/skin	4	4
Extra nipple	3	2
Nevus/blood vessel	3	6
Miscellaneous	6	4
Total	190	100

NFS, not further specified.
[a] From Neave 1967.
[b] Including 1 chromosomal aberration, NFS.

Hospital 1992, Berkowitz et al. 1993). Down syndrome, 10 of which occurred, being due to a chromosomal aberration (Lejeune et al. 1959, Gardner et al. 1973), obviously cannot be the responsibility of maternal diabetes. When these and the other disqualified conditions listed in Table 12.1 were omitted, the malformation frequency became 5.8% in the index infants and 1.4% in the controls, a more realistic but still appreciable difference (this ignores that the frequency in the controls was appreciably lower than usual, no doubt indicating inadequate examination). All percentages given below (except where indicated) will be for corrected malformations, that is, the total minus the disqualified ones.

Questions Raised by Perinatal Mortality

A matter relevant to the question at hand, though not given special attention by Neave, was the malformation frequency in dead offspring. As was usual in that era, perinatal mortality was greatly increased in the diabetic pregnancies, 16.6% versus 3.7% in the controls, and a large disproportion of the total malformation load occurred in the dead infants, index and control.

As repeatedly stated in the present work, it is widely accepted that the frequency of major congenital malformations at birth is approximately 3%, and this has not markedly fluctuated over the years since good records have been kept (Warkany and Kalter 1961, Kalter and Warkany 1983). The percent of perinatal deaths that is malformed is much larger than this, and to repeat, in contrast with the relative constancy of the overall figure, has progressively grown as the rate of perinatal mortality from the many causes of fetal and neonatal death that have proved controllable has continuously fallen (Kalter 1991).

In keeping with the usual finding, the frequency of congenital malformations in the perinatal mortalities in Neave's sample of diabetic pregnancies was significantly larger than the overall one (17.2% versus 5.8%), as it was in the controls (14.7% versus 1.4%). The malformation figures for all deaths and for stillbirths and neonatal deaths separately, as well as for survivors, are listed in Table 12.2.

Various noteworthy facts are revealed by Table 12.2. Conforming to what had often been found by investigators at that time, the frequency of malformations in the diabetic perinatal mortalities was not significantly greater than that in the controls (17.2% versus 14.7%). This resemblance was perhaps brought about by both groups being autopsied equally often. Compelling evidence that autopsy made a difference is the fact that in the index cases the malformation frequency in autopsied specimens was significantly larger than in those not so examined, showing

Table 12.2 Corrected Congenital Malformation (CM) Percentages in Stillbirths, Neonatal Deaths, and Survivors[a]

	Diabetic Group (70)	Controls	*P*
Stillbirths	24/232 (10.3)	4/34 (11.8)	> .05
Neonatal deaths	50/198 (25.2)	10/61 (16.4)	> .05
Survivors[b]	75/2162 (3.5)	23/2497 (0.9)	« .001

[a] From Neave 1967.
[b] Liveborn minus neonatal deaths.

that close inspection resulted in greater uncovering of malformations. (This fact refers only to the uncorrected malformation frequencies, since details enabling omission of inadmissible defects were not given for autopsied and unautopsied infants separately.) Unfortunately as well, perinatal mortality and autopsy rates were not stated for the hospitals individually, so differences in malformation rate between them that might have stemmed from such variability could not be revealed.

Incidentally, an indication that autopsy rate was not necessarily a measure of the quality of examination of the dead control infants was the fact that the malformed perinatal mortalities comprised a significantly larger proportion of all malformed infants in the diabetic group than in the controls, again despite the autopsy rates in the two groups being approximately equal. A final entry in Table 12-2 must be pointed out. Although the malformation frequency was not significantly different in index and control perinatal mortalities, it was significantly greater in the index survivors than in the controls. This fact can perhaps be looked upon (as inferred in the Hagbard 1956 study noted later in this chapter) as meaning that maternal diabetes caused an increase only of less serious abnormalities of the sorts that may present ambiguities in diagnosing; not ignoring the even greater likelihood that the controls were not as well examined as the index infants.

Racial Considerations

Race also had some relevance. Overall, 12.7% of the diabetic women surveyed were nonwhite, predominantly black, although the proportions in the different hospitals varied greatly, ranging from 1.2% in the Boston Lying-in Hospital to 75.6% in the Cincinnati General Hospital. Since race markedly affects the frequency of several different congenital malformations (Altemus and Ferguson 1965; Ivy 1968, Erickson 1976, Christianson et al. 1981, Polednak 1986, Chávez et al. 1988), it is possible that variability of the pregnancy outcomes was related to many of the hospitals having a large nonwhite patient load or by associated factors. Actually, this matter divided the hospitals into two almost discrete kinds: five with a large mean percentage of nonwhite diabetic pregnancies, 41.2%, and five, with only 2.3% nonwhite, a huge statistically significant difference ($P \ll .001$).

Table 12.3 Corrected Congenital Malformation Frequency in White and Nonwhite Diabetic Pregnancies in 5 Hospitals with Largest and 5 With Smallest Nonwhite Diabetic Patient Population

% Nonwhite Population	Pregnancies (w)		% Congenital Malformations					
			Index Group			Control Group		
	White	Nonwhite	White	Nonwhite	Total	White	Nonwhite	Total
41.2	408	286	3.4	7.0	4.9	1.2	1.0	1.2
2.3	1854	44	6.1	6.8	6.1	1.5	4.5	1.5
Total 12.7	2262	330	5.6	7.0	5.8	1.4	1.5	1.4

Based on Neave's 1967 data.

The malformation frequencies in these two groups of hospitals are presented in Table 12.3. In hospitals with a large percentage of nonwhite patients, 3.4% of white and 7.0% of nonwhite infants were malformed, and in hospitals with a small percentage of nonwhite patients, the respective frequencies were 6.1% and 6.8%. That is, the malformation frequency in white infants in hospitals with predominantly nonwhite patients was significantly lower ($P<.05$) than in hospitals with predominantly white patients, whereas that of nonwhites in the two types of hospital did not differ. Unhappily, what was different about hospitals with many and few nonwhite patients that gave these results was left unanswered. But the outcome cannot be ignored, pointing as it does to a further source of heterogeneity, which lowers confidence in the interpretation given to the overall results.

Biases in Research

Neave discussed several difficulties he encountered in pursuing his research that may have distorted the analysis. His original intent, for the purpose of statistical validity, was to collect records of a sample of at least 3000 births of diabetic women. This goal was not met because some births later had to be excluded for various reasons: birth weight less than 1000 g, plural and out-of-hospital delivery, maternal misdiagnosis, indefinite or no diagnosis, insufficient information, lost records, mismatching or no matching with controls. All told, these exclusions led to a 14% deficit. No information about the omissions was given.

Bias of another sort may have introduced a different complication. An important bit of evidence that pointed to congenital malformations being increased in the diabetic pregnancies rested on Neave's refutation of what he called "observer bias." Recognizing this ubiquitous difficulty—which he characterized as follows: "Offspring of diabetic mothers often present formidable clinical problems.... There is no question that these infants are preferentially treated and that the chances of observing and recording malformations are greater [in them] than in the offspring of nondiabetic mothers"—he attempted to negate it by determining the frequency of malformations that were likely to be easily recognized because of being "grossly evident" and hence not subject to this bias. These defects, too, he found occurred almost twice as frequently in index as in control infants; and thus he felt that this bias, and other possible ones that he enumerated, had not influenced the recorded data. But these findings were contradicted by other data offered by him, namely, that the frequency of these conspicuous types of malformations in perinatal mortalities in the index group was not different from that in the controls. It is difficult to know how to reconcile these apparently contradictory findings, found in other studies as well.

One malformation of special importance, sacral absence, because it has been thought to be part of a specific diabetic embryopathy, must again be given some particular attention, though interestingly it was not included in the list of defects considered exempt from observer bias. Two infants with total sacral absence occurred in the index births in the Boston Lying-in Hospital, and one with absence only of the coccyx in the Johns Hopkins Hospital, all three being perinatal mortalities.

Indirectly, through the former two cases, a question arose about the adequacy of the search of the hospital records made by the abstracters hired to perform this task. Though Rusnak and Driscoll (1965) recorded three children with this condition as born to diabetic women at the Boston Lying-in Hospital between 1952 and 1964, only one of them was among the cases included by Neave; and Neave's second Boston case, born in 1956, was not one of those described by Rusnak and Driscoll. Apparently also absent from the records of index births made available to Neave was the symmelic infant noted by Gellis and Hsia (1959) and Driscoll et al. (1960). One is left therefore with the suspicion that, since relevant records were possibly overlooked or erroneously included, others pertaining to children malformed and not malformed may have been similarly mishandled.

MULTICENTER STUDIES

Until the 1980s multicenter studies were relatively modest in size and made no pretense of surveying anywhere near the entire population of a region. In time, however, as the number of units cooperating in these studies grew, they began to overlap in sweep and were often indistinguishable from those that intended to cover the entire populations of their respective geographical areas. The latter, the strictly population-based studies, will be discussed later in this text.

To begin at the beginning, the perspective of the earliest multicenter studies, which did not even know they were multicenter studies, reflected their time by paying little or no attention to congenital malformations (Miller et al. 1944, Peel and Oakley 1949, Medical Research Council 1955). The first authors cited obtained data from the records of three hospitals in New York City, New Haven, and Boston, the second, by questionnaire from 26 hospitals and hospital-based centers in Great Britain and Ireland, and the third, from nine British diabetes centers. They all dealt almost exclusively with the relation of a number of maternal and treatment variables to the predominant concern of the day, the high level of perinatal mortality, and showed by their almost total neglect of malformations how little influence they considered such conditions to have on this problem. This was remedied by the next study of this sort.

An Early Swedish Study

This study consisted of a comprehensive analysis of records of diabetic pregnancies delivered in 1948–1954 obtained from the obstetric departments of 21 general hospitals located in many parts of Sweden (Hagbard 1956, 1961). Most of the patients had been insulin treated for several years. Information on a total of 472 children weighing at least 1000 g at birth or from pregnancies proceeding beyond 28 weeks were collected. As was usual for the time, a large number, 36.3%, were stillborn or died in the first postnatal week.

The impact of congenital malformations on this outcome, it is obvious from the space allotted to these conditions—a bit more than one of the 180 pages in the entire 1956 monograph—was not thought of much importance. Yet such abnormalities were found in 6.4% of the offspring, and the list of the defects provided by the monograph in a table revealed that for the most part they consisted of the major varieties and represented various systems and parts. But which of them occurred in the mortalities was not designated. And this is of significance, since an unusually large proportion of the defective offspring, 63.3%, were found among the perinatal mortalities, leaving the remaining defects, for the most part probably of the less serious sorts, in 4.1% of the survivors.

Almost nothing was said of the way these abnormalities were detected, aside from the children usually being treated as premature and therefore carefully watched for the first 5 days of life, and most perinatal mortalities, except for a few macerated stillbirths, being autopsied. The protocol from hospital to hospital apparently varied, as did the patient representativeness, but this was not detailed. The need for a control apparently was never entertained.

Large Studies

The rationale for multicenter study of reproductive outcomes of diabetic pregnancy should not be merely that it is the means of collecting the large number of subjects that may be needed to come to grips with difficult questions and their statistical analysis. The prime purpose, I would say, is to reach for greater representativeness of pregnant diabetic women at large, something not to be expected of patients referred to specialized clinics and large hospitals, who usually constitute a biased assortment of this population. To the extent that investigators were alert to the dangers of misinterpretation presented by selection factors, and their success in minimizing them, the findings of multicenter studies are credible. It might be argued, of course, that population-based studies would have an even greater advantage in this respect, a proposition examined in Chapter 13. Many multicenter studies have been conducted in recent years. Some of the more important ones are described here.

The Collaborative Perinatal Study

The mother of all multicenter studies was the Collaborative Perinatal Study sponsored by the then National Institute of Neurological Diseases and Blindness of the U.S. National Institutes of Health (Berendes and Weiss 1970, Niswander and Gordon 1972). It was a grand scheme whose purpose was to provide knowledge of the relation between pre- and perinatal factors and subsequent aberrant neurological development. To achieve this goal, 14 university-affiliated medical centers were recruited to collect the required obstetric and pediatric information. The study continued for 7 years, ending in December 1965, with the final registration of 55,908 women and their pregnancies.

Of that number about 39,200 were included in the first overall report of the study (Niswander and Gordon 1972, pp. 239–245). Of course, even this quite large number included relatively few pregestational diabetic women, altogether 254, which gave the appreciable, perhaps excessive, prevalence of 6.5 per 1000 pregnancies. Only two pregnancy outcomes were mentioned, and these only perfunctorily, perinatal mortality and neurological state at 1 year of age. The rate of the former in diabetic pregnancies was 14.4%, which was nearly four times that in nondiabetic pregnancies. White and black pregnancies were not different in this respect, perhaps because the black women included in the study were of urban origin and probably relatively well off socioeconomically (Berendes and Weiss 1970). Incidentally, the perinatal mortality rate in pregnancies of women found abnormal on a glucose tolerance test was not significantly different from that in nondiabetic women.

More complete analyses of the voluminous data that dealt with aspects relevant here appeared in later years. From Boston came a report about newborns of diabetic mothers that was part of the Collaborative Study, but exactly how it fit into it was not made clear (Hubbell et al. 1965). In an article that inquired into the etiological bases of cardiovascular malformations, such abnormalities in the offspring of diabetic women were noted to have a frequency of 2.5%, which was about three times that in those of nondiabetic women (Mitchell et al. 1971b). This large figure, however, was based on examination "undoubtedly...more complete in some centers than in others," by pediatric cardiologists and other interested physicians, of children with definite or suspected congenital heart disease up to the age of 1 year (Mitchell et al. 1971a). Thus, this frequency cannot be compared with the rate of such defects discovered only in the perinatal period, the period as previously explained, of concern here, because the frequency found at birth is well known to be significantly augmented by the emergence or recognition of abnormalities during postnatal months and years (eg, Neel 1958, McKeown and Record 1960, Mellin 1963, Hakosalo 1973, Klemetti 1978, Hoffman and Christianson 1978, Christianson et al. 1981), even taking into consideration the deaths at various postnatal ages of some malformed children (McDonald 1961, Hardy et al. 1979, Myrianthopoulos 1985). This matter will be adverted to again below, when it will be seen to have made for imponderabilities in analyzing an even wider range of observations (Chung and Myrianthopoulos 1975b).

Another fact bringing confusion to Mitchell et al.'s (1971a) paper is that it labeled 786 women as "diabetic," a far greater number than the 254 so reported by Niswander and Gordon (1972). This enlargement gave the unusual prevalence rate of about 14 per 1000, which undoubtedly means that as well as pregestational diabetic pregnancies those with gestational diabetes and abnormal glucose tolerance were included, a conjecture supported by Naeye (1979).

A pathology study of all autopsied deaths in the Collaborative Study unfortunately did not specify the results from diabetic pregnancies (Froehlich and Fujikura 1969). In a study that did do so (Naeye 1979) 5 of 46 (10.9%) stillbirths and neonatal deaths from 652 diabetic pregnancies (the large number again owing to the inclusion of glucose intolerant as well as insulin-independent pregnancies) had congenital abnormalities, a frequency not different from that reported in perinatal mortalities in those years (Kalter 1991). A vast effort to utilize the data of the Collaborative Study to examine the teratogenic potential of drugs found that 13 of 333 (3.9%) children of diabetic mothers had malformations, a frequency considered to indicate a relative risk of 2.2. But again this figure was inflated by the children being periodically examined during their first 4 years of life (Heinonen et al. 1977, pp. 31, 430), as well no doubt as being based on inadequately examine controls. Mention of the outcome of diabetic pregnancies elsewhere in this book was unclear.

In addition to the partial information given in the papers cited earlier in this chapter, several detailed reports were published of the findings of the Collaborative Study that pertained to congenital malformations generally and to those in offspring of diabetic mothers in particular. It is not amiss to recall that the Collaborative Perinatal Study (which later was also sometimes called the Collaborative Perinatal Project) was a prospective investigation of the etiology of neurological and sensory disorders of children detected during the first 7–8 years of life.

Very complete accounts have appeared of the great variety of congenital malformations encountered in the entire number of children (Myrianthopoulos and Chung 1974, Chung and Myrianthopoulos 1975a, Myrianthopoulos 1985, Hardy et al. 1979). The presentation in the last of these (pp. 292–293) is especially revealing, since it gave the number of children with each listed abnormality who were diagnosed in the nursery and at 1 year of age, and hence vividly demonstrated the greatly increased frequency that the protracted period of examination resulted in.

A full report of the malformations in the offspring of diabetic mothers enrolled in the Study was made by Chung and Myrianthopoulos (1975b). Unfortunately, the study's design and intent and the authors' penchants negated any great usefulness the findings may have had for the present monograph. In one respect it was an advance, since it differentiated between the several forms of diabetes, but continued to contain a main hindrance: the numbers and types of abnormalities noted were those diagnosed throughout the first year of life. But it also had other problems. Though one can agree with the authors (Myrianthopoulos and Chung 1974) that the division of malformations into major and minor is sometimes arbitrary, still there is much consensus as to what is one or the other, and in this paper this consensus was quite often disregarded—over half of the cases with abnormalities that were listed as major are generally considered minor or dubious. (The extent to which this practice can influence outcomes was articulated when Klemetti 1978 found "a trebling of…frequency if the definition is made wider than strictly structural malformations to include minor deviations and functional disturbances.") Another bias was introduced by adding to the study a large number of diabetic pregnancies (far more in fact and probably of greater disease severity than the study sample) from the Joslin Clinic. For these reasons, as well as because it was impossible to learn which defects were found neonatally and which discovered later, in the children of the diabetic and nondiabetic women, the roughly doubled frequency of "major" malformations recorded in the former can be of no help in assessing the question of the teratogenicity of pregestational diabetes.

Other things undoubtedly also damaged the study's usefulness for the purposes relevant here. The number of women contributed by the participating centers was very uneven. Almost 42% came from just two of them—the Boston Lying-in Hospital, and the Pennsylvania Hospital in Philadelphia (Niswander and Gordon 1972). This maldistribution probably led to a serious bias as far as the ascertainment of congenital malformations is concerned—variability in racial composition, which ranged from 0% white in New Orleans to 97.6% white in Buffalo (Myrianthopoulos and Chung 1974), although the overall sample that was analyzed for the relation between maternal diabetes and congenital malformations was fairly evenly divided in this respect (Chung and Myrianthopoulos 1975b). Nevertheless, these wide disparities among the participating institutions and the undoubted differences in patient selection and malformation diagnosis, plus the matters mentioned in the previous text, fatally weakened the applicability of the data so laboriously collected and analyzed to the question of concern here.

A United Kingdom Study

Through obstetric and other personnel of a large number of hospitals throughout the United Kingdom, 773 women with pregestational diabetes, almost 90% insulin treated, who gave birth in 1979–1980 were identified (Lowy et al. 1986b). A questionnaire survey was used to gather information about them and their offspring. The perinatal mortality rate, 5.6%, though far less than it had been in former years, was still nearly four times that for all babies in the United Kingdom at that time.

Major congenital malformations, when the two with Down syndrome were omitted, occurred in 4.0%. This was probably an exaggeration, since it included some with uncomplicated talipes, patent ductus arteriosus, and ventricular septal defect. The perinatal mortalities accounted for nearly 42% of all the malformations (13/31); that this was probably an underestimate was indicated by the malformation frequency in stillborns being far less (12.0%) than in neonatal deaths (55.6%), which as was often the case probably meant that many of the former were not or could not be autopsied.

The malformations affected many parts, although the authors felt that some of them were "relatively specific," especially those of the heart and great vessels (which included, as noted, an unspecified number of offspring with patent ductus arteriosus and ventricular septal defect) and certain central nervous system defects. But no instance of anencephaly and only one of spina bifida was mentioned, which is strange since these central nervous system defects had a relatively high frequency in many regions of the United Kingdom (could this have been due to prenatal identification and selective abortion?) Of interest, because of their notoriety, but given no special attention by the authors, was the occurrence of three cases of sacral absence (the manner of whose diagnosis was unmentioned) and two of holoprosencephaly. In addition, minor malformations (defined as those "unlikely to interfere with the baby's life") were noted in 22 babies, but whether they were associated with the major ones was not mentioned. An attempted analysis of the relation between first-trimester blood glucose level and malformation incidence had no useful outcome, mainly because major and minor malformations were not considered separately.

Confidence in the extent to which the surveyed women were representative of the overall pregnant diabetic population was clouded by two facts. First, only 38% of the 474 hospitals from which information was requested participated in the study. Second, on average, less than one pregnant diabetic woman was reported for every 1000 pregnancies, though this varied geographically from 0.3 to 1.9 per 1000 (such wide variations may be common; they were also noted in the many hospitals of an American metropolitan area [Miller 1965]); whereas pregestational diabetes has usually occurred in about 5–6 per 1000 pregnancies (Niswander and Gordon 1972, Kalter and Warkany (1983). Finally, it appears that the outcomes of the pregnancies comprised only those that were "fully analysed," though this term was not explained.

The NIH Diabetes in Early Pregnancy (DIEP) Study

The National Institute of Child Health and Human Development contracted with five US medical centers to engage in a collaborative study of malformation and fetal loss in diabetic pregnancy (Mills et al. 1983). It was considered that by recruiting women before conception, long-standing and hitherto unsatisfactorily answered questions regarding these outcomes could be addressed (Mills et al. 1983). The study was conducted in 1980–1985 and the results published soon after (Mills et al. 1988a,b).

The original plan was modified later, and malformations in offspring of women entering the study early were compared with those of women entering late (an apparently unforeseen happening), instead, as originally planned it seems, of making the comparison with a group not collected concurrently (Mills et al. 1983). Thus of the 626 insulin-dependent diabetic women, 347 entered the study "early," that is, before (86%) or within 21 days of conception (14%), and 279 others after this time. This may explain why controls were obtained only for the early-entry group.

Malformations were usually diagnosed only on the third day after birth by trained examiners guided by a checklist of defects, but other diagnostic methods, such as ultrasonography and radiography, were additionally used when an anomaly was suspected. The frequency of admissible major congenital malformations in the "early-entry" group was 3.7% (or 2.3% if the isolated ventricular septal defects are omitted; the argument for doing this is presented in Chapter 14) and 7.2% (or 6.1% if again the venricular septal defects are omitted) in the late-entry group (the former an apparently large difference but one barely statistically significant). Remarkably, the controls had a frequency of major congenital malformations of only 1%, and no explanation was offered for this unrealistically low level.

The increased frequency in the early-entry group (vis-à-vis the control) was not considered to be related to mean blood glucose and glycosylated hemoglobin levels during early pregnancy, a conclusion departing from conventional thoughts about glycemic control and maldevelopment, and severely criticized, as will be seen later in Chapter 15, where these topics are extensively dealt with.

Questions regarding the design and communication of the study must be explored. Putting the outcome of the study into doubt and negating much of the purposes of such investigations, both the diabetic and control subjects were highly selected. The former, recruited "by means of public appeals as well as through the medical system," were apparently healthier than usual, since any with hereditary teratogenic tendencies themselves or in first-degree relatives or diabetes in the latter were excluded, as were those being treated with potentially teratogenic pharmaceutical drugs for various diseases or disorders (all of which causes one to wonder at the authors' apparent surprise that the subjects took so few drugs, and the probably unwarranted extrapolation from this revelation [Simpson et al. 1989]). The controls, employees of corporations, medical centers, and prepaid health plans, were highly motivated volunteers whose pregnancies were planned.

Next, the discrepancy between the number of diabetic women entering the study early who spontaneously aborted (as reported by Mills et al. 1988a; discussed in Chapter 3) and the number continuing their pregnancies was not explained. Last, the number of perinatal mortalities (usually well examined, as we have learned) and the malformations occurring in them were not specified. The aspects of the study concerned with the relation between abnormal prenatal development and glycemic control in early diabetic pregnancy (Mills et al. 1988b) and with fetal growth delay (Brown et al. 1992) will be addressed in Chapter 15.

Four Recent Studies

A prospective nationwide study was conducted in 1982–1985 at 36 participating regional and county hospitals in Sweden (Hanson et al. 1990, Hanson and Persson 1993). The 557 registered women were calculated to constitute 80% of the total number of type 1 diabetic pregnancies in the country during the years of the study. Partly counterbalancing this great advantage of surveying what was undoubtedly a quite representative sample of such pregnancies was the drawback of the pregnancies being able to be followed only from the time the women were enrolled in the study, the median time of which was 9 weeks of gestation. This may have been the reason for the rather low frequency of spontaneous abortions of 7.7%. Still this was very close to the 7.2% in the randomly chosen nondiabetic control pregnancies. Despite the women receiving the best medical care of the day the perinatal mortality rate continued to be over four times that occurring in the general population. A total of 4.2% congenital malformations was found at examination on the day of birth and at discharge from the hospital, but over half of the abnormalities were of minor varieties, leaving 2.0% major, compared with 1.0% in the controls (none of which was specified in either group).

A California multicenter program, encompassing 19 clinical units in 8 perinatal regions, during 1986–1988 registered 572 pregestationally diabetic women, 8.0% before conception and 53.3% in the first trimester (Cousins 1991c). The fraction of the total of such pregnancies in the state during this time that this number may have comprised was not noted. The findings of this ambitious effort were disappointing, since its many numerical discrepancies and other inadequacies made it difficult to interpret the perinatal mortality and congenital malformation data.

A nationwide program conducted in 46 diabetes centers in France in 1986–1988 enrolled 320 pregnancies of pregestational diabetic women, which was about 25% of all known diabetic cases (Gestation and Diabetes in France Study Group 1991). In the unaborted pregnancies, the frequency of malformations was 5.2%; but the data are equivocal since the malformations were not defined, their diagnosis not described, and those found not individually named.

A multicenter study conducted in Denmark in 1976–1990 by the 11 hospitals in Northern Jutland registered all pregnancies of type 1 diabetic women in the county, consisting of 328 consecutive and unselected pregnancies of 205 women (Nielsen and Nielsen 1993). The great majority of the births occurred in the main obstetric hospital, at Aalborg. Spontaneous abortions occurred before the end of the 12th week of gestation in 11.1% of the otherwise uninterrupted pregnancies (none of the interruptions being occasioned by suspicion of malformation). In the remaining pregnancies, 4.3% died perinatally, apparently not different from that expected for the region; all were autopsied and one found multiply malformed. Seven survivors had cardiac malformations and one major and six minor skeletal malformations. The rate of major malformations in all, therefore, was 3.5% (9/255).

13

POPULATION-BASED STUDIES

INTRODUCTION

In determining the frequency of a characteristic in a group of individuals—large or small—to ensure that the result is a true reflection of the entire population, the study group should be as similar to the entire population in all conceivably relevant attributes as possible. It is not easy to satisfy this requirement. Most of the studies this monograph is concerned with—hospital-based studies—were conducted at special hospitals or diabetes clinics, that is, facilities whose patients were often directed to them because of complications needing care beyond the usual; thus, they were not a cross-section of all pregnant diabetic women. Therefore, whatever may have been found with regard to the consequences of the disease in such women may be suspected of not truly reflecting the outcomes in all its sufferers. This uncertainty may have been further increased by the limited number of subjects that such studies almost always contained, regardless of the size of the facility and the length of the study. In fact, the longer they ran, the more heterogeneous the study groups may have been, making extrapolation even more hazardous.

Two ways of possibly reducing this unreliaility, and yielding more valid interpretation, have been made use of. One of these—multicenter studies—as seen in Chapter 12, tried to do this by enlarging the sample, thereby possibly producing more statistically acceptable conclusions. What this methodology obviously did not eliminate is the problem of unrepresentativeness: although the aggregated number of subjects may have been much greater than most centers could collect alone, they were still in almost all instances largely composed of nonrandomly selected women.

The goal of population-based studies on the contrary is to survey the entire population of subjects in a geographical area, which would fulfill the purpose completely. But studies of diabetic pregnancies of this sort have had their own brand of problems, since they relied on sources of information—public health and vital statistics certificates recording births and deaths, alone or sometimes supplemented by various hospital records—which often proved to be deficient in important details regarding both mother and child. Exemplifing such difficulties are overall studies of congenital malformations (eg, Knox et al. 1984, Greb et al. 1987, Calle and Khoury 1991, Snell et al. 1992, Stone 1992).

Population-based studies nevertheless can provide insights not otherwise obtained. Such efforts proceed along two paths—from alleged cause to supposed effect or vice versa. Thus, in the examples provided below, the investigations started either with diabetic pregnancies to see whether they resulted in congenitally malformed offspring more often than did nondiabetic pregnancies or with malformed offspring to learn whether more of their mothers were diabetic than those of nonmalformed offspring. The first type is called a cohort study, and the second a case-control study. In both cases, the key ingredients are unbiased collection of the subjects and suitability of the controls.

Cohort studies of the outcome of pregnancy in diabetic women have sometimes relied on information obtained from vital statistics documents, supplemented to improve the search for diabetic pregnancies by cross-references to hospital records of births and deaths and other sources of data. And sometimes, when the study was confined to a limited region, they have relied on information obtained from all or most of the hospitals in the region. The latter thus became magnimulticenter studies and were often beset by some of the difficulties inherent in more conventional multicenter studies.

COHORT STUDIES

Early Birth Certificate Studies

Certificates of live birth and fetal and infant death in 1958–1959 from the New York City Department of Health furnished information that indicated that the offspring of diabetic women had a frequency of congenital malformations, as recorded within 48 hours of delivery, of 8.3% compared with 1.5% in those of nondiabetic women (Erhardt and Nelson 1964). The authors aptly commented on the necessity of "any surveillance system [having] definite stipulations [as to inclusion and exclusion of abnormalities]...so that comparison of data from place to place or from time to time may be possible." Unhappily, evaluating their own findings was made difficult by the defects being listed rather unspecifically, so that beyond those that were clearly inadmissible it could not be judged whether others were also dubious. The certificates did not specify the type of diabetes, but its prevalence, 2.5 per 1000, when compared, for example, with the 6.6 rate found in the Collaborative Study during the same era (Niswander and Gordon 1972) indicated that perhaps not all diabetic women were so identified on the documents. These deficiencies, plus the obviously inadequate control data, render any conclusions regarding the diabetic pregnancy outcome precarious.

A similar survey of birth certificates—of live births only—in Hawaii in 1956–1966, uncovered far smaller frequencies of malformations, still larger in diabetic than in nondiabetic pregnancies, 1.8% versus 0.9% (Goodman 1976). The low frequency in the former may have been due to the dilution of the outcome by the inclusion of gestational diabetic and glucose intolerant pregnancies, but it is not likely to have been significantly affected by only live births having been surveyed. However, even this low rate was magnified by including defects that could not be attributed to maternal diabetes: a Down and rubella syndrome, as well as several other inadmissible defects, omitting which reduced the frequency to 0.87%, almost identical with that (an unrealistically small one) in the nondiabetic pregnancies.

A Norwegian Study

A pioneering population-based study made use of the legal requirement in Norway that every offspring of 16 weeks' gestation or more be registered at 7 days after delivery (Jervell et al. 1980). From such records for 1967–1976, several noteworthy data were gleaned. A total of 1035 births to diabetic women occurred, nearly 55% of them in larger hospitals. As elsewhere, this interval saw a great decrease in the perinatal mortality rate—from 17.7% to 6.1%. Finally, a malformation frequency of 4.4% was noted in diabetic pregnancies compared with 3.0% in all births, with the excess accounted for by cardiovascular and central nervous system abnormalities.

Judging these findings was difficult, since the defects in the 45 abnormal offspring were not completely spelled out and their association with perinatal mortality was unclear. Two things impaired the credibility of the results. In most of the women, the diabetes was definitely present before pregnancy, but how many of these were insulin-dependent was unknown, since this fact was not included on the registration record. And the prevalence of diabetic pregnancy was low, 1.6 per 1000. This could have had various explanations, especially undernoting of diabetes cases as well as low overall diabetes prevalence.

An Australian Study

Population surveys of the association of maternal diabetes and congenital malformations in western Australia were harmed, perhaps mortally, by several faults (Stanley et al. 1985, Bower et al. 1992). Through a notification system using information gathered by midwives, it was found that 427 confirmed diabetic women gave birth in 1980–1984. Auxiliary to this were hospital records, which disclosed diabetes type, and a congenital malformation registry, linkage with which identified malformed offspring of diabetic women. That the population surveyed consisted of two distinct groups, Australian Aborigines and nonaboriginal individuals, was shown, if by nothing else, by the 18 times greater proportion of pregestational diabetics in the former who were not insulin-dependent. No doubt the explanation for this difference is that Aborigines were prone to precocious insulin-dependent type 2 diabetes, resembling in this respect the Pima Indians discussed in Chapter 6. This was also supported by the almost seven times greater prevalence in them of what was called gestational diabetes, but which apparently was mostly glucose intolerance.

Analysis of the congenital malformation findings was made difficult by their not being listed specifically and by the unclear tabulation of the results. This was remedied by the enumeration that Dr. Carol Bower kindly sent me of the abnormalities in the 39 affected children born during these years, which indicated that the conditions in 13 of the children were diagnosed at postneonatal ages up to 3 years and that 8 of the remaining children had inadmissible defects (congenital hip dislocation, hypospadias, trisomy 21, congenital hypothyroidism) and one was misdiagnosed. Of the 39, 15 occurred in Aborigines, for a frequency of 15.3%; that in nonaborigines was 7.3%. The supplied listing did not note which of the defects were diagnosed at birth and which later; hence congenital abnormality frequencies could not be calculated for either group.

The Swedish Congenital Malformation Registry

Motivated by the thalidomide catastrophe (Lenz 1961), Swedish medical authorities set up a national system of intense surveillance of congenital malformations in 1964 for the purpose of prompt warning of the presence of new environmental teratogens (Källén and Winberg 1968). Fortunately, up to the present little evidence of such a presence has been detected (Källén 1987a, 1989a). But another of the uses to which the registry has been put—examining the possible effects on offspring of maternal diabetes, among other maternal diseases—has furnished some positive results, but none that has as yet been other than sparsely published (Källén 1987a,b, 1989b). Dr. Bengt Källén, however, was kind enough to send me a more detailed account of these results, for the years 1978–1981 (Källén, personal communication 1985).

Congenital malformations have also been registered in Sweden by the Medical Birth Register, which has enabled the identification of these and other pregnancy outcomes in women with selected diseases and various problems. It has accounted for more than 99% of the births in the 50 hospitals in the country (Källén and Winberg 1968). In 1978–1981, it recorded 379,516 births, of which 1512 were of women with diabetes, giving a prevalence of 4.0 per 1000 births (Källén 1985), about what was often found elsewhere during this period. But this was considered to be higher than usual, an excess believed to be due to dilution with "25% of cases which do not fulfill the criteria of what is usually called diabetes…." From this, it was further reasoned that the pregnancy outcome risks that the study discovered probably were underestimates in the same proportion. The prevalence data cited for many other countries undermined this opinion, however.

The Swedish Register of Congenital Malformations noted 35 malformed offspring in the 1512 diabetic pregnancies, whereas the Medical Birth Register recorded 116. This difference and perhaps other questions may be explained by the fact that the quality of the information the former reported "ultimately depends on hospital-based records [and such] information varies from hospital to hospital" (Bakketeig et al. 1984). Among the 116, considering only those with malformations Källén called "significant," that is, excluding numerous minor or uncertain ones, the list provided by him showed that 56 offspring (3.7%) of the diabetic mothers were malformed. This frequency was more than twice the 1.6% recorded among the entire population for such malformations. The latter figure should be looked upon skeptically for the usual reasons. More acceptable are comparisons, for example, of abnormalities in perinatal mortalities or of specific well-defined abnormalities. In a study of the latter sort, dealing with limb reduction defects, Källén (1989b) found a frequency in the offspring of diabetic women considerably increased over the usual rate in Sweden. Others, however, have found an unimpressive relation between maternal diabetes and these conditions (Polednak and Janerich 1985) or none at all (Czeizel et al. 1983).

Comparing malformation frequencies in perinatal mortalities, obviating as it does many imponderabilities, should make for greater crediblity, as recognized when it was said that dealing with "dead and autopsied offspring…probably increases the reliability of the description" (Källén and Winberg 1974). Such a comparison provided no support for the overall finding, however, because, although the diabetic perinatal mortality rate was more than three times the overall one, the frequency of malformations in these deaths (24.4%, 10/41) was not statistically significantly different from that in the entire population surveyed (20.0%, 617/3101).

A Washington State Study

In this statewide study, pregnancies of women with diabetes in 1979–1980 were identified through birth and fetal death certificates supplemented by maternal and infant records from 89 hospitals and birthing centers, totaling about 95% of all Washington State births in this period (Vadheim 1983, Connell et al. 1985). By the use of both vital statistics and hospital records, it was believed greater completeness of case identification and accuracy of recording of diabetes would be ensured. The importance of the hospital material was shown by a preliminary study of births in 1975–1979, which indicated that less—perhaps far less—than 50% of diabetic pregnancies were recorded as such on the vital statistics certificates. There was also a close positive relation between the rate of such pregnancies and obstetric unit size, with the five Regional Perinatal Centers contributing the greatest proportion. This, plus the fact that only 38 of the hospitals reported any diabetic births at all, probably pointed to an important source of the underreporting. The control consisted of pregnancies of nondiabetic women, information about whom was randomly collected from birth and death certificate files. Their suitability for this task will be discussed later in this section.

During the 2 years of the definitive study, residents of Washington State had 133,246 deliveries of greater than 20 weeks' gestation, 266 of which were by pregestationally diabetic women, for a prevalence of 2.0 per 1000. Realizing that this was significantly less than the rate often found elsewhere, Vadheim proposed several possible reasons for it, but considered the most likely to have been underreporting, combined possibly (though to me unconvincingly) with a lower overall diabetes prevalence.

About 25% of these pregestational diabetics did not require insulin, which was a much larger percentage, for example, than the 11% found by Lowy et al. (1986b). This disproportion may partly have been caused by equating class A with gestational diabetes (Vadheim 1983). Hence, it is likely that some of the non–insulin-requiring women were not pregestational diabetics, and thus the prevalence was actually even less than 2 per 1000. Also separately ascertained were women with gestational diabetes, denoted class A or A/B, that is, not requiring or requiring insulin, respectively. The prevalence of this type of diabetes was 2.9 per 1000, far lower than has often been the case, again suggesting underdiagnosis or underreporting.

It may partly have been because congenital malformations were only one of many sorts of offspring morbidities consequent upon maternal diabetes that the wide-ranging study (Vadheim 1983) was concerned with, that numerous inconsistencies and inadequacies regarding malformations crept into it. Certainly also because it depended on sources of data of variable quality, it should not have been unexpected that the analyses would be unsatisfactory. Having essentially an epidemiological thrust, the study gave much attention to its design and to the classification of diabetes in pregnancy and less to considering the possible incompleteness and unreliability of the civil and hospital records the survey was based on.

These data, as presented in two discrepant tables (Vadheim 1983, pp. 120, 132), showed that the frequency of major congenital malformations in the offspring of pregestational diabetic women was 13.0% (33/253) or 13.9% (28/201), significantly greater than that in the nondiabetic controls (1.8%, 15/838). Many attempts were made to explain the increased risk in the overt diabetic cases, larger than was found by most other studies. But among them the likelihood that the number of malformed case children was inflated in the ways noted in a following paragraph and that the number in the controls was underreported were unmentioned. Nor was the bias mentioned that records of deaths up to the age of 1 year were included in the calculation.

Inspection of the detailed list of case infants with alleged major congenital malformations appended to the thesis revealed in fact that many of the defects were not major, possibly not due to maternal diabetes, or even present in the cases, since findings in controls may have crept into this list. There was also some confusion about offspring numbers. The total with major malformations of pregestational diabetic women, as noted above, was 33 in one table, 28 in another, and 48 in the list in the appendix. But included in the last were 14 with minor and other ineligible abnormalities (Table 13.1) as well as 10 women with an undesignated condition, who might have been controls.

It is worth looking closely at one set of the malformations listed in the Appendix. This consisted of five instances of the caudal regression syndrome and two of sacral absence, three of the seven in gestational and four in pregestational births—an unusually large number of this family of rare abnormalities to be found in so relatively small a sample of cases. Some of the descriptions of the defects may offer a clue to this abundance. One of the sacral ageneses was listed—presumably copied verbatim from the original record—as follows: "Hypoplastic lower extremities, with flexion contractures of ankles (sacral absence)," which in all probability means that the person originally diagnosing the abnormalities, mindlessly following the

Table 13.1 Congenital Malformations Excluded as Relevant, Listed as Major by Vadheim 1983

Wide midline space in upper gingival ridge
Coloboma (otherwise unspecified), a familial trait?
Long philtrum
Micro sigmoid colon
Minimal spanning of eyelids, simian crease right hand
Small cleft in alveolar ridge
Mild hypertelorism, long philtrum, poorly formed upper lip; abnormal hair whorl, very questionable microcephalus
Second-degree hypospadias, left simian crease
Trisomy 21
Sandifer syndrome (torticollis)
Trisomy 18
Familial facial/foot syndrome
Concave ribs, bony protruberance, left parietal-temporal area, unusual meatal skin tag
Probable Goldenhar syndrome, complex congenital heart disease, probable fetal alcohol syndrome

misconception of the day, interpreted the lower-limb defects in his patient as being equivalent to sacral absence. Could any of the others have been similarly misunderstood? The second was described as consisting of "sacral agenesis and caudal regression," together with facial asymmetry, and other abnormalities, leaving an unclear picture. One of the five instances of caudal regression syndrome was accompanied by urogenital and other defects, including polysplenia, and another by imperforate anus. The remaining ones were called "classical," a designation not without ambiguity. Only one of the seven occurrences, in an infant of a noninsulin-dependent mother, was lethal, but whether the infant was autopsied was not noted. Since no definition or description was given of what "caudal regression syndrome" was considered to consist of, doubt must remain that it was tantamount in these cases to the defect thought to be specific for diabetic embryopathy, especially since three of the seven instances were in infants of gestational diabetic women, in whom the frequency of congenital malformations is not increased (Kalter 1998). Such indefiniteness was not uncommon; most authors were equally vague in designating this state. For example, Ramos-Arroyo et al. (1992), in a table listing malformations included "caudal dysgenesis," and in the text revealed that this meant "agenesis or hypoplasia of the femur, sacrum and/or lower vertebrae," a truly mixed bag and truly and hopelessly confusing any attempt to relate a specific embryopathy with the maternal disease.

It was hoped that the Washington State perinatal mortality data would be informative and compensate for the overall inadequacies of the study. With respect to the perinatal mortality rate itself, there was little difference between the pregestational diabetic and control pregnancies, 11.6% versus 8.4%. But because of missing or questionable information, the facts regarding malformations were disappointing. The malformation frequency in the diabetic mortalities was significantly larger (50%, 14/28, in Vadheim 1983; 42.8%, 12/28, in Connell et al. 1985) than in the controls (7.1%, 5/70), but this wide difference was suspicious for several reasons. First, none of the stillbirths, which composed a significantly larger proportion of the control than of the diabetic mortalities, apparently was autopsied, and in reverse a larger proportion of the diabetic than control neonatal mortalities was autopsied. As for the autopsies, differences no doubt prevailed from hospital to hospital in the attention given those with and without special problems.

Last, outweighing other considerations, the question of the validity of the composition of the control intruded. The pregnancies of the diabetic women took place in 38 of the nearly 90 hospitals in the state (Connell et al. 1985), whereas those of the control women, being a random selection from the vital statistics documents, apparently occurred in all or nearly all the state's hospitals. Furthermore, 79% of the diabetic women gave births in just 16 of the 38, the largest and best-equipped hospitals, those in which it can be safely assumed that the offspring of women referred for special treatment received the closest attention. For all the reasons mentioned, no great trust can be put in the supposedly increased congenital malformation frequency in diabetic pregnancies found by this population-based study.

A Northern Ireland Study

The Northern Ireland study was an ambitious attempt to collect data on the outcome of all known pregnancies of insulin-dependent pregestational diabetic woman delivering in the 17 obstetric units in Northern Ireland in 1979–1983, all but 4 of which had diabetic births (Traub et al. 1987). Information was obtained from various hospital-based sources, but since none was found to be completely accurate, various means of tracing and cross-referencing were used to ensure that documentation of diabetic pregnancy was reliable. The patients were not randomly distributed among the medical facilities, but disproportionately attended the five regional diabetes referral units, especially the major one at the Royal Maternity Hospital in Belfast, which served 55% of all the identified diabetic pregnancies in the period surveyed. Throughout the country during these years there were 139,250 deliveries, including a total of 221 pregnancies of 187 diabetic women, for a prevalence of 1.6 per 1000, quite low compared with other findings, which may indicate that, despite its diligence, the search for diabetic pregnancies fell short. Agreeing, the authors commented, "It is disappointing that current record systems seem to be so inadequate...."

Fifteen offspring of diabetic mothers had major congenital malformations (not individually named, but consisting of neural tube, renal, and cardiac defects), for a total of 7.4% (15/204 not spontaneously aborted). No nondiabetic controls being collected, comparison was made with the overall population malformation frequency—2.5%, unaccountably thought to be one of the highest in the world. However, when survivors were considered separately from mortalities (8 of 12 of which were malformed), their malformation frequency was 3.6%, little different from that in well-examined newborn infants.

Comparisons between those delivered at local hospitals and those referred to the Royal Maternity Hospital at some time during pregnancy or attending the latter throughout pregnancy were of interest. The two groups did not differ in frequency of spontaneous abortion, but did so slightly in frequency of perinatal mortality (7.0% and 4.4%, respectively) and more so in that of malformation (10.5% and 3.3%, respectively; not a statistically significantly difference, however). It is conjectural whether it was nevertheless related to the more diligent examination the special hospital may have afforded.

The patients referred during pregnancy to the major center had a higher incidence of complications of diabetes and attended this main Northern Ireland teaching center for management of severe problems that could not be dealt with at local hospitals. The history of those cared for at this facility from early in their pregnancies was not noted, but there can be little doubt that in a city with a population exceeding 300,000 in the 1980s (Paxton 1987) women with special needs were funneled there. Despite 70% of the latter group receiving some form of preconception counseling and achieving modest reductions in blood glucose level (contrasted with none who received such counseling in the peripheral hospitals), there was no improvement in the pregnancy outcome in the group as a whole.

The Hesse Study

As in the Northern Ireland study, the Hesse study drew on the records of so many hospitals and covered so large a percentage of the population that it was practically equivalent to a conventional population study (Lang and Künzel 1989). The total number of 1982–1986 births on which it was based, 113,128 children, comprised about 78% of all born during this period. Through the omnibus term "diabetes mellitus" 446 diabetic pregnancies were identified, some probably large, but an unknown number of which were not the pregestational form. Congenital malformation data were also vague and nonspecific, the total being 2.8% in diabetic cases and 0.5% in controls. A computerized sheet listing 15 or more individual malformations, not specified, however, in the article, supposedly guided the diagnosis, but this aid seems not to have been used. The only thing to say for this project is that even a large population sample all by itself is not in the least a guarantee of definitive results.

The Maine Diabetes in Pregnancy Program

Through a regional network of private and hospital-based physicians 160 pregestational diabetic women who had 185 pregnancies in 1987–1990 were located (Willhoite et al. 1993), which, it is of interest to note, far exceeded the 94 births to such diabetic women recorded on Maine vital records for these years. Based on the number of live births in the state in this period, as reported by the National Center for Health Statistics, the number registered by the program gave a prevalence of approximately 2.7 per 1000 pregnancies, less than often found elsewhere. As in the Washington State study, a larger proportion of the cases was noninsulin-dependent than has usually been found in hospital-based studies.This may mean that physicians participating in the program mistakenly designated some women as pregestational diabetics or that the program captured a wide variety of diabetes types.

Nine offspring in all were congenitally malformed, but the overall abnormality rate could not be calculated because the number of pregnancies coming to term was not stated; nor was the number of malformations occurring in the mortalities. No control was obtained. A primary purpose of the program was to establish an educational forum that would provide pregnant diabetic women with preconception counseling and care. In this it had limited success, however, since only about one-third of the women received such counseling. Only one of the malformed offspring was born to women who received preconception couseling, and, according to the authors, this was not a significantly lower frequency than in the others. These results are considered further in Chapter 15, which deals with attempts to prevent malformations by counseling before or early in pregnancy.

An Iceland Study

Since 1974, all diabetic patients in Iceland have been cared for at the National University Hospital in Reykjavík, the only established diabetic clinic in the country. This centralization enabled a validated prevalence of 1.4 per 1000 of type 1 diabetes to be established most recently, the lowest of any Nordic country (Hreidarsson et al. 1993). It also permitted all pregnancies of diabetic women in Iceland to be identified; in 1981–1990 there were 86 such occurrences, 66% of whom were type 1 and 34% type 2, glucose-intolerant, or gestational diabetics. In all of these there were two fetal anomalies, both cardiac: one occurring in the two perinatal mortalities, the other successfully surgically repaired. Assuming the worst case—that both malformed children were offspring of the 57 type 1 diabetic women—the frequency of the abnormalities was 3.5%, close to that expected for populations as a whole. Perhaps this survey done in a small island nation has come closest to a definitive answer to a perplexing question. It might have been clinched had a control been included.

CASE-CONTROL STUDIES

Earlier Studies

Case-control studies, a population-based examination of the association of maternal conditions and congenital malformations, have a relatively young history. The earliest such study of diabetic pregnancy appears to have been conducted in 1965–1973 by the Finnish Register of Congenital Malformations, which examined the prevalence of "diabetes mellitus" and various infectious diseases and other problems in women who gave birth to infants with central nervous system malformations (Granroth 1978).

Based on the finding that 1.5% of the 710 cases of all central nevous system defects occurred in offspring of women with diabetes and that none of the controls was diabetic, it was considered that the defects were significantly associated with the maternal condition. Two facts weakened this conclusion: first, over one-third of the abnormalities on which it was based were hydrocephalus and microcephalus, two defects, as noted above, of mixed etiology and vague diagnostic criteria; and, second, the Finnish registry required the notification of all malformations detected not only at birth but during the first year of life (Saxén et al. 1974), greatly diminishing the usefulness of the outcome for evaluating defects present at birth.

What can be considered a novel variation of the case-control approach was taken by Matsunaga and Shiota (1980). They examined 3474 well-preserved, undamaged abortuses induced for sociomedical reasons, as permitted by Japanese law (Nishimura et al. 1968). The women undergoing the procedure were apparently a random sample, and the morphological condition of the embryos was unknown to the gynecologists performing it. Six of the abortuses came from women with "diabetes mellitus," seemingly a low incidence of the disease, until it is recalled that Japan has a low prevalence of insulin-dependent diabetes (Patrick et al. 1989, WHO Multinational Project 1991). Only one of the "diabetic" abortuses had a malformation, a myeloschisis, which was a frequency not significantly different from that in the entire sample.

In a study at the Children's Hospital in Philadelphia of 150 children with myelomeningocele and 22 with anencephaly, the mothers of none of the former and one of the latter was an "overt" diabetic (Eunpu et al. 1983). This was fewer than expected, according to a calculation made by the authors.

More Recent Studies

Baltimore Washington Infant Study

Recent case-control studies were generally more ambitious than the few earlier ones. Typifying them was the Baltimore Washington Infant Study (BWIS). This was a widespread survey of live-born children with congenital cardiovascular malformations (CVM) for the purpose of investigating their association with maternal diabetes (Ferencz et al. 1987). The malformed children were identified by searching the records of 53 hospitals in Maryland, the District of Columbia, and five northern Virginia counties, supplemented by hospital pathology and vital statistics death records. The malformations of concern were those identified at birth or confirmed before 1 year of age by autopsy or various diagnostic procedures performed at six pediatric cardiology centers. From these numerous and diverse sources 2568 infants with CVM were enrolled in 1981–1987, but after omitting those for whom no information regarding maternal diabetes, etc, was available and for other reasons, there remained 2259 (Ferencz et al. 1990).

Information regarding maternal health was acquired by interviewing the mothers of the malformed children and those of a randomly selected control group in their homes at unstated times after the births, at which time it was recorded whether or not they were diabetic or had diabetes apparently from before or only during the index pregnancy. These statements were not confirmed medically. Significantly more case mothers claimed to be pregestational diabetics than did controls (1.5% versus 0.5%), indicating an association of maternal diabetes and the malformations. Gestational diabetes was also increased in the former, but not significantly. An analysis of individual types of CVM indicated that only a few were significantly increased (double outlet right ventricle, truncus arteriosus, tetralogy of Fallot, ventricular septal defect), whereas many others were not.

The study had several shortcomings, which detracted from its impressiveness, the most serious and obvious one being its entire reliance on unconfirmed maternal recall at unstated, perhaps delayed, times after birth. As the authors admitted, this probably led to "misclassification of true overt and gestational diabetes." At least as serious is the well-known difficulty, as McKeown (1988) put it, that "...mothers who have had an abnormal child report a higher frequency of many occurrences than mothers whose children are normal" (p. 104). Possible evidence that this did happen was the elevated frequency of many sorts of CVM in children of gestational diabetic mothers.

Perinatal mortality is another concern here. Some of the abnormal cases died perinatally and were diagnosed postmortem; but the proportion of all cases that these composed was not stated. CVM have been found in 1.5–2.7% of perinatal deaths (Hoffman and Christianson 1978) and formed a sizable proportion of all such defects found perinatally. Since a large percentage of infants with congenital CVM may die in infancy without their condition being recognized (Abu-Harb et al. 1994), it is likely that many malformed infants failed to be included in the study under discussion.

Once again, findings at postneonatal ages were included, which makes for difficulty, since a significant proportion of CVM are found in later months of infancy (eg, Hoffman and Christianson 1978). In an earlier BWIS report, Ferencz et al. (1985) themselves reported that 80% of septal defects were diagnosed after the first month of life. Although the practice of considering older ages may be necessary for depicting a fuller picture of the situation, it debases the value such studies may have for clarifying the larger problem that this monograph was grappling with.

Finally, and most strangely, malformed offspring with abnormalities whose etiology was more or less clearly known to have nothing to do with maternal diabetes were not excluded from consideration, as was properly done in other case-control studies described in the following paragraphs. These included various recognized syndromes, and especially those with conditions due to chromosomal aberrations, accounting for 4.7% and 12.1% of the entire sample, respectively. Failure to exclude the latter is particularly egregious, since Down syndrome is so often associated with congenital CVM, especially ventricular septal defect (Park et al. 1977, Hyett et al. 1995). This failure badly weakened any conclusion about the relation of diabetes and the malformations that the study claimed.

Swedish Cardiovascular Malformation Study

Another such study of heart defects was based on data recorded in 1981–1986 by two Swedish registries, the Registry of Congenital Malformations and the Child Cardiology Registry existing at four specialty centers (Pradat 1992a). The focus was stillborn and live-born children with major congenital CVM, usually identified by clinical signs in the first postnatal week, by special diagnostic procedures or at autopsy within the first year of age. Infants with known chromosomal aberrations were excluded from consideration.

Cases were compared with nonmalformed matched controls of normal birth weight surviving the neonatal period randomly selected from the Medical Birth Registry. The various case and control maternal characteristics examined for their possible association with the malformations were also discovered from this registry. This source noted that 22 of the 1324 case and 17 of the 2648 control offspring had mothers with "diabetes mellitus," giving an odds ratio of 2.7. The author regarded this as a "strong correlation" with the disease, but found that the association was significant only for septal defects. Judging from the 6.4 per 1000 prevalence of the maternal condition in the controls, it is likely that the diabetes ascertained was of the pregestational variety.

Two difficulties with the study impaired its helpfulness for the purposes of this work. The number of case perinatal mortalities and their malformation frequency, and the number of the 22 cases with diabetic mothers diagnosed after the neonatal period, were not stated. The significance of the results per se will be evaluated in a section in Chapter 16 devoted to the studies in which children of diabetic mothers were followed up postnatally.

CDC Congenital Renal Disease Study

An investigation bearing a remote likeness to a case-control study can be mentioned here. Data gathered in 1970–1984 by the Birth Defects Monitoring Program (BDMP) of the Centers for Disease Control (CDC), used primarily to examine the temporal trend of renal absence and renal dysgenesis, were used incidentally to search for associations of these conditions with an unstated number of maternal conditions or exposures. In this way it was found that "maternal diabetes" was noted in the records of 20 of 709 infants with the former of these abnormalities, suggesting that they were associated (Stroup et al. 1990).

The things that can be criticized about this study are legion, besides the vagueness of the designation of the maternal illness. The BDMP being a "passive system" was based on newborn hospital discharge diagnoses made by physicians and other staff that were not routinely checked for accuracy; thus, renal abnormalities other than those of concern may have been included inadvertently. In addition, some infants with Potter syndrome and perhaps with other conditions of recognized or suspected etiology were probably included as well. Not all hospitals that were contacted participated, and not all records requested were received. Maternal history was abstracted from the infants' medical records, a source open to incompleteness and inaccuracy. The resemblance of the study to a case-control one, however, totally breaks down because, since the search for associations seems to have been almost an afterthought, there was no control. Clearly, no credence can be given to the study's finding regarding the association of these renal conditions and diabetes.

Atlanta Study

This study, casting a wider net, considered all "serious or major" malformations in children born in resident hospitals in the five-county metropolitan Atlanta area in 1968–1980 (Becerra et al. 1990). Among the 333,637 live births, 7133 were finally diagnosed as malformed by 1 year of age. This material had originally been gathered for a different purpose—to assess the risk of US Vietnam veterans for fathering children with congenital malformations—and the study may have suffered to some extent from the constraint that the original investigation was under to "be completed as quickly as possible" (Erickson et al. 1984a).

Information regarding many aspects of maternal health before and during the index pregnancy was obtained from mothers of the malformed and matched control children by telephone interview, 2–3 years after the births (Erickson et al. 1984b). Not all parents were located or cooperated, and for only 4929 case and 3029 randomly selected control mothers, about 70% of the eligible individuals in each group, were interviews completed. Participation was lower for nonwhite than white mothers, who formed one-third and two-thirds, respectively, of all births.

Medically validated insulin-dependent, presumably pregestational diabetes was noted in 26 case and two control mothers (Becerra et al. 1990, Khoury, personal communication 1994), giving therefore a very significant relative risk ratio of 7.9. Based on the overall malformation rate found in metropolitan Atlanta in 1968–1980 of 2.3% cited by Becerra et al. (1990), this risk thus implied an 18% malformation frequency in offspring of diabetic mothers, far more than even the most convinced and enthusiastic believers in the teratogenicity of diabetes had ever averred in recent times. Even larger risk ratios were calculated for certain specific malformations, especially of the central nervous and cardiovascular systems, even though the authors stated that these infants were not "particularly prone to a characteristic pattern of defects."

The numbers of insulin-dependent diabetes in case and control mothers previously noted gave prevalences of 5.3 and 0.7 per 1000, respectively, the former being about that found in the population at large and the latter falling far short of this expectation. Since ratios are based on two numbers, if one of them is suspect the ratio is untrustworthy. Positive replies by case mothers to the question, "At any time before [date of index birth] were you ever diagnosed as having diabetes or sugar diabetes?" were medically validated; negative replies by the control mothers were not. The authors defended this inconsistency by asserting that the possible underascertainment of insulin-dependent diabetes should have been negligible; but then they themselves explained it by the absence of routine intensive diabetes screening of the area's population during the study period.

It must be recalled that both parents were interviewed and that the interviews consisted of an inordinately large number of questions, expected to take 45 minutes (Erickson et al. 1984b). This was undoubtedly a burden to all, but without doubt the questions were considered more burdensome and intrusive by parents of normal than those of malformed children and, understandably, were probably answered less patiently, fully, and accurately by the former than the latter. Even the case mothers may have felt put upon, which may explain the finding of far smaller frequency of gestational diabetes than expected to be reported by them.

Other problems and weaknesses besetting the study can also be mentioned. Control mothers were selected from birth certificates of children "without defects"; the accuracy of these documents with regard to the recording of malformations has frequently been found wanting (eg, Gittelsohn and Milham 1965, Mackeprang et al. 1972, Hexter and Harris 1991). The case infants included stillbirths as well as live births; the controls only live births. An unstated number of the malformed case infants were diagnosed postneonatally, as revealed by the list of defects given by Erickson et al. (1984a); there was no opportunity for doing so in controls. This list also revealed that a substantial number of the defects were not major malformations or had a known or probable etiology. The relative risks were based principally on occurrence of individual malformations, not on that of malformed infants. Reflections on this procedure will be found just below.

Miscellaneous Studies

In a study of births in two Belgrade University obstetrical clinics in 1986–1988, 591 children were born with congenital malformations. Omitting minor malformations and those of genetic etiology left 113. Two of their mothers had "diabetes" during pregnancy compared with none of the controls, a nonsignificant difference (Ananijevic-Pandy et al. 1992).

In a Spanish case-control study, minor malformations and those due to single genes and chromosomal aberrations were included in the analysis (Ramos-Arroyo et al. 1992). The study, part of a collaborative study of congenital malformations that monitored about 10% of the live births in the country, was based on births in 1976–1985 in 38 mostly mid-sized hospitals located in different parts of the country. During this period 10,087 infants were discovered to be malformed in the first 3 days of life. This was 2.0% of the total born, a low figure, especially since a large proportion of the malformations—nearly 40%—were minor types, strongly indicating that the local physicians making the diagnoses overlooked an appreciable percentage of the malformations. The ascertainment of maternal insulin-dependent diabetes was equally poor, the prevalence in mothers of case infants being 1.1 per 1000 and in controls 0.2 per 1000. This 5.5-fold difference was meaningless, however, if only because it was reckoned on the total of all malformations.

The odds ratio for major malformations alone was larger, 8.7, but still misleading, of course, because of the severe underascertainment of the maternal condition, especially in the controls. Similar analyses were made for specific malformations, as done in the Atlanta study, which means that the unit of the analysis was the individual abnormality, one by one, and not the abnormal infant.

Even if the scheme of the study had been impeccably constructed, this type of analysis is illegitimate and distorts the results for the following reason. If maternal diabetes is hypothesized to be teratogenic, then all the otherwise etiologically unassignable malformations in malformed children of diabetic women (and nearly 50% of them reported in this article were multiply malformed) must be assumed to have the same etiology; thus, it is the child and not its individual abnormalities—not to mention exaggeration of statistical significance owing to sample size inflation—that must be the unit of analysis of the strength of the association.

A case-control study of the relation of congenital hydrocephalus to maternal diabetes was conducted in Alsace, with the aid of a registry of births occurring in 1979–1987 (Stoll et al. 1992). Omitting cases of hydrocephalus due to chromosomal aberrations and part of recognized syndromes, 76 instances discovered within the first year of life. Three of their mothers had "diabetes," as did two of the mothers of the matched controls, an insignificant difference.

A malformation surveillance program at the Brigham and Women's Hospital in Boston in 1972–1974 and 1979–1990 found insulin-dependent diabetes in the mothers of 11 of 147 (7.5%) offspring with neural tube defects (Holmes 1994). How many of these women had pregestational diabetes was not stated. No control was obtained. The prevalence of these defects in the 123,489 births in these years was 1.2 per 1000, rather low for a presumably largely white patient load in an area in which a significant part of the population has a greater-than-average proneness to these abnormalities (Naggan and MacMahon 1967).

It may not be inappropriate to note one final article here. A retrospective study of 22 families each with a child with sacral absence found a 5% recurrence rate and a similar one of association with (an undesignated type of) maternal diabetes (Magnus et al. 1983), making it equally likely (or unlikely) that the condition had a genetic as an environmental provenance. These authors also cited reports of an association of this sacral abnormality with paternal diabetes, for which evidence of teratogenicity has never been found (eg, Koller 1953, Rubin and Murphy 1958, Chung and Myrianthopoulos 1975b, Theile et al. 1985). Apropos of this study, it is relevant to note the virtual nonexistence of studies of the frequency and type of congenital malformations that exist in the families of women with diabetes.

14

SPECIFIC CONGENITAL MALFORMATIONS

Among persons who harbor no doubt that diabetes and malformations are associated, some have held that the disease is associated with an increased frequency of all congenital malformations, whereas others believe the increase is limited to some particular ones, especially or even entirely. The former school was represented by Pedersen (1977), although somewhat equivocally, when he said "No specific defect is peculiar to diabetes, but severe congenital heart disease and skeletal deformity are characteristic" (p. 196). The latter school, less hesitantly, has favored a number of abnormalities, among them, of course, caudal dysplasia, but also holoprosencephaly, neural tube defects, and cardiovascular malformations. This chapter will look into these assertions.

CAUDAL DYSPLASIA

Introduction

Many studies have reported caudal abnormalities in offspring of diabetic women. One or another form of such conditions was mentioned in 58 articles that I identified—nearly two-thirds of European origin and one-third American, the earliest from over 50 years ago (Peel and Oakley 1949). This leaves many more in which there was no such mention (but more of this later). Increased awareness of the assumed association of these conditions with diabetes no doubt accounted for the fact that more than 50% of the publications mentioning it and 75% of the American ones have appeared since 1980.

It has aptly been said that it is "difficult to make a good case for caudal agenesis as a diabetic embryopathy mainly because of the poor definition of the syndrome..." (Chung and Myrianthopoulos 1975b). Ever since Duhamel (1961) included malformations of the lumbosacral spine as an element in his "syndrome of caudal regression," the use of this term has been confused and abused. As explained elsewhere in this work, Duhamel defined this syndrome as including not only defects of the vertebrae, but also in "variable proportion anomalies of the rectum, of the urinary and genital systems...and of the lower limbs." This scheme was the culmination of his attempts to explain the frequent association of anorectal with other abnormalities, especially of the lower vertebral column (Duhamel 1959, 1961), which led him to theorize that since these were the very abnormalities found most often in sirenomelia they must form a syndrome of graded and variable content. Opposing the extension of this theory to diabetic pregnancy is the common observation that in sirenomelia the sacrum, though often dysplastic, is seldom absent.

Thus, contrary to the attempted revision of the nomenclature (eg, Welch and Aterman 1984), it is sacral absence that is the specific defect of the so-called caudal dysplasia syndrome, if such a syndrome exists at all. Nevertheless, Duhamel's concept has left the residue of making the analysis of the conjectured association of diabetes and sacral abnormalities difficult.

The source of this difficulty is that many of the nonvertebral malformations—anal, femoral, and so on, said to be part of the caudal dysgenesis syndrome ("...an absolutely obnoxious term in my opinion" [Benirschke 1987]) has each by itself often been taken as denoting it. Thus, when, as is often the case, infants of diabetic women are labeled as having the syndrome or one or another of its variant designations, without clear-cut description of the abnormalities that are present, it is impossible to know whether sacral absence, the malformation thought by Benirschke (1987) and others to be "characteristic for the offspring of maternal diabetics," was truly present or not. The few crystal-clear examples of the misuse invited by this term only hint at other such instances masked by vague and imprecise terminology.

The syndrome has been equated with "...reduction defects of the legs with or without agenesis of the lower segments of the spinal column..." (Soler et al. 1976). An infant said to have caudal dysplasia was thus described, "Une radiographe post mortem montre qu'il existe 6 vertèbres lombaire; *le sacrum est normal* [emphasis added], ainsi que le reste du squelette" (Kubryk et al. 1981). Others mislabeled had severe defects of the lower limbs (Assemany et al. 1972), femoral and humeral defects and fistulae on the sacrum (Bergstein 1978), and bilateral femoral hypoplasia alone (Hitti et al. 1994). Two of the many further examples of the potential confusion caused by such imprecision will be cited, to illustrate the widespread misinterpretation it encourages.

Amendt et al. (1974) observed six instances of what were called "caudal regression," of which only three had sacral absence, and the others defects of the pelvis alone or combined with vertebral defects. Likewise, Ballard et al. (1984) observed three of "caudal dysplasia," only one of which had sacral absence, another unspecified sacral vertebral abnormalities, and the last defects of the long bones of the legs; Miodovnik et al. (1988) observed three of "caudal dysplasia," in none of which was it explicitly said that the sacrum was absent. Finally, of the three instances of sacral dysplasia noted in 1950–1974 in children of diabetic women at the diabetes clinic of the General Hospital in Birmingham, England (incidentally, as was often the case, identified neonatally no doubt only because they were multiply and lethally malformed), only one apparently lacked sacral vertebrae, although this fact was detailed in one report (Malins 1979) but not another (Soler et al. 1976). Thus, the designation sacral or caudal regression or dysgenesis or dysplasia does not necessarily mean that there was sacral absence.

Nor have animal experimenters, out of their depth, been immune to this misconception. In one instance, hindgut malformations, one of the many types of abnormalities induced in mice by the potent vitamin analogue retinoic acid, was equated with caudal dysplasia, which, compounding the misconception, was then erroneously stated to be associated with gestational diabetes (Alles and Sulik 1993). With far greater justification, thymic absence induced in mice by excess vitamin A (Kalter and Warkany 1961) was considered completely analogous to a human condition, the DiGeorge syndrome (DiGeorge 1968, Lammer and Opitz 1986), a rare affliction with immunological consequences (Warkany 1971, pp. 739–740).

Therefore, if the proposition that caudal abnormalities are associated with maternal diabetes is to be seriously examined, only clear-cut instances of sacral absence must enter into the consideration. It is also to be remembered that absence of the sacrum fails to be discovered in the neonatal period in a large proportion of affected children (Van Dyke et al. 1995) because of absence of external indication, and only first comes to medical attention months or even years later, when urological and other difficulties surface. Such late-detected instances cannot be included in an analysis of phenomena found at birth. For example, the case of sacral aplasia presented by Manzke et al. (1977) was supported by a radiograph of a 5.5-year-old child, making it obvious that the condition was only diagnosed at an advanced age.

Reports of Caudal Abnormalities

The facts, as they are, can now be put into focus. All told, 86 offspring with caudal abnormalities were mentioned in the 58 articles just noted, for a prevalence of 5.6 per 1000 births. In Europe, this rate did not vary over time, remaining at about 6 per 1000, whereas in America it rose from 1.9 in the years before 1980 to 8.7 per 1000 afterward (Table 14.1).

However, only 32 of the 86 offspring (37%) were categorically stated to have sacral absence, and the age at which the condition was first diagnosed was not always clearly stated. Of the 32, about 17% died perinatally, at least 31% survived the neonatal period, and the fate of 52% was not mentioned at all. Assuming then, based on these figures, that about half of these deaths were detected neonatally, it may be estimated that over the years in both regions together the mean prevalence of the condition at birth was about 4.4 per 1000. (At this point, it is important to be reminded that the estimates arrived at here and above failed to take into con-

Table 14.1 Frequency of Caudal Abnormalities in Offspring of Women With Pregestational Diabetes (per 1000 Births)

Era	Europe		America	
	Articles	Frequency[a]	Articles	Frequency[a]
< 1980	22	37/6147 (6.0)	5	6/3200 (1.9)
≥ 1980	16	22/3440 (6.4)	15	21/2403 (8.7)

[a] Number with caudal abnormalities/total (%).

Of the number abnormal in Europe, 9/37 and 6/22 and, in America, 5/6 and 12/21 were explicitly designated as having sacral absence, although in most instances the means of diagnosing the condition were not stated.

sideration the reports of malformations in several thousand offspring of diabetic women in which, whether because they were overlooked or not present, no such spinal malformations were mentioned.)

What is known of the frequency of sacral absence in the general population, especially that discovered at birth, with which this tentative figure may be compared? Very little. In a search of nearly 1 million birth registrations in Czechoslovakia in 1961–1964, five cases of "agenesis" of the lower spine were located (Kučera and Lenz 1967), a low frequency it seems. The fact that these registrations recorded an overall malformation frequency of only 1.4% and that not all instances of the spinal malformation are detected at birth nevertheless make the figure hardly credible.

A survey of stillbirths and live births in Spanish hospitals since 1976 uncovered frequencies of 4.5 and 0.2 per 1000, respectively, of "caudal dysgenesis (any degree)" (Martínez-Frías et al. 1994). But these figures cannot be taken seriously, since the surveyed conditions included "urinary, genital, and/or anal anomalies, and/or those with lumbosacral spine defects (including the most severe anomalies of the caudal region such as sirenomelia)...."

That most children with such conditions survive the neonatal period was indicated by only one instance of sacral absence being found in 2145 autopsied perinatal mortalities (Holmes et al. 1976). A radiological analysis of the spines of 700 children of postneonatal ages examined in 1940–1955 gave a more realistic assessment: four had absent infralumbar vertebrae, for a frequency of 5.7 per 1000 (Shands and Bundens 1966), about 30% more than the exaggerated one calculated for diabetic births previously noted.

It is appropriate to mention that the undoubtedly overblown frequency of sacral absence occurring at birth calculated above is a far cry from the estimate made years ago—over 200 times greater—of lower spinal abnormalities in children of diabetic mothers (Passarge and Lenz 1966), an estimate still uncritically cited years later (Feigenbaum et al. 1996). My deduction, plus the data in the few publications relating to the population frequency of sacral absence in perinatal mortalities and older children, despite their relative exiguity, point to the unlikelihood of this malformation being more common in the offspring of diabetic women.

The major source of the belief that it is associated with diabetes comes from case reports of their concurrence. But case studies do not prove relationships. "The most that a case study can show is that a proportion of cases of a type of defect have occurred after exposure to some factor such as disease or medication of the mother during early pregnancy. It does not show that exposure has occurred in a higher proportion of cases than of all pregnancies and therefore cannot be regarded as proof that this exposure is even a risk factor for the defect, let alone a cause" (Leck 1993).

CENTRAL NERVOUS SYSTEM MALFORMATIONS

Introduction

The congenital central nervous system (CNS) malformations, anencephaly, meningocele/encephalocele, and spina bifida, sometimes considered together under the heading neural tube defects (NTD), have often been said to be among those that are especially increased in the children of diabetic women. All are detectable at birth, but anencephaly, consisting as it does of degenerated brain tissue perched above an incompletely formed cranium, and usually accompanied by distorted facial features, is markedly conspicuous and especially unmistakable, particularly since it is invariably lethal before or soon after birth (Lemire et al. 1978).

Because of these features, anencephaly has gotten much attention, and extensive information regarding its worldwide distribution and prevalence is at hand. Also provoking and enabling such investigation no doubt is the harsh reality that in many parts of the world anencephaly is among the most common of the major congenital malformations. This, plus the extraordinary variations in its frequency—racial, ethnic, temporal, socioeconomic, geographic, plus the as-yet unexplained fact of its being far more common in newborn girls than boys (Elwood and Elwood 1980, Little and Elwood 1991)—have piqued the interest of geneticists, epidemiologists, and many others in anencephaly for many decades (Penrose 1957).

These variables undoubtedly are relevant to the possible relation of anencephaly and maternal diabetes, but except for geography and an occasional mention of ethnicity or race, information regarding them was all but totally ignored in the multitude of publications dealing with the pregnancies of diabetic women. Even such elemental facts as the sex of anencephalic infants or occurrence of NTD in previous pregnancies or other close family members were almost never mentioned. Thus, the possible impact of these variables on the frequency of the malformation was closed to analysis.

Anencephaly being the most glaring of the NTD makes it almost impossible to overlook, unlike abnormalities of the lower spinal cord and thus no doubt is seldom unregistered in hospital and vital records. Furthermore, although many anencephalics are stillborn (Martin et al. 1983, Sadovnik and Baird 1985) and many of these are macerated (Mufarrij and Kilejian 1963), even in these instances the defect seems to be readily identified. For these reasons, as well as because it is the most common of the NTD, anencephaly is the one whose putative association with maternal diabetes is primarily considered here.

It can be taken for granted that especially in diabetic pregnancies, closely monitored as they usually are, the conspicuousness and lethality of anencephaly ensure that in virtually every case it was noticed and recorded. Therefore, in determining its frequency all reports of pregestational diabetic pregnancies were considered, not only those in which malformations—CNS or others—were noted and enumerated, but those as well in which it was explicitly stated or could be taken as implied that no malformations were found; with only those excluded that noted malformations but did not specifically name them.

Prevalence of Anencephaly

All Births

The outcomes were calculated both for all births and for perinatal mortalities. The data for the former show that the mean rate of anencephaly in offspring of

Table 14.2 Frequency of Anencephaly (With or Without Spina Bifida) in Diabetic and Overall Births in Europe and America Before and Since 1980 (per 1000 Births)

	Europe	America
	Diabetic Births[a]	
Before 1980		
UK + Ireland	16/3822 (4.2)	–
Boston	–	5/1319 (3.8)
Other	24/7371 (3.2)	12/5452 (2.2)
Since 1980		
UK + Ireland	9/1794 (5.0)	–
Boston	–	3/432 (6.9)
Other	14/4386 (3.2)	17/5264 (3.2)
	Overall Births[a, b]	
Before 1980		
UK + Ireland	7.6	–
Other	1.1	–
America	–	2.9
Since 1980		
UK + Ireland	2.8	–
Other	0.9	–
America	–	1.5

[a] Number of anencephaly/total births (%).
[b] Calculated from information given by Little and Elwood 1991.

diabetic women over the nearly 6 decades since about 1940 was 3.6 per 1000 in Europe and 3.0 per 1000 in America (Table 14.2). This table discloses several notable things. First, the frequency in Europe hardly differed in the years before and since 1980, whereas in America it increased (almost entirely owing to data from Boston), despite the considerable widespread population declines in this malformation that occurred in the last couple of decades (Mathers and Field 1983, Yen et al. 1992). Boston, as noted, had a higher frequency than other American areas, and one wonders whether this may have been due to the highly select patient sample attending the Joslin Clinic or to the large Irish component in the population of this city. Second, the frequency of anencephaly in the United Kingdom and Ireland was much greater than in the continental European countries surveyed, conforming to the former being generally a high-rate region and the latter a lower-rate one (Penrose 1957, Dolk et al. 1991, Little and Elwood 1991).

These figures may be compared (see Table 14.2) with population statistics derived from a summary of published worldwide estimates of the prevalence of NTD from before 1980 and more recently (Little and Elwood 1991). The more recent ones have certainly been distorted by failure to include defective specimens diagnosed and eliminated prenatally (EUROCAT 1991, Limb and Holmes 1994). Some of the decreased occurrence in the overall population in recent years has also been attributed to nutritional supplementation during pregnancy (Oakley et al. 1994), but how much of the reduction can be accounted for by this factor, by improved socioeconomic conditions, and by the recurring temporal swings NTD are subject to are still open questions. It is not to be overlooked, however, that diabetic births have apparently not shared in this overall decline, although early metabolic care of diabetic women is a major effort in their recent management.

The mean population prevalences conceal much intraregional variation, but they seem to indicate that diabetic pregnancy has been associated with higher frequencies of anencephaly than have occurred in the general population. This reading must be accepted cautiously, however, since several considerations may challenge its reliability. In addition, for example, to "nonuniformity in the duration and diligence of case ascertainment" (Borman and Cryer 1990), most of the overall prevalences were based on population series, whereas the data from diabetic pregnancies came from hospital series, which leaves the door open to the possibility that the excess in the latter was partly due to biases stemming from referral and self-selection of diabetic women. For example, familial occurrence of NTD, known to be associated with increased risk of recurrence (Little and Elwood 1991), may have led to the high level of anencephaly detected in diabetic women prenatally screened by the alphafetoprotein assay (Milunsky et al. 1982). Absence of details about the women and their histories and how they came to be cared for at a large Boston hospital, however, make this speculative.

Finally, although the data from diabetic pregnancies were based on relatively large numbers recorded over the decades, they were most certainly only a small percentage of all such pregnancies during these years. In the US alone with 3.5–4 million births annually, in the last 40 years there were about three-quarters of a million births to pregestationally diabetic women. The conclusion is unavoidable that the diabetic pregnancies that entered into published series were undoubtedly a selected and intensively observed set, and as such their outcomes must be suspected of not being entirely representative.

Perinatal Mortalities

Uncertainty that may still linger can be lessened by another calculation: that of the frequency of anencephaly in perinatal mortalities in diabetic pregnancies reported since 1940. Only reports of series of pregnancies were analyzed in which the occurrence of perinatal mortality was explicitly noted and in which all the malformations were named. This may give a more definitive picture of their frequency (Table 14.3). As usual there was a clear inverse relation between the frequency of perinatal mortality and that of anencephaly. As the former decreased over the years, in Europe and America, the latter increased in both regions, reaching levels of 12.0% and 3.8%, respectively.

Table 14.3 Frequency of Anencephaly in Diabetic Perinatal Mortalities (PNM) in Europe and America Before and Since 1980

	Europe		America	
	% PNM	Anencephaly/PNM (%)	% PNM	Anencephaly/PNM (%)
< 1980	19.1	47/2448 (1.9)	18.3	14/1307 (1.1)
≥ 1980	5.5	27/224 (12.0)	7.2	10/262 (3.8)

Again, overall population data with which to compare these figures are scarce. Those from an assessment of the fetuses of 12,620 high-risk pregnancies of various sorts referred over a 4.5-year period may be useful (Manning et al. 1985). Two percent of the pregnancies were of insulin-dependent diabetic women (which is about four times the overall prevalence of the condition and illustrates the selective proclivities of large medical centers). Ninety-three of all the offspring were perinatal mortalities (0.7%), and 15 of them had anencephaly, a frequency of 16.1%. The number of the mortalities that occurred in the diabetic pregnancies and the number of these that were anencephalic were not stated, but omitting the probable number of the latter reduced the frequency of the malformation in the nondiabetic remainder to 15.2%, indicating that the frequency in the diabetic mortalities was not excessive.

Can these high-risk pregnancies be suitable for comparing with diabetic ones? Yes, because these supposedly high-risk Canadian pregnancies, it turns out, had a lower mean perinatal mortality rate than did the white population of the US during a comparable period ((Powell-Griner 1989). Thus, it is legitimate to take the anencephaly frequency in mortalities as representative of the overall population and to conclude that the frequencies in the most recent diabetic pregnancies were not out of line with them.

CARDIOVASCULAR MALFORMATIONS

Introduction

Infants of diabetic women were reported to have an increased frequency of congenital cardiovascular malformations (CVM); these in fact were usually their most common abnormalities. Vexing questions have confounded these observations, however, frequently because of difficulties of ascertainment and multiplicity of malformation type—in distinction in both regards to defects of the CNS. As Kenna et al. (1975) commented: "...congenital heart disease is...possibly the most difficult group of defects to ascertain with any accuracy...[because many] affected infants show no abnormal symptoms or signs at birth...[and] 'congenital heart disease' is not a single entity, but comprises a large number of anatomically distinct lesions..."

General CVM Prevalence

Congenital malformations of the heart and great vessels are among the most common congenital malformations in all babies, not only in children of diabetic mothers. Years ago they composed about 10% of all congenital malformations (Rowe et al. 1981, p. 110), but later rose to perhaps 20% or more (eg, Roth et al. 1987) and to about 40% in all neonatal and infant deaths associated with malformations (Berry et al. 1987, Kalter 1991).

Their reported frequency has varied greatly, however, for several reasons in addition to uncertainties of ascertainment. Studies have sometimes considered only live births and thus excluded the appreciable number in stillbirths (Hoffman 1990). Because CVM are not all detected at birth, the cumulative frequency has varied with the length and diligence of postnatal follow-up. In addition, time has brought more refined diagnostic methods, which have yielded larger estimates (Anderson 1991). No doubt these new procedures, as well as more intensive and longitudinal efforts, allowing the detection of types and degrees of abnormalities once less apparent, led to the increases discovered, usually up to 1 year of age but also beyond, from 3–5 per 1000 live births in most past studies (Rowe et al. 1981, p. 111) to 8–10 per 1000 and more found lately (Hoffman 1990, Meberg et al. 1994). These prevalences will be of particular interest later in this work, when the health of older children of diabetic women is discussed.

Ventricular Septal Defect

All types of CVM are not equally numerous. Almost invariably the most prevalent one is ventricular septal defect (VSD), once composing about one-quarter to one-third of all CVM (Hoffman and Chrstianson 1978, Anderson 1984), and more recently as much as 45–57%, almost certainly due to surged recognition (Spooner et al. 1988, Anon. 1994, Meberg et al. 1994). Indeed, it is likely that the increase in the total frequency of CVM may be due in large part, if not entirely, to the great jump in that of VSD (Newman 1985, Fixler et al. 1989, Martin et al. 1989). This was made especially obvious by Meberg et al.'s (1994) finding of no significant increase between 1982–1985 and 1986–1991 in any CVM but VSD.

Alhough it was unclear earlier whether this "epidemic" of VSD, as it was called (Layde et al. 1980), was an artifact due to refined diagnosis, the evidence now clearly indicates that the increase was indeed due to the detection of small, isolated septal defects (Laursen 1980, Newman 1985, Spooner et al. 1988, Martin et al. 1989, Fixler et al. 1989, Anon. 1994, Meberg et al. 1994), of the sorts largely overlooked by past, less precise methods of diagnosis. It must not be neglected, however, that most of these are of the sorts that close spontaneously in a large proportion of cases and hence are without physiological consequence (Evans et al. 1960, Mitchell et al. 1967, Anderson et al. 1984). In a recent period this "repair" occurred in almost 70% by 1 year of age (Meberg et al. 1994)!

But the cumulative rate of CVM is not the item of interest here. It is instead the frequency discovered in the neonatal period, since it is during the first days and weeks that the majority of children of diabetic women were examined for congenital defects.

CVM in Perinatal Mortality

Concrete information about the frequency of CVM in the neonatal period comes from perinatal mortalities, but this source presents ambiguities tied to inconsistent stillbirth definition and variable rates of perinatal mortality and autopsy. Data of this sort in addition are relatively few, especially with the decrease in the rate of autopsy in recent years. Nevertheless, it is clear that the CVM frequency in mortalities is appreciable. Studies of stillbirths and neonatal deaths—all or almost all of which were autopsied—noted a mean of 3.5% and

12.5%, respectively (Richards et al. 1955, Mitchell et al. 1971a, Kenna et al. 1975, Hoffman and Christianson 1978). These and the other few data revealed a combined background frequency of about 6–8% in perinatal mortality for the years before 1980. Information of this sort for later years appears not to exist or at any rate was not found (see Table 14.4).

CVM in Surviving Offspring

Population studies have yielded only indirect and very uncertain indications regarding the newborn period, especially since they arrived at widely variable estimates of the proportion of CVM diagnosed neonatally—eg 36–66% (Hoffman 1987, Stoll et al. 1989).

Information regarding "survivors" (defined here as live births less neonatal deaths, diagnosed neonatally) is even scarcer than that for perinatal deaths. Few articles were found that contained data permitting calculation of the frequency of CVM explicitly diagnosed in survivors. For such information, records of congenital malformations in birth certificates, especially of CVM, are unreliable, being notoriously faulty.

Even estimates derived from examining infants were seriously flawed (Hoffman 1968, 1987). One apparently carefully conducted survey found the frequency in survivors to be about 5 per 1000 (Hoffman and Christianson 1978), just about the same as the 6 per 1000 found in infants diagnosed by 1 year of age during earlier decades (Richards et al. 1955). One study, however, noted that 11.3% of infants with CVM died in the postneonatal period (Mitchell et al. 1971a), which may mean that some ascertained frequencies of CVM were serious underestimates.

Fortunately, data regarding the frequency of CVM in surviving offspring, though not copious, were published in the last 15–20 years. Moe and Guntheroth (1987), in Seattle, noted 49 infants with an unequivocal diagnosis of VSD in 10,476 live births in 1981–1986, of whom at least 47 survived the neonatal period, that is, 4.5 per 1000 for this one type of CVM alone, the only one reported. From this it can be extrapolated that the overall CVM frequency in survivors was about 9 per 1000. Spontaneous closure occurred in 45% of these cases by a mean of 12 months. From somewhat ambiguous figures reported by Stoll et al. (1989) in Strasbourg, it can be deduced that CVM was noted in 489 surviving infants diagnosed by the first week, in 105,330 live births during 1979–1986 (4.6 per 1000). Meberg et al. (1994), in Oslo, noted 224 infants with CVM in 22,810 live births during 1982–1991, perhaps 92% of whom survived the neonatal period (9.0 per 1000). About 57% of the total were VSD, that is, about 5.1 per 1000. Again, a large percentage—over 69%—closed by the first year. A recent study (Hyett et al. 1999) of the association of nuchal translucency and major CVM in 29,154 karyologically normal fetuses of 10–14 weeks of pregnancy found a rather lower overall prevalence, 1.7 per 1000 pregnancies. This in itself was an overestimate, since it included a number of fetuses diagnosed after intrauterine death. I append a comment of the authors, namely, that "...the overall prevalence of major cardiac defects in such a group of fetuses (about 2%) is similar to that found in pregnancies affected by maternal diabetes mellitus...."

MATERNAL DIABETES AND CARDIOVASCULAR MALFORMATIONS

Several epidemiological studies previously discussed paid particular attention to the association of CVM and maternal diabetes (Mitchell et al. 1971a, Ferencz et al. 1990, Pradat 1992a). Having been conducted or participated in by pediatric cardiologists, they presented a full enumeration and description of the types of CVM found. But because of the nature of such studies, the frequencies they reported were based on abnormalities diagnosed at various, sometimes extended, childhood ages. Hence, they cannot entirely serve the principal purpose of this inquiry, namely, to determine whether the frequency of malformations found in the neonatal period was greater in the children of diabetic women than in the general population. For this purpose, information about children examined at birth or in the earliest weeks afterward must be used, that is, reports of hospital series of diabetic pregnancy, in which such information, though sometimes imperfect, may be found.

Perhaps in an early attempt to grapple with such questions, Kučera (1971a, compiling the information given in a large number of reports of hospital-based series, found that heart anomalies were about five times more common in diabetic pregnancy than in a large population sample. But, as he well noted, the validity of this wide difference was imperiled by numerous confounding factors, which may have led not only to overestimating the former frequency but also to underestimating the latter. Even more to the point, from the facts given above that the frequencies of CVM differ so greatly in perinatal mortalities and survivors, we can see that total findings do not address the question validly (Table 14.4).

CVM in Diabetic Pregnancy Mortalities

Seven studies of CVM in diabetic perinatal mortalities in the 1940s to 1960s noted frequencies of 4–14%, with a mean of about 10% (Rowe et al. 1981, pp. 675–680). Fuller information regarding this period yielded a mean frequency of about 7–8%, which was about the same as the frequency at the time in the overall population (see Table 14.4). As much as possible, this item is based only on autopsied diabetic mortalities. Population data for a comparison for the more recent period were not found.

Because the CVM frequency took the marked increase in recent years just described, Table 14.4 not only presents data for perinatal deaths and survivors separately, but also for earlier and later years, as far as possible. The doubling it reveals of the CVM frequency in diabetic mortalities in recent years in Europe and America was no doubt largely the outcome of the overall increase in the congenital malformation frequency that followed upon the reduction in offspring death (Kalter 1991). Whether widened diagnosis may also have contributed is unknown.

CVM in Diabetic Pregnancy Survivors

Comparison of survivors of diabetic and population pregnancies was readily made for the earlier period, but data for the later one were scarce; only two,

Table 14.4 Congenital Cardiovascular Malformation (%) in Diabetic and Population Perinatal Mortalities[a] and Survivors

	Europe		America	
Offspring	< 1980[b]	≥1980[b]	< 1980[b]	≥ 1980[b]
		Diabetic Births		
SB	2/176 (1.1)	2/44 (4.5)	6/155 (3.9)	5/73 (6.8)
ND	29/343 (8,4)	7/27 (25.9)	32/293 (10.9)	16/87 (18.4)
PNM	36/344 (10.5)	4/28 (14.3)	10/150 (6.7)	7/24 (29.2)
Total	67/863 (7.8)	13/99 (13.1)	48/598 (8.0)	28/184 (15.2)
Survivors[c]	75/4717 (1.6)	45/2047 (2.3)	17/1370 (1.2)	35/1316 (2.7)
		Population		
SB	92/2078 (4.4)	–	60/1676 (3.6)	–
ND	187/1046 (17.9)	–	88/1163 (7.1)	–
Total[d]	305/3231[e] (9.4)		148/2839 (5.2)	
Survivors	415/190,236 (0.2)[f]	(0.5–0.9)[g]	176/60,153 (0.3)[f]	(0.9)[h]

SB, stillbirth; ND, neonatal death; PNM, perinatal mortality.
[a] Patent ductus arteriosus omitted.
[b] From 84, 56, 55, and 40 articles, respectively, published in these years.
[c] See text for definition.
[d] From Richards et al. (1955), Mitchell et al. (1971b), Kenna et al. (1975), Bound and Logan (1977), Hoffman and Christianson (1978).
[e] Including perinatal mortality not otherwise specified
[f] From Harris and Steinberg (1954), Leck et al. (1968), Feldt et al. (1971), Hoffman and Christianson (1978).
[g] Based on data in Meberg et al. (1994) and Stoll et al. (1989).
[h] Moe and Guntheroth (1987).

possibly three, relevant reports were identified (Moe and Guntheroth 1987, Stoll et al. 1989, Meberg et al. 1994). The findings show that surviving offspring of diabetic pregnancies had a CVM frequency greater than that of the general population in both Europe and America. But to the extent that the sparseness of the more recent data made interpretation possible, the differential appeared to have narrowed in the former region but to have remained the same in the latter (see Table 14.4).

It may be that this regional difference was due to temporal changes that occurred to a greater extent in one region than the other. While the population CVM frequency increased in later years to approximately the same extent in both regions, from 0.2–0.3% to 0.9%, the diabetic CVM frequency increased only slightly in Europe (1.6% versus 2.0%) and much more so in America (0.9% versus 2.9%). What the difference may be due to is unclear, but zealousness of diagnosis, as noted, cannot be disregarded in interpreting these data.

No persuasive analysis could be made of the type or types of CVM that might have accounted for the increased frequency in diabetic pregnancy, since the number of cases was small and the number in which the defects were specified were few. In the latter, many consisted of VSD, apparently amounting to a larger frequency than occurred in the general population (Hoffman and Christianson 1978). It must not be forgotten, however, that the frequency of VSD in all live births is quite substantial, amounting in the latest findings to 3.5–5.1 per 1000 (Moe and Guntheroth 1987, Meberg et al. 1994, Graham and Gutgesell 1995).

As recent findings have shown, intense examination of children leads to elevated discovery of CVM, so the apparent excess of CVM in surviving children of diabetic women may also have resulted in part from such close attention, especially in America. In any case, VSD, the predominant lesion, has long been considered to have little clinical importance, since "most cases are clinically insignificant" (Carlgren 1959) and "with small defects, the clinical course is benign" (Graham and Gutgesell 1995). Furthermore, many sooner or later close spontaneously (Anderson et al. 1984, Moe and Guntheroth 1987, Meberg et al. 1994, Tegnander et al. 1995).

The temporal increase in the CVM frequency in survivors, in contrast with that in the mortalities, was inconsistent, being statistically insignificant in Europe but more real in America. This difference may have been due to VSD forming a larger proportion of CVM in the latter, resulting, as in the general population, from earlier and more intense diagnosis of smaller defects (Bound and Logan 1977, Laursen 1980, Spooner et al. 1988, Fixler et al. 1989).

The CVM picture in diabetic births may thus be summed up as follows. For the perinatal mortalities the data clearly showed that there was no increased occurrence of such malformations. In fact in the earlier period some population groups had larger frequencies than did the diabetic cases, and the increase in later years was probably the by-product of the greatly lowered mortality rate. The record for CVM diagnosed in the neonatal period in survivors was inconsistent, being apparently increased only in America, possibly indicating that the latter was largely due to more intense diagnosis, especially of VSD, which compose a significant percentage of all CVM.

Prenatal Diagnosis

This section ends with a summary of the findings regarding CVM in the fetuses of pregnant diabetic women examined during the mid-second trimester by echocardiography. From the late 1980s to the time of this writing, several such studies were conducted to detect and diagnose malformations, especially CVM, in diabetic women.

Eight such studies of women with insulin-dependent diabetes, probably mostly of pregestational origin, were identified (Gomez et al.1988, Pijlman et al. 1989, Wheller et al. 1990. Greene and Benacerraf 1991, Brown et al. 1992, Maher et al. 1994, Albert et al. 1996, Smith et al. 1997). Another three studies not separately presenting findings from women with types 1 and 2 and gestational diabetes, or explicitly naming the diabetes of their subjects, will be ignored. A total of 1533 fetuses were examined and CVM diagnosed in 52 of them (3.4%). Two of the reports failed to name all or most of the heart defects found; when their findings as well as the inadmissible or questionable conditions were omitted, the frequency was reduced to 1.9%.

Seventeen screening programs of nearly 150,000 mostly low-risk and unselected patients in 1991–1997 reported frequencies of prenatally diagnosed CVM with a mean of 0.66%, but with the astonishingly wide range of 0.14–1.6% (Kirk et al. 1997). These are the figures against which the diabetic risk is to be judged. The calculated risk is almost three times the mean found by the survey. Although this suggests that diabetic pregnancy poses an increased fetal risk for CVM, without full information regarding the pre- and perinatal mortality fate of abnormal fetuses, which was missing in the articles along with controls and vital maternal data, a valid comparison with the situation in surviving neonatal offspring is not possible.

A few incidental findings should be noted. Not all the defects were successfuly detected prenatally. Not all the defects were considered structural or "critical" (ie, probably requiring surgical or medical intervention), as evidenced by the fact that in one study only 25 of 47 abnormal fetuses were said to have structural defects (Wheller et al. 1990) and in another only 40 of 143 were considered as probably requiring surgical repair (Tegnander et al. 1995). The interesting fact was also revealed in one study that none of the mothers with defective previous offspring had recurrences (Meyer-Wittkopf et al. 1996). Finally, none of the mean glycemic levels, measured in three studies, was statistically significantly greater in women with abnormal fetuses than in the others.

15

PREVENTING CONGENITAL MALFORMATIONS

Soon after the beginning of the insulin era, it became a firm tenet that the children of pregnant diabetic women were at increased risk of developing congenital malformations. Addressing this consensus, the causes and prevention of these abnormalities have been the subject of countless scholarly publications. From early on, innumerable etiological factors—genetic, metabolic, and teratological—were considered as the possible basis of this risk (eg, Gabbe 1977, Simpson 1978). But for prevention the most promising path to pursue seemed the metabolic one, since, as was reasoned, "If perturbations in the maternal metabolic milieu...cause anomalies in offspring, then strict diabetic control should lower the anomaly rates..." (Ober and Simpson 1986).

HYPERGLYCEMIA AND CONGENITAL MALFORMATIONS

No doubt it was the great progress in reducing the perinatal mortality rate in diabetic pregnancy, and the vision of its not far off normalization, that gave rise to the expectation of also lowering the frequency of malformations. Attributing the former to good control of diabetes during pregnancy held out the promise that the latter could be similarly overcome. Clear evidence indeed soon appeared that control—that is, keeping the maternal blood glucose level at near-normal limits—succeeded in lowering the mortality rate (Karlsson and Kjellmer 1972).

Another success this study claimed was that by lowering the blood glucose level the congenital malformation frequency had also been reduced. But several things invalidated this claim. Some of the malformed children were apparently diagnosed postneonatally; women with gestational diabetes were included in the study, obviously because it was not well understood at the time that the malformation frequency is not increased in children of women with this form of diabetes (Kalter 1998). The perinatal mortality rate decreased significantly in the later of the two periods surveyed—one of apparently closer metabolic control—but the malformation frequency did not. But the ultimate misunderstanding so far as malformations are concerned was to concentrate on the blood glucose level in the last weeks of pregnancy, when it could no longer have been related to abnormal embryonic development.

Table 15.1 Relation Between 1st-Trimester Glycemic Level and Congenital Malformation in Diabetic Pregnancy

	% HbA_1 ($\bar{v}$ ± SD; n)							
Authors	MCM	mCM	Nonmalformed	*P*	%HbA_1	n	%MCM	%mCM
Jovanovic et al. 1981	–	–	9.7	–	–	–	–	–
Miller et al. 1981	9.5 ± 1.0 (15)	–	8.4 ± 1.6 (111)	~.02	< 8.6	58	3.4	–
					8.6–9.9	35	22.8	–
					≥ 10.0	23	21.7	–
Reid et al. 1984	–	–	–	–	< 8.0	58	3.4	1.7
					8.6–9.9	44	11.4	2.3
					≥ 10.0	25	24.0	4.0
Ylinen et al. 1984	9.6 ± 1.8 (11)$^+$	9.3 ± 1.9 (6)	8.0 ± 1.4 (131)$^+$	$^+$.02	< 8.0	63	3.2	1.6
					8.0–9.9	62	8.1	4.8
					≥ 10.0	17	23.5	11.8
Key et al. 1987[a]	–							
Stubbs et al. 1987	12.5 ± 2.2 (7)	–	–	–[b]				
Miodovnik et al. 1988	12.4 ± 2.8 (9)	–	10.2 ± 2.0 (134)	> .05	< 2 SD	29	0	–
					2–4 SD	45	6.7	–
					> 4 SD	69	8.7	–
Rose et al. 1988	12.4 ± 2.4	–	–	–	–	–	–	–
Greene et al. 1989	13.2 ± 2.7 (14)$^+$	10.6 ± 3.0 (6)*	9.9 ± 1.9$^\times$	$^{+ vs *}$> .05	< 9.1	176	0	1.1
				$^{+ vs \times}$< .001	9.1–12.0	46	10.9	4.3
					> 12	28	32.1	7.1
Lucas et al. 1989	10.3 ± 1.8 (8)$^+$	10.3 ± 2.7 (6)	8.9 ± 2.3 (79)$^+$	$^+$> .05	< 9.2	45	8.9	–
					9.2–11.1	26	23.1	–
					> 11.1	16	25.0	–

Table 15.1 ***continued***

Authors	% HbA_1 ($\bar{v}$ ± SD; n) MCM	mCM	Nonmalformed	*P*	%HbA_1	n	%MCM	%mCM
Hanson et al. 1990	9.8 (10)	9.1 (11)	–	> .05	< 10.1	460	1.1	1.5
					≥ 10.1	31	16.1	12.9
Nielsen et al. 1990	–	–		> .05[c]				
Shields et al. 1993	8.0 ± 1.2 (20)	–	7.9 ± 1.8 (155)	> .05				
	8.5 ± 1.2 (8 CVM)							
Rosenn et al. 1994	11.5 ± 2.3	–	10.3 ± 2.0	> .05		–	–	–
Greene et al. 1995[d]	–							

MCM, major congenital malformations; mCM, congenital malformation.

a Congenital malformation data of offspring of women with type 1 and 2 diabetes were presented collectively. Despite having significantly different mean HbA_1s, "pregnancy outcomes in Type I and II diabetic patients were similar."

b The median HbA_1 of women bearing children with major malformations was not statistically different from that of mothers with minor malformed children.

c The authors considered all 20 malformations as major.

d Mean HbA_1 (7.1) for mothers of major and minor malformed children were presented collectively; not significantly different from those of the nonmalformed.

An apparent clue to where attention should have been focused instead came from the startling insight that "malformations in infants of diabetic mothers occur before the seventh gestational week" (Mills et al. 1979). This pronouncement, novel to many diabetologists, led many investigators to direct their attention to maternal blood glucose in the earliest weeks of pregnancy. Recognizing at the same time that a longitudinal perspective was called for, the investigations turned to the recently discovered entity, glycosylated hemoglobin, to provide that view.

Glycemic Level and Malformation

Since the late 1970s, about a dozen reports have appeared of studies that examined the relation between the frequency of congenital malformations and the level of glycosylated hemoglobin (HbA_1) in the first trimester of pregnancy of diabetic women (Table 15.1). A preliminary one noted that the HbA_1 levels in the mothers of three congenitally malformed children were among the five that exceeded the range for the well-controlled diabetics (Leslie et al. 1978), which suggested that excessive glycemic level was associated with maldevelopment.

A more definitive study, of a larger group of diabetic women, found a significantly higher mean HbA_{1c} level in mothers of malformed than in those of nonmalformed children, and a rough dose-response relation between glycemic level and malformation frequency (Miller et al. 1981). Similar results were obtained by others in this period (Jovanovic et al. 1981, Reid et al. 1984, Ylinen et al. 1984). In the Ylinen study, however, the odd observation was made that mothers of children with minor malformations as well as those with major ones had significantly elevated glycemic levels. In the light of the fact that minor malformations are not increased in diabetic pregnancy, this seems difficult to explain. Other paradoxes followed.

With further studies, the picture became cloudier. As Table 15.1 indicates, in all but one of the later reports, the relation between glycemic level and malformation rate was statistically insignificant or at best of borderline significance. In two studies, of cardiovascular malformations and microcephaly, as in those of total malformations, no association was found with maternal glycemic level (Shields et al. 1993, Greene et al. 1995). Compounding the uncertainties of analysis was contamination of the data in some cases by inclusion of defects not major and of diabetic women not pregestationally insulin dependent.

Furthermore, others shared the earlier puzzling observation of similar mean glycemic levels in mothers of children with minor and major malformations (Greene et al. 1989, Lucas et al. 1989, Hanson et al. 1990), and underscoring its reality was the finding of a dose-response relation between minor malformation frequency and glycemic level (Reid et al. 1984, Ylinen et al. 1984, Greene et al. 1989, Hanson et al. 1990). One may offer the explanation that a nonspecific common factor underlies the relation between glycemic level and both major and minor malformations, in which case hyperglycemia and major fetal maldevelopment are not directly related.

It should be noted that the proportion of the diabetic women with the highest glycemic levels, at the right end of a skewed distribution, was far larger in hospital-based studies, with a range of 11.2–48.2% and a mean of 20.2%, than in a population study, with a mean of 6.2% (Hanson et al. 1990). This indicates that women attending—usually referred to—diabetes clinics early in pregnancy were more severely affected than diabetic women generally. But despite this relative diabetic severity, there was little unambiguous evidence of an association of glycemic level and congenital malformation.

One can ask: should it be surprising that studies pursuing the leads of earlier ones often largely contradict them? It is after all only positive findings that are followed up, which then sometimes turn out to have been deceptive.

PRECONCEPTION CONTROL AND MALFORMATION

Early Temporal Comparison Study

Studies in which congenital malformations were associated with poor metabolic control during early pregnancy were complemented by others that took what appeared to be the logical step of attempting to reduce their occurrence by instituting rigorous control before conception. An early indication that undertaking a regimen of this sort might be efficacious came from comparing the outcomes of pregnancies of diabetic women served by different hospitals in the Copenhagen area (Pedersen and Mølsted-Pedersen 1978). Compared were women attending two hospitals for many years and thus presumed to be in good glycemic control with those attending another hospital, few of whom had ever been cared for at a hospital.

The comparison was partly undermined, however, by the fact that the two groups of women were not entirely mutually exclusive. Other faults were that the congenital malformations were not listed and were defined obscurely to begin with. Owing to all of these, the results were vague and inconclusive. Inexplicably, they were considered to be positive and the proposition reasonable (Anon. 1980). Thus, others were encouraged to study the possibilities of preventing malformations by metabolic control from before conception.

Edinburgh "Pre-pregnancy Clinic" Study

One group had already taken on this challenge. Beginning early in 1977 a "pre-pregnancy clinic" was begun in Edinburgh, one of whose goals was to "obtain optimum diabetic control at the time of conception" (Steel et al. 1980). At intervals over the next decade, reports appeared of the outcome of the pregnancies of the diabetic women who attended the clinic and of those who failed to do so. By the time of the latest report to date, pregnancies of 143 insulin-dependent diabetic attenders and 96 nonattenders had been studied (Steel et al. 1990). The results were impressive. Two of the offspring of the former women (1.4%) and 10 of the latter (10.4%) had major malformations, a statistically significant difference, indicating that preconception metabolic control had been successful in reducing their frequency.

Before accepting this conclusion, one needs to examine the methodology of the study. As Steel et al. (1990) agreed, the two groups—attenders and nonattenders—

were not randomized, a logistical and ethical impossibility, of course. But this is the least of the "randomization" problems, a greater one being concerned with how the two groups were created. Various means were used to announce the imminent establishment of a clinic whose purpose would be to counsel diabetic women contemplating becoming pregnant. All insulin-dependent women aged 14 to 40 registered in the Diabetic Department of the Edinburgh Royal Infirmary were sent personal letters on two occasions inviting them to attend this clinic. It was advertised in notices displayed in the department and in the clinic newsletter; colleagues were asked to refer "appropriate" patients; it was brought to the notice of young women during personal contact at the diabetic units of the Infirmary and the Hospital for Sick Children (Steel et al. 1982, 1984a,b). The final number of 143 women attending the pre-pregnancy clinic were hence mostly self-selected, had planned pregnancies, and were highly motivated. They were informed of the importance of optimum diabetic control before conception and throughout pregnancy, and means, where not already practiced, were instituted to ensure this.

The second group, the 96 not attending the pre-pregnancy clinic, included patients of the Diabetic Department not enrolled because of ignorance of the clinic's existence or no desire to attend and others not originally department patients (these amounted to 87, leaving 9 unaccounted for). Sixteen of the 96, however, were seen in March 1976 to February 1977, that is, before the pre-pregnancy clinic came into existence (Steel et al. 1980, 1982); therefore, they and their three malformed offspring (Steel and Johnstone 1992) should not have been included among the offspring of the "legitimate" nonattenders. Also improperly included were the four babies whose malformations were not recognized until after the first few weeks of life, including a one with a sacral agenesis diagnosed at the age of 3 years (Steel et al. 1982, Steel and Johnstone 1992). It is necessary to exclude these four, among other things, because no assurance was given that all the children were closely followed up for this length of time.

Omitting these seven offspring, all of whom were borne by the nonattenders, and the 16 incorrectly included nonattenders, leaves the following malformation frequencies: 2/143 (1.4%) in the attenders versus 3/80 (3.8%) in the nonattenders: $\chi^2 = 2.6$, $P > .05$.

Thus, even without considering the highly prejudicial methodology of the study, there was no significant difference in the congenital malformation frequency in the two groups of women. This was so despite the significantly lower first-trimester glycohemoglobin level in the attenders. Still, it would have been of interest to know some undivulged facts, such as the mean levels in the mothers of the malformed and nonmalformed offspring in the two groups and the relation of minor malformations to these levels.

Karlsburg Study

Another diabetes center studying the effect of preconception glycemic control on prenatal maldevelopment was located in Karlsburg in what was then the German Democratic Republic. This hospital, attended at the time by about half of all pregnant diabetics in the country, was charged with caring for those with special risk during pregnancy. Two goals of the diabetes program were to teach monitoring of basal body temperature to fix the date of conception and to achieve optimal metabolic control before conception and during early pregnancy. Fairly detailed reports were made of the 620 insulin-dependent women delivering in 1977–1983 (Fuhrmann et al. 1983, 1986). Only 184 of the women were willing to take part in the very demanding schedule of preconception hospital visits and the metabolic and dietary regimen; these entered the hospital before 8 weeks of pregnancy. The remaining 436 women did not submit to the regimen and entered hospital and began intense metabolic control later than this time. About 84% of the former and far fewer of the latter had normoglycemia during the early weeks of pregnancy. Glycosylated hemoglobin was not assayed.

A total of 17 offspring had major congenital malformations diagnosed in the first 3 weeks of life, 2 from the preconception-controlled women and 15 from the late-entering ones; at least 5 of the latter defects were questionable. Either omitting or including the inadmissible defects gives frequencies that were not statistically significantly different (2/184, 1.1%, versus 10/436, 2.3%; or 1.1% versus 3.6%).

Although, because the glycemic control program failed to affect the frequency of malformations, the analysis need go no further, other elements will nevertheless be discussed to note differences between the two groups of women, as an illustration of possible biasing factors that must be recognized and discounted if such efforts are ever to attain legitimacy.

The two groups obviously greatly differed in the desire to undertake the strenuous metabolic and dietary requirements of the program—less than 30% doing so. In part, this may have been because of the great distances some women had to travel from their home for the frequent consultations and lengthy preconception hospitalizations that were sometimes imposed. Acceptance of these conditions suggests inordinate motivation. This self-selecting quality may have been due to the early registrants having had poor perinatal outcomes in previous pregnancies twice as often as the late registrants (Fuhrmann 1982, Fuhrmann et al 1983, 1986). Other features by which the two groups may have differed, such as age, education, and so on, as noted by Steel et al. (1990) in their groups, were not mentioned.

National Institutes of Health Study

Patient self-selection can introduce potent biasing factors. Numerous personal characteristics prompt diabetic women to seek preconception care or respond to various approaches advertising such programs and to maintain the often arduous discipline imposed by them (Janz et al. 1995). A minority of insulin-dependent diabetic women, even in areas offering these programs, seek or participate in them or receive any care or counseling before pregnancy (Gabbe and Landon 1989, Holing et al. 1998). Women getting such attention differ in many ways from those failing to do so. The possible importance of the background and motives of those who do should not be minimized in evaluating the outcome of studies wishing to understand the bases of their findings. Until such influences are sorted out, there can be no definitive resolution of the question of the basis of the favorable pregnancy outcome found in some preconception studies.

A study that set out to meet this challenge was an ambitious multicenter collaborative effort, discussed in part in Chapters 3 and 12, conducted prospectively in 1980–1985 under the auspices of the U.S. National Institutes of Health (NIH) (Mills et al. 1983). The large sample number needed to answer the question satisfactorily could only be supplied, it was felt, by a joint effort of this sort. This study was one of the rare ones that included a nondiabetic control group. Its purpose, however, was to act as a contrast to the diabetic women in the spontaneous abortion part of the study (Mills et al. 1988b) and had no relevance to the one under discussion (Mills et al. 1988a).

The plan, as usual, was to recruit insulin-dependent diabetic women before conception who would be monitored to ensure early diagnosis of pregnancy. And although the majority of the subjects were indeed enrolled before they conceived, others (24.1%) only entered the study up to 21 days following conception. Both, however, were considered collectively and called the "early-entry group." Also studied was a late-entry group, diabetic women enrolled after 21 days following conception. No uniform standard for diabetic management of the early-entry group was imposed on the several centers participating in the study, and no metabolic data were obtained for the late-entry group.

To ensure uniformity, all children were examined for congenital malformations on the third postnatal day only. The frequency of all malformations in the children of the early-entry group (4.9%) was statistically significantly smaller than that (9.0%) in the late-entry group. But if the defects in both groups that are minor or dubious are omitted (labial fusion, paraurethral cyst, and strawberry hemangioma in the early-entry group; clubfoot, inguinal hernia, cryptorchidism, and Hirschsprung disease in the late-entry group; see Table 2 in Mills et al. 1988a) the frequencies are reduced to 4.0% and 6.8%, respectively, and are no longer significantly different. It should also be noted that five of the abnormalities in the early-entry group and three in the late group were ventricular septal defects, defects that very often close in later infancy (eg, Tegnander et al. 1995), whose significance and fate could hardly be determined by a single early postnatal examination. Omitting them would further lessen the statistical significance of the difference in malformation frequency of the two groups.

Also analyzed were glycemic levels in weeks 5–12 of early-entry women who did and did not have malformed children, which revealed that at no time during these weeks did the former have significantly higher mean levels of glycosylated hemoglobin than the latter, nor were different degrees of hyperglycemia associated with malformation frequency.

For the sake of argument, let us accept the interpretation of the malformations made by the 12 examiners of the children at the five different centers collaborating in this study and, using this liberal outlook, try to see whether the plan of the study succeeded in its goal of analyzing the separate putative roles of maternal self-selection and strict periconceptional diabetic control in leading to a favorable effect on pregnancy outcome in diabetic women.

Unfortunately, as might have been foreseen, this goal was a chimera from the beginning, since motivational factors could not be avoided. One clear bit of evidence of this was the fact that early-entry (or preconception-counseled) women were significantly older than the late-entry ones (incidentally similar phenomena were seen in many like studies [Goldman et al. 1986, Steel et al. 1990, Rosenn et al.

1991, Willhoite et al. 1993, Holing et al. 1998]) and undoubtedly pointed to their greater concern because of untoward outcomes in previous pregnancies, such as had been documented by Fuhrmann et al. (1986), for example.

Mills et al.'s (1988b) finding of no correlation between glycemic level and malformation frequency raised a small storm of protest. A *Lancet* leader writer (Anon. 1988), echoing the conventional wisdom, asserted that "there is unquestionably an increased incidence of major congenital abnormalities in the infants of diabetic mothers." Thus, in comparing the malformation frequency in the early- and late-entry groups, he or she, accepting the reported malformation data, pronounced that the "findings are in complete accord" with received gospel, which totally missed the point, since what Mills et al.'s negative judgment came from was not a comparison of these two groups but of the women in the early-entry group who did and did not have malformed children.

Other critics, whose letters all appeared in the Sept. 8, 1988, issue of *Lancet* (vol. 319, pp. 647–648), had a variety of complaints, none of which seriously undermined Mills and colleagues' findings. Another charged that since comparing the mothers of malformed and nonmalformed offspring was not a primary aim of the study, it was improper to make such a post hoc analysis (Skyler 1989). But a reading of the paper outlining the NIH study design (Mills et al. 1983) reveals nothing that debars retrospective analyses and indeed mentions an example of when such will be carried out.

Much was also made of the fact that the frequency of malformation in the early-entry group was higher than that in the control, which was interpreted to mean that the metabolic control of these women was suboptimal. The foundation of this point can also be challenged by returning to Mills et al.'s Table 2, in which the strange discovery is made that none of the total of eight abnormal children of the 389 control women had a major congenital malformation (with the possible exception of one with a condition vaguely labeled an "anatomical brain lesion"). It is clear that these children were not as thoroughly examined as were the children of the diabetic mothers, or they were a most unusual group; thus, no argument can be based on the supposed difference in malformation frequency between them.

Miscellaneous Preconception Control Studies

An Israel study of 52 insulin-dependent diabetic women succeeded by preconception metabolic control in reducing the glyohemoglobin levels to near normal (Dicker et al. 1987). Its effectiveness in controlling malformations, however, was precluded by none occurring in either the diabetic or control group. Unfortunately, details regarding the definition and diagnosis of malformations were lacking.

A 3-year multicenter California study aiming at preconception glycemic normalization of diabetic women registered only 27 diabetic women (Cousins 1991c). None of them had malformed children, in contrast to 347 pregestational diabetic women enrolled some time after conception, 23 of whose children had congenital malformations. The conditions were not enumerated, preventing analysis of their admissibility. Nothing was said about how they were diagnosed, but in addition to fatal and surgery-requiring abnormalities, significant psychological conditions were defined as major defects. First-trimester glycosylated hemoglobin levels were measured, but data were not presented for women entering the program before and after conception. Little of any clear value seems to have come out of this study.

A more modest study from California was clearly presented (Kitzmiller et al. 1991). By means of announcements in various media, word of mouth, or physician referral, diabetic women were recruited in 1982–1988 to participate in a program of preconception instruction and rigorous glycemic control. Diabetic women who were already pregnant were similarly registered for metabolic management at different times during gestation, nearly half of them at as early as 6–8 weeks, but many as late as 21–32 weeks. About 65% of the women in both groups were insulin-dependent. An apparent selection bias was made evident by the fact that the former group, though of approximately the same age as the latter, had an earlier disease onset.

Congenital malformations were found in one offspring of the 84 women in the preconception group with viable pregnancies and 12 of the 110 women in the postconception group. Omitting inadmissible abnormalities leaves none in the first and nine in the second. Four of the latter were ventricular septal defects (only one of whose mothers had a glycohemoglobin level above 10%). All surviving children were reexamined at 1 year of age, but it was not stated how many of the septal defects were still present at that time.

There was a stepwise increase in the frequency of the accepted major malformations in the postconception group with increased maternal glycohemoglobin level, but predominantly the increase was beyond the 10.6% level. There were no data regarding the glycemic state of the postconception groups in the earliest weeks of pregnancy, but such information would have helped in interpreting one of the malformations, holoprosencephaly, since it arises as early as at 5 weeks of gestation (Müller and O'Rahilly 1989).

The data indicated a possible relation between hyperglycemia in early pregnancy and fetal maldevelopment (it is noteworthy, though, that in an earlier study of a management program instituted in the first trimester, conducted by one of the authors of this article [Jovanovic et al. 1981], no major or minor congenital malformations were found). It is unfortunate that the possible existence of more anterior etiological factors, which were hinted at in studies finding simultaneous association of major and minor congenital malformations with hyperglycemia, was overlooked by this study in not recording all minor congenital malformations.

A study designed to optimize the glycemic state of diabetic women planning to become pregnant was conducted in Cincinnati in 1984–1989 (Rosenn et al. 1991). After a large number of women removed themselves from the program, perhaps finding the regimen too difficult to comply with, 28 randomly selected pregnancies of the remaining women—some of whom had entered the program more than once—made up the preconception study group. A similarly selected group of 71 pregnancies of diabetic women that enrolled within 9 weeks following conception made up the control. The mean glycohemoglobin level of the control at the first prenatal visit was significantly higher than that of the study women, despite which the malformation frequencies in the infants of both were similar and very low. No satisfactory explanation was attempted for this result, which seemed to contradict strongly held beliefs.

A statewide program of preconception counseling for pregestational diabetic women was conducted in Maine in 1987–1990 (Willhoite et al. 1993). During this time, 185 pregnancies (64% type 1, 35% type 2) were reported by 150 counselors (physicians, nurses, and others), 62 in women seen before conceiving, predominantly in a nonhospital setting and 123 not (percentages with type 1 and 2 diabetes in each group not disclosed). Major congenital malformations were reported in one child of the former group and eight of the latter, a suggestive but not statistically significant difference. No metabolic data were included. The abnormalities were not all fully described, and the methodology of their diagnosis was not mentioned.

These failings call for a brief aside. Much naïveté regarding fetal maldevelopment was also true to one extent or another of some of the studies discussed in this section, and others elsewhere above, in glaring contrast to the frequent abundance of detail about the diabetic state and metabolic management of the patients, unbalanced approaches that obviously stem from the predominant professional interests of the investigators. But this neglect often diminished the value of the studies in the eyes of a teratologist.

The completeness of the ascertainment of diabetes accomplished by the Maine statewide program must be considered. Publications of the National Center for Health Statistics indicated that during the 4-year period of the program 76,072 live births occurred in Maine. According to the expectation of about five pregestational insulin-dependent diabetic births per 1000 pregnancies not including perinatal deaths, there should have been approximately 335 such pregnancies in these years, almost three times more type 1 diabetic pregnancies alone than were the subjects of the report. A shortage of this size must have implications regarding representativeness and selection of subjects.

TEMPORAL TRENDS

Several studies were made that compared pregnancy outcome in two periods in which different management of diabetic pregnancy was practiced or presumably practiced. For example, studies at the Birmingham Maternity Hospital extended over many years, in the course of which it is likely that management improved. As expected, as the rate of perinatal mortality decreased during this time, the frequency of lethal congenital malformations increased significantly, but the rate of all malformations also did (Soler et al. 1976). The latter, however, was clouded by the inclusion of various minor and other inadmissible defects (see Table 11-1) and so cannot be credited. The comparison between the two periods made by Ballard et al. (1984) was discussed earlier. In a report from the Mayo Clinic, a chart depicting pregnancy outcome over a 30-year period showed that the frequency of congenital defects increased decade by decade, from about 8–15% (Lufkin et al. 1984), whereas that of the control remained constant at about 2–3%. The specific data for these periods were not given, and nearly half of all the malformations listed in the diabetic cases were minor or otherwise inadmissible.

An extensive set of observations in Copenhagen over the 20 years 1967–1986 noted a constant 7–8% of major congenital malformations in the first 15 years and a decline in the last 5 years to 2.7% (Damm and Mølsted-Pedersen 1989). This gratifying outcome was thought to be due to improved diabetic care and metabolic control during the latter years, which were facilitated by the high frequency of planned pregnancies in that period.

This belief seems to be contradicted, however, by the data presented, which showed that the mean glycohemoglobin levels before 13 weeks of pregnancy in women with planned and unplanned pregnancies were very much alike (7.1% versus 7.3%), even though the malformation frequency in the former was significantly less than in the latter and there was no correlation between HbA_{1c} and malformations. The glycohemoglobin similarity should perhaps have been expected, since the outpatient department of the Copenhagen Diabetes Center had given advice for optimal metabolic control since 1976. The improved malformation record therefore continued unexplained, but may possibly be expained by the later inclusion of infants of less that 1000 g birth weight, since lighter babies are at reduced risk for malformations (Kalter 1991). The presentation of weight-specific data regarding malformation frequency would have been useful in examining this possibility.

A report comparing 1971–1977 and 1978–1985 noted that in the first period no women were enrolled in a "systematic preconception program," whereas in the second 18% were (Tchobroutsky et al. 1991). There was no difference in the malformation frequency between the two periods, however, perhaps because the number enrolled was insufficient to have made any impact. Also, the efficacy of the program in controlling blood sugar was not documented.

A MATTER OF PUZZLEMENT

Despite the findings detailed in this chapter, it is repeatedly and dogmatically echoed "that there is no doubt that congenital malformations occur more frequently in the offspring of diabetic mothers...[that] studies of glycosylated hemoglobin during the 1st trimester have demonstrated a significant relationship between poor metabolic control in diabetic pregnancy and the likelihood of congenital malformations" and, destroying the entire set of beliefs, that diabetic pregnancy is teratogenic in animals (Coustan 1998), citing for the last asseveration experimental studies that had been discredited in an obstetrics journal itself (Kalter 1997). Which misapprehension the penultimate chapter in this book should lay to rest.

It is always the lazier course merely to follow where others lead, but which, as the sheep found in Hardy's *Far From the Madding Crowd,* often leads to peril.

16

EARLY AND LATE STUDIES: PRENATAL AND FOLLOW-UP

FETAL GROWTH DELAY

Most fetal problems associated with diabetic pregnancy—perinatal mortality, congenital malformations, macrosomia, preterm birth—are prominent and have long been recognized. In contrast, another presumed manifestation of diabetic pregnancy, retarded prenatal growth, is covert and perhaps was for that reason only recently brought to attention.

It was uncovered fortuitously in the course of an ultrasound study. In searching for the possible early prenatal origins of neonatal overgrowth in offspring of insulin-dependent diabetic women, Pedersen and Mølsted-Pedersen (1979) noted instead that many early fetuses were considerably smaller than normal and reasoned that the delay was probably of embryonic origin. Furthermore, the smallest of the retarded fetuses weighed significantly less at birth than others and seemed at increased risk of malformation. Confirmatory reports strengthened this indication, and for good measure noted that small fetal size was correlated with maternal first-trimester glycemic state (Pedersen and Mølsted-Pedersen 1981, Pedersen et al. 1984, Tchobroutsky et al. 1985, Visser et al. 1985).

Growth-retarded fetuses were not restricted to insulin-dependent diabetic pregnancies, however, but also occurred in those of class A diabetics, that is, in noninsulin-dependent pregestational diabetes and even in gestational diabetic women (Sutherland et al. 1981). These findings call for a new interpretation, since they must mean that the growth delay in and of itself could not be related to fetal maldevelopment; because, as was often noted elsewhere in this work, malformation frequency is not increased in class A or gestational diabetes. Thus, if retarded growth and risk of maldevelopment are associated, this must be due to both being the outcome of antecedent or ancillary conditions, as Little et al. (1979) and Spiers (1982) suggested.

But an even more fundamental doubt was raised, that of the accuracy of the observation of delayed fetal growth itself, based on the likelihood of mistaken dating of conception owing to inaccurate estimation of ovulation (Little et al. 1979, Steel et al. 1984b, 1995).

Sad to relate, but too common merely to be a curiosity, the provocative early findings and the attractive theories they fathered were not long afterward refuted by sonographic studies in early pregnancy. Cousins et al. (1988), employing rigorous obstetric dating criteria, relative to controls, found no delayed fetal growth in insulin-dependent diabetic pregnancies; Reece et al. (1990), comparing diabetic and nondiabetic pregnancies, found no statistically significant difference in size and growth rate of the early fetal head; and Brown et al. (1992) found no difference in early fetal growth rate between diabetic and nondiabetic pregnancies. Note that in all three of these studies, nondiabetic pregnancies were included, controls, in such investigations at least, if not in other sorts, having correctly been considered mandatory for credible interpretation.

FETAL DETECTION OF MALFORMATIONS

The prenatal visualization of congenital malformations became truly effective with the development of real-time ultrasonography. This permitted many different structural abnormalities to be detected in the second trimester (Campbell and Pearce 1983, Hegge et al. 1990) and incidentally provided the possibility of altering the prevalence of some of these conditions at birth by fetal elimination (Julian-Reynier et al. 1994).

Such sonographic studies in diabetic pregnancies were prompted by the finding of early fetal growth retardation. Up to the present, relatively few have been made (Szabo et al. 1986, Gomez et al. 1988, Pijlman et al. 1989, Greene and Benacerraf 1991, Brown et al. 1992, Albert et al. 1996), and their purpose has varied—to provide obstetric guidance, maternal counseling and choice, and to examine the relation of maldevelopment to fetal retardation, glycemic control, and alphafetoprotein level. But they have accomplished little, perhaps because they were beset by the familiar inadequacies and failures: biased ascertainment, no control (an even more than usual necessity in prenatal studies, as realized by those conducting the studies described in the previous section), and lack of discrimination between true major malformations and minor and otherwise questionable ones.

Prenatal detection of cardiovascular malformations is discussed in Chapter 14.

FOLLOW-UP OF CHILDREN

We leap from features of embryos of diabetic women to postnatal physical and developmental characteristics of their children, especially congenital malformations, height and weight, neurological state, and intellectual ability. Children of various ages beyond infancy, usually of early school age, were examined or their parents questioned about these matters.

Congenital Malformations

Almost all the earliest follow-up studies and many of the later ones took malformations discovered at various older ages for their outcome subject.

Malformations or deformities were defined variably; and interestingly, when they included controls, the children of diabetic men and prediabetic women were used for this purpose (Koller 1953, White et al. 1953, Claye and Craig 1959, Dekaban 1959, Hagbard et al. 1959). The largest study, part of an early multicenter project, gathered data through questionnaires sent to mothers (Hagbard et al. 1959). If even a generous view is taken of what constitutes a deformity, the total frequency of the defects discovered in the neonatal period and afterward was not significantly larger in the children born after the women developed diabetes than in those born before, that is, in the prediabetic period. The same nonsignificant difference occurred in a study from a nearby country (Hiekkala and Koskenoja 1961).

In the next decade, two relatively large studies following children for many years found abnormality frequencies of 8–9%, respectively, but included as major defects various inconsequential abnormalities (Breidahl 1966) and found no difference from the control (Farquhar 1965, 1969b).

Degen et al. (1970) were surprised, they said, to find no additional pathologies, physical or neurological, in children examined at ages 1–13 years. White (1971), amplifying an earlier report (White et al. 1953), noted that the frequency of congenital anomalies was almost identical in the older children of diabetic women and diabetic men. Essex et al. (1973) cited an unpublished doctoral dissertation (Watson 1970) that noted that the frequency of malformations in children of diabetic women was not statistically different from that in a control group. A Danish study reported that 4.9% of a large number of children of diabetic women examined at 15–26 years of age had major malformations and 6.2% minor ones (Yssing 1975). The study lacked controls and none of the abnormalities, an appreciable proportion of which was said to run in the families, was named. Other studies apparently found no additional malformations in children of various ages beyond those discovered at birth (Amendt 1975, Stehbens et al. 1977, Cummins and Norrish 1980). Similarly, in another study, children followed up for 1–27 years, discounting dubious conditions, had a maximum of 3.2% malformations (Schwaninger 1973).

Cardiovascular malformations (CVM) were the subject of a study of children examined at several ages up to 7 years (Rowland et al. 1973). All together, 19 cases were diagnosed (3.8%), 14 of which had occurred in perinatal mortalities. Which defects were present in the latter unfortunately was not stated, since four of them—three ventricular septal defects and a patent ductus arteriosus—were conditions that often vanish in time. Nevertheless, the frequency of CVM was far greater than the usual population rate.

A doubt lingers whether at least some of this excess was related to the mothers of the children being a highly select sample of diabetic women attending the Joslin Clinic and the children themselves undergoing intensive serial examinations when "signs or symptoms suggesting heart disease prompted referral" to the hospital for evaluation. This doubt might have been quelled had a proper control been employed rather than the wholly inappropriate one. In an early study, of the physical and mental development of 123 children of diabetic women, only one child with a malformation (a CVM), was found (Fredrikson et al. 1957).

A late study found 15% malformations during a 3-year follow-up in the children of insulin-dependent diabetic women, about twice that in controls (Sells et al. 1994). Some of the abnormalities were obviously already present in neonates, but the age at which others, like ventricular septal defects, were discovered was not mentioned. This is an important consideration, since this condition very often spontaneously closes by 1 year of age (eg, Moe and Guntheroth 1987). It was not clear therefore whether the frequency at older ages was different from that at birth. This study was an offshoot of the Mills et al. (1988a) multicenter study, and some of the other doubts about the congenital malformation findings will be found in a previous chapter where the latter is discussed. Finally, it may be mentioned as apropos to this section that dental development was found to be delayed in one study (Amendt 1975) but normal in another (Adler et al. 1977).

Height and Weight

The children of diabetic women in the past were very often excessively heavy at birth (Hsia and Gellis 1957), and in fact this serious complication, macrosomia, is not uncommon even today. Since birth weight may influence postnatal growth (see Bergmann et al. 1984 for citations), among the questions about the prognosis of children of diabetic women awaiting resolution was whether and how neonatal and later size were related, although the question was rarely put in these explicit terms, Instead, for the most part investigators simply sought to establish whether later height and weight were within normal limits or not.

The diverse findings at best reflect the absence of a standard approach to the question. It was found that at various later ages the children (often as compared with national standards of the time and place) were taller and heavier than normal (White et al. 1953), shorter but heavier (Hagbard et al. 1959), of normal height and weight (Komrower and Langley 1961), normally distributed in height (Hiekkala and Koskenoja 1961, Farquhar 1969a, Amendt 1975), often above the 90th percentile for height and weight (Breidahl 1966), and tended to be heavier than normal (Weitz and Laron 1976). Most recently again they were found significantly taller and heavier, which, since it was not true of the children of diabetic fathers, was concluded to be evidence of the lasting effect of intrauterine environmental factors on later body build (Bergmann et al. 1984).

Also, to compound the confusion, some children proportionately large at birth were significantly heavier and taller at 4 years of age than others not large or disproportionately large at birth (Jährig et al. 1993), and others, obese at birth, but of normal weight and length at 1 year of age, had increased weight and height at later ages, effects that were correlated with various maternal and fetal characteristics (Silverman et al. 1991). In this study, the outcome in children of women with gestational and type 1 diabetes were reported collectively; how this may have vitiated the observations is unclear. (This commingling also damaged any validity other studies may have had [Rizzo et al. 1994, 1995, Yamashita et al. 1996]).

If the majority wins, then greater height, at times accompanied by greater weight, comes closest to the consensus, but discordant findings cannot be discounted. A definitive examination of the question is still awaited, one that will be discriminating in its choice of mothers whose children are to be longitudinally followed, will take an agreed-upon approach, and that for comparison will not rely entirely on sometimes outdated and inappropriate population standards.

Neurological Development and Intelligence

It is not surprising that the birth traumas and neonatal morbidities children of diabetic women often experienced, and still occasionally experience, led to asking whether these events had long-term psychological and related consequences. In fact, many follow-up studies of such children were directed to these considerations. Here, too, not surprisingly the results were mixed, probably because as it hardly seems necessary to reiterate, most of the studies were beset by the usual shortcomings of limited sample size, diverse follow-up procedures, varied and seldom entirely appropriate "controls"(and others well enumerated by Goldstein et al. 1991) and hence that some investigators found an increased incidence of mental and neurological impairment and others did not.

The pioneering effort of this sort (only a brief summary of which as far as can be determined was ever reported) found that at examination at 6 months to 15 years of age, 86 of 91 children of "diabetic" women had "developed perfectly normally, mentally and physically," and of the four others still alive, two had "oligophrenia," one diabetes mellitus, and the last a congenital heart lesion (Pedersen and Schondel 1949).

An early greatly detailed study, a Swedish multicenter project, gave negative results (Hagbard et al. 1959), but another large-scale survey, the Collaborative Study, found that children of diabetic women with ketonuria during pregnancy had a mean IQ of 93, significantly less than the score of 102 of children of mothers without ketonuria or the 101 of controls (Churchill et al. 1969). Curiously, the reduction was true of children of class A mothers as of more severe degrees of diabetes. Later studies, however, noted no relation between maternal ketonuria and IQ nor any abnormal neurological development or diminished IQ in children of insulin-dependent or gestational diabetic women. On the contrary, in some studies the majority had IQs over 100 (Persson et al. 1984, Persson and Gentz 1984, Silverman et al. 1991). Most recently, significant IQ impairment was found at about 4 years of age; the data, however, coming from children of mothers with insulin-dependent, noninsulin-dependent, and gestational diabetes all mixed together, cannot be taken seriously (Yamashita et al. 1996).

Applying other criteria of intellectual and neurological development, most older studies reported deficits to one extent or another (Francois et al. 1974b, Haworth et al. 1976, Manzke et al. 1977, Stehbens et al. 1977), but not all (Watson 1970), whereas almost all the more recent ones found little or no such outcome (Cummins and Norrish 1980, Hadden et al. 1984, Olofsson et al. 1984, Ornoy et al. 1994, Rizzo et al. 1994, Sells et al. 1994, Kimmerle et al. 1995). One dissenting voice found that children who had been growth-retarded as early fetuses performed worse on certain developmental tests than controls and thus that children of diabetic women were at risk of psychomotor developmental problems (Petersen et al. 1988, Petersen 1989). Considering the possibly flawed means of relating fetal size and age mentioned above, this finding, too, may be suspect. The other noted an inverse relation between IQ and maternal lipid metabolic factors in late pregnancy (Silverman et al. 1991). Another noted a positive correlation, of psychomotor development at 6–9 years with maternal late trimester beta-hydroxybutyrate, a measure of maternal metabolic state, but, as mentioned, it was flawed by not considering children of mothers with insulin-dependent and gestational diabetes separately (Rizzo et al. 1995).

Discrepancies in the relation between features in children and maternal states, such as that of cognitive ability and toxemia, might have been due to the recent great reduction in severity or occurrence of that maternal condition (Cordero and Landon 1993). But it is not likely that anything of this sort can explain the wide variability found in congenital malformation frequency and type.

A COMMENT

A striking means of commenting on these studies of the later consequences of being born to insulin-dependent pregestationally diabetic women and by indirection on much of the diabetes work discussed in this work until now is to compare their execution with one generally similar to them: an investigation of the putative developmental consequences in children of women who had hypertension during pregnancy (Ounsted et al. 1984). The sine qua non for validity of studies of human reactions to given situations is that the subjects be a fair sample of the entire group from which they are drawn and that the experimental procedures be strictly defined.

In the words of the statistician-philosopher Ronald Fisher (1934), "It is a statistical commonplace that the interpretation of a body of data requires a knowledge of how it was obtained. Equally, it is usually understood that the conclusions drawn from experimental results must rest on a detailed knowledge of the experimental procedure actually employed." These requirements were met by the Ounsted study: the ascertainment of the pregnant subjects was detailed and the maternal risk situation and the means of evaluating the developmental state of the children were strictly defined.

On the contrary, in the diabetes studies the primary essential ingredient of a representative sample was ignored or unestablished, and the second sometimes flouted, with the collective inclusion of pregnant women with different types of diabetes—insulin-dependent, noninsulin-requiring, and gestationally diabetic women, as well as some whose diabetes type was not specified at all.

In the hypertension study, the follow-up procedure consisted of ascertaining the relation between numerous maternal factors and the intellectual state of children of a specific age as evaluated by standardized tests. The former included social class, birth rank, maternal smoking status, preeclampsia, spontaneous or other delivery, breast or bottle feeding, birth weight for gestation age, fetal distress, and various others, all of which affected the several test scores in different ways, some being associated negatively, some positively, some not at all.

Again, by contrast, the diabetes studies were directed toward diverse ends diversely investigated. Of course, they were not conducted by one group at one period of time. That explains and should in part excuse the heterogeneity of their findings and their consequent overall inconclusiveness. But it does not excuse the great majority of them neglecting the consideration of many factors that may have been relevant in their studies, especially serious obstetric problems that often attend diabetic pregnancies—hypertension, ketoacidosis, preterm delivery, and so on (Cousins, 1987, Beaufils 1990, Siddiqi et al. 1991). Thus, what is not yet satisfied is the need for an indisputable answer to the question of what can be expected to be the physical and mental development of children of mothers with type 1 diabetes, the form of diabetes that is most worrisome.

Solace can be taken, however, in the findings of the hypertension study, since all in all they indicated that "children who survive a highly adverse intrauterine environment with subsequent complications at delivery and in the neonatal period are no more likely to have developmental problems in childhood than those whose early biographies had been much less hazardous."

17

DIABETIC PREGNANCY IN ANIMALS: I

It is reasonable to believe that human beings and other animals share propensities and adverse responses to diseases. If this is so, human diseases may be advantageously studied by turning to animals afflicted with conditions mimicking them, that is, by the use of so-called animal models. Pregestational insulin-dependent diabetes is one of these conditions, presenting not entirely resolved problems, which have been felt would benefit from animal investigation.

It is to the unraveling of unanswered questions left in the wake of the widely accepted belief that this type of diabetes leads to congenital malformation that much of the experimental investigation discussed in this and the next chapter has been directed. These studies have depended on the existence of diabetes in laboratory animals, the several kinds of which, both experimentally induced and spontaneously occurring, have provided opportunities for investigating in the laboratory many aspects of this complicated disease in association with pregnancy.

The original method of producing diabetes experimentally—partial or total pancreatectomy—in this case in dogs, was, as is well known, the one that led to the discovery of insulin (Banting and Best 1923). The surgical method was also the earliest one used in pregnant animals, but with variable success in producing the disease. Pregnant animals were sensitive to the procedure, and many aborted or died, outcomes often still occurring in modern work (Hultquist 1950).

EXPERIMENTALLY INDUCED DIABETES

In what was perhaps the last study using surgery, female rats were operated on at various times during pregnancy, and insulin was then administered to most of them (Hultquist 1950). Almost half died soon after, and in nearly half of the remainder all conceptuses perished. Many offspring reaching term died, especially those with excessive birth weight; the latter occurred particularly after surgery during midpregnancy. In other cases, birth weight was reduced. Such inconsistent, apparently contradictory, results continued in later studies.

In this as in many other early studies, almost undivided attention was given to offspring survival and weight, not surprisingly since these were among the features of most concern in pregnant diabetic women in those days. Malformations were regarded as contributing relatively little to these problems, which seemed to have been confirmed by this rat study, since only one offspring in several hundred had a congenital defect—a cleft palate.

Alloxan

Even before Hultquist's study, pancreatectomy had already been replaced by a simpler, less traumatic way of inducing diabetes, by injecting the diabetogenic chemical alloxan, the first one with this property to be discovered (Jacobs 1937, Dunn and McLetchie 1943). The second one, steptozocin, followed after about 25 years (Rakieten et al. 1963); these, plus to a lesser extent spontaneous, hereditary forms of the disease (Rerup 1970, Salans and Graham 1982, Bone 1990), provided the techniques and material for pursuing in vivo studies of the fetal effects of diabetes in pregnant animals.

Alloxan causes diabetes by destroying beta cells of the pancreatic islets. But it also has the unwanted consequence of causing kidney damage. The latter is reversible however, while the islet injury is long-lasting or even permanent. A difficulty arises because although the nephrotoxic effects are generally caused by larger dosages than the diabetogenic ones, the dose ranges overlap, making it necessary to adjust the dosage to minimize one sort of damage while causing the other. The consequent need to moderate the dosage of alloxan limits the severity and duration of the diabetes it induces. This problem is more acute in some species than in others; for example, in rats the overlap is great (Lukens 1948). Until streptozocin came along, however, alloxan was the only chemical diabetogen available.

Two further features of alloxan are to be noted. First, it has an extremely short half-life at physiological temperature and pH. No doubt because of this characteristic, although it induces diabetes by all routes of administration, alloxan is most effective, needing smaller dosages, when given intravenously (iv). Second, sensitivity to its diabetogenic property varies widely within and between species (Rerup 1970, Lukens 1948, Martinez et al. 1954, Cohn and Cerami 1979). The meaning of this fact as concerns prenatal development has been little appreciated.

Studies of the effects of alloxan-induced diabetes on reproduction and pregnancy, made mostly with rats, began very soon after the discovery of the chemical's remarkable property. It was injected not only at various times during pregnancy, but most often before or soon after conception, when it frequently caused infertility, whole-litter resorption, and increased stillbirth, as it also did in females with extremely elevated blood glucose levels. Treatment later in pregnancy mostly caused increased fetal mortality, but the viability of surviving offspring was little impaired.

Gross congenital abnormalities did not occur in the earliest studies (eg, Miller 1947), except for an instance of a tail defect and a unilateral cataract (Bartelheimer and Kloos 1952) and some histological abnormalities of dental tissue (Kreshover et al. 1953). [Years later reduced tooth size, but no other abnormality, was found in late fetuses of rhesus monkeys with induced diabetes (Bennett et al. 1981).] Deviations from normal offspring weight and size, in either direction, were infrequent. Insulin, when given, prevented much of the untoward effects. Many of these studies were summarized by Angervall (1959).

Rats continued to be the subject of these studies for about the next 20 years, but progressively less so during the latter half of this interval. Most had the same assortment of outcomes—infertility, abortion, increased offspring death, inconsistent effect on newborn weight, and apparently no gross malformations (Angervall and Stevenson 1960, Lawrence and Contopoulos 1960, Lazarow and Heggestad 1970).

A few major and minor fetal abnormalities occurred in a small number of later studies. In one, Wistar females received 160 mg/kg (here and below this refers to female weight) alloxan intraperitoneally (ip) on the 8th day of gestation, that is, during embryogenesis (Takano and Nishimura 1967). (Where necessary, gestation datings have been revised to make the day of positive mating the first day of pregnancy.) It was given at this time because in preliminary trials, as others had also observed, earlier treatment largely prevented continued pregnancy. A small percentage of the surviving late fetal offspring of females with persistent diabetes had externally detectable malformations—microphthalmia, exencephaly, and cleft palate or cleft lip and palate; internal inspection in addition revealed many with cataract and hydronephrosis. Examination of the skeleton in specially prepared specimens revealed a few conspicuous abnormalities, but none of absence or delayed development of the lower vertebrae. The significance of this will emerge subsequently.

Contrary to these results, only trivial external abnormalities occurred in a very low frequency in rats of a different stock, Carworth Farms, given 175 mg/kg alloxan subcutaneously (sc) some weeks before mating (Ward and Readhead 1970). Also different was the occurrence of many instances of supernumerary rib, a condition usually considered an indirect outcome of disturbed developmental homeostasis consequent upon maternal stress or toxicity (Khera 1994). But there were no lower vertebral defects. Nor were gross abnormalities found in late fetal offspring of Albino Farms rats administered 100 mg/kg alloxan on the 10th day of gestation, only an occasional rib and sternebral absence, but no other skeletal abnormality (Ellison and, Maren 1972).

Varying in an important detail from the studies described above was one done by Deuchar (1977). She gave Wistar rat females 60 mg/kg alloxan iv on the 10th day of pregnancy, and—this is the difference—examined offspring just 2 days later, that is, at an embryonic stage, and found a few with nonclosure (as became clear later, undoubtedly delayed closure) of the neural folds and distortion of one or more heart chambers. Older fetuses were not examined. Other studies in which early-stage prenatal offspring were the subject of examination will be noted in this and the next chapter.

Finally, Wilson et al. (1985) gave Wistar females 200 mg/kg alloxan ip on the 7th day of pregnancy and examined the offspring at two near-term ages, the 21st and 22nd days of gestation (rat gestation length is 22–23 days). All told, 16.5% and 27.2%, respectively, of fetuses from females with moderate and severe hyperglycemia had a wide variety of internal and external congenital malformations, although each was only 2–4% in frequency. These percentages are not statistically significantly different from each other, that is, severity of hyperglycemia was unrelated to malformation frequency. This is in distinction to the decreased ossification of sternebrae and caudal vertebrae in the younger, the 21st-day, fetuses examined, which occurred in frequencies proportional to the severity of the maternal diabetes. This situation was exceedingly transient, however, since fetuses just 1 day older had a largely normal ossification pattern. The authors thus suggested that the skeletal deficiencies "represented delayed ossification which became less striking later in gestation."

In sum, first, in only two of the five above-described alloxan studies did major congenital malformations occur; second, relatively few offspring had such abnormalities; and, third, the abnormalities were diverse and without any pattern that could be discerned to compose a "syndrome." In addition, there were some minor or other defects, especially at certain skeletal sites, which probably represented retarded development.

Another matter also apropos to diabetes teratogenicity was only mentioned incidentally, namely, variability of the animals to the diabetogenicity of the injected chemical. For example, in the two articles in which relevant data were given (both using the commonly used Wistar rat), alloxan caused diabetes in only about half of the females; the others remained nondiabetic or were only moderately or very briefly diabetic. In another, also using Wistar rats, only those becoming diabetic were used, but the proportion they composed was not specified.

It appears to me that in evaluating the malformation picture, neglecting the outcome of pregnancy of animals resistant to one extent or another to the diabetogenic effects of alloxan is like (in studies of diabetic women) not considering the pregnancies of those with less severe degrees of diabetes and hence biases the interpretation. The importance of such omitted material is supported by studies revealing that level of hyperglycemia and teratological outcome were poorly correlated.

In the 1960s, as rats lost popularity, perhaps in part because of the largely unimpressive teratological results obtained with them (earlier it had been concluded that alloxan diabetes does not adversely affect the fetal outcome "unless it impairs the general health of the mother" [Ferret et al. 1950]), they were replaced by mice. And indeed the mouse studies, at least later, did provide a contrast in this regard.

But an earlier extensively described experiment with mice had no great success in causing malformations (Koskenoja 1961). Single sc injections of 200 mg/kg alloxan to mice of a commercial breed before conception or at various times during gestation induced severe or mild diabetes, depending on whether the females were fasted or not preceding the injection. In both groups, a significant fraction of the pregnant females died or aborted, but their surviving offspring, except for a few runts, appeared normal at birth. The only abnormalities were anomalies of the iris and lenticular opacities. The latter, however, only appeared in offspring some weeks after birth; breeding trials indicated they may have been due to the diabetes facilitating a genetic tendency. The occurrence of similar synergisms is recounted in later pages

Other studies had some greater success. In the earliest of these, unpedigreed Phipps Institute colony female mice received 100 mg/kg alloxan iv on one of the 9th through 14th days of gestation (Watanabe and Ingalls 1963). Near-term survivors had gross malformations varying in composition according to the day treated, the great majority cleft palate and most of the remainder digital ectromelias. A different condition (agnathia), found in pilot studies, illustrated but not described in this article, occurred after alloxan injection in the first week of pregnancy, that is, before implantation. This malformation occurred in other studies as well.

The only skeletal abnormality noted, and that in a small number of instances and only after the latest day of treatment, was wavy rib, which especially because it is usually transient is not considered a true abnormality (Kast 1994). No other skeletal defect occurred, including impaired or retarded growth of the lower vertebral column. Skeletal changes were also few in another study from the same laboratory (Endo and Ingalls 1968). In connection with the comment made earlier, it is relevant to note that all the externally malformed offspring were borne by only 22 of the 90 surviving diabetic females bearing fetuses. The mean blood glucose level of these 22 relative to that of the others was not stated.

Different results occurred in another study. Late fetal offspring of ddS mice given 200 mg/kg alloxan ip on the 9th or 10th day of gestation had relatively modest overall malformation frequencies, the majority of which were limb defects, but of different sorts than seen previously (Takano et al. 1965). The limb defects occurred after treatment on both days, but cleft palate (of which there were a few) only after injection on the later day. Both studies thus had treatment time-related consequences, which pointed to direct effects of the administered chemical (this topic will be returned to below). Not mentioned was the proportion of treated mice that carried the malformed offspring and their relative glycemic status.

Experiments in which injection was made before or soon after the time of conception appeared to exclude the likelihood of alloxan itself, rather than its diabetogenic effect, being the teratogenic impulse. In one such study, ICR mice were given 200 mg/kg alloxan sc on the first day of gestation (Takano and Nishimura 1967). Late fetal offspring of the persistently diabetic females (about 75% of all) were malformed more often than those with transient glycosuria, 7.2% versus 1.9%, an impressive but nevertheless not a statistically significant difference. The external malformations were predominantly of the neural tube. (Several cleft palates also occurred, but with a frequency not significantly different from that in the control group.) By far the most common, however, were several types of internal abnormalities—cataract, microphthalmia, and hydronephrosis; the first was noted previously (Bartelheimer and Kloos 1952, Koskenoja 1961) as well as later in an excellent histo-ontological study (Giavini and Pratti 1990), an undeniable consequence of the direct impingement of elevated maternal blood glucose on a fetal structure.

In another such study, female CF1 mice were given 50 mg/kg alloxan iv 3 days before mating (Endo 1966). As usual after preconception or early postconception treatment, only a small minority of animals had successful pregnancies, and only about a third of these had malformed offspring. The overall malformation rate was small (7.8%), and again the spectrum of abnormalities varied from that noted previously: agnathia, seen only rarely in other studies, was by far the most common defect, with craniorachischisis and other neural tube defects lagging behind.

The teratological outcomes of pre- and early postconception alloxan treatment thus consisted almost entirely of neural tube and possibly facial malformations, types distinct from the limb defects predominating following administration of alloxan during the period of embryogenesis. This difference therefore raises the possibility that although the former set of malformations emanated from the diabetogenic action of the alloxan, the latter were due to its immediate effects on the embryo.

This study brought further attention to a consideration integral to teratological research, that is, the dose-response relation, translated in diabetes studies into the relation between the severity of the maternal hyperglycemia and teratogenicity rate. In this study, the relation was a loose one, since although the mean blood glucose level was significantly higher in females with than without malformed fetuses, the distributions of the levels overlapped widely, so in effect it could not be predicted whether a given female with a particular blood glucose level would bear abnormal offspring or not. It appeared therefore that either hyperglycemia was not the sine qua non of the malformations or subsidiary elements modulated the teratogenic response.

This problem was only partly resolved by a study in which insulin was also administered (Horii et al. 1966). Unpedigreed Phipps stock mice received 80 mg/kg alloxan iv on the fourth day after conception, that is, prior to implantation, and beginning 30–36 hours later 0.4 U Lente insulin every 12 hours until the 16th day of gestation. Controls got alloxan only. Blood glucose level was checked at various times during pregnancy. Controls had offspring with a malformation frequency of 5.0%, with neural tube defects and cleft palate predominating and insulin-supplemented females offspring with 0.2% malformations.

Insulin thus prevented malformations, but the basis of this action was clouded. This was because while in the insulin-treated females the blood glucose level was greatly reduced, in the noninsulin-treated ones the mean level during midpregnancy in females bearing normal offspring was virtually identical with that in females bearing malformed offspring. These seemingly irreconcilable results can again only be interpreted as meaning that hyperglycemia alone cannot be responsible for malformations induced in diabetic mice and thus that alleviation of the hyperglycemia was not by itself responsible for their prevention, conclusions also reached on the basis of various lines of reasoning by the authors themselves.

Almost all the studies previously described, as well as those described later in this chapter, have one notable feature in common: low overall malformation frequencies compared with those often induced in experimental teratology studies. The reason for this may be the following. If, as was suggested (Horii et al. 1966), the malformations stemmed from "extensive disturbance of metabolic homeostasis" and if malformation frequency were related to degree of such disturbance, any greater degree of the latter—as would be caused by even larger doses of alloxan—would be lethal to most pregnant females (as was noted in early investigations of the dose-resonse relations of the chemical [Lukens 1948] and in others cited above) and would thus close the door to greater malformation frequency.

This possible explanation of at least of some of the limitations of the teratological consequences of induced diabetes is reminiscent of early studies of the teratogenicity of nutritionally deficient diets. In the days before vitamin antagonists existed, such experiments required a balance to be achieved between a degree of malnutrition so extreme as to impair growth and development of animals and one permitting them to mature, maintain fertility, and produce surviving congenitally malformed offspring (Warkany and Nelson 1941).

Streptozocin

With the advent of the 1970s, with few exceptions, alloxan virtually ceased being used in studies of the effects of diabetes on reproduction and fetal development, being replaced by streptozocin (STZ). This came about because of the advantageous features the latter offered: more specific beta cell toxicity, reduced nephrotoxicity, generally larger margins between diabetogenic and general toxic and lethal dosages, and no or reduced need of insulin for greater maternal survival. What was thus enabled was easier and more specific induction of degrees of diabetes, which was expected to facilitate teratological study (Junod et al. 1967).

As in the early reproduction studies with alloxan, the rat was the favorite species for STZ experiments. And as with the older chemical, in the many reports of such studies made with STZ in the last 30 years or so, the record of the induction of congenital malformations has been most inconsistent. The number reporting them is outweighed by those clearly asserting their absence or failing to mention malformations at all. Since the object of these studies varied, it is uncertain whether offspring were expressly inspected for malformations in all of them, although conspicuous abnormalities would probably not have been overlooked. This large number must be taken as signifying the overall negligible teratological potential of STZ-induced maternal diabetes in animals.

Matched against this preponderance are the relatively few studies in which congenital malformations were noted. A feature of importance, already alluded to, is the prenatal age at which the offspring were examined, since the fate of abnormalities diagnosed at younger prenatal ages will afford insight into their etiology. In most of the studies, the diabetic females were killed 1–3 days before expected term, and their offspring were at late fetal stages when examined. In a small number of studies, on the other hand, the animals were killed during midpregnancy or thereabouts and the offspring examined at embryonic or early fetal stages. The significance of observations at early and late stages are interdependent, however, and must be described and discussed together.

The first teratology study of STZ-induced diabetes, it turned out, was one of the few in which abnormalities occurred (Deuchar 1977). Wistar female rats were given 40–45 mg/kg STZ iv some days before or on the day of conception and their fetuses examined on the 14th or 21st day of gestation. Abnormalities in the younger ones consisted of variable degrees of failure of the neural tube to close and distortion or reduction in one or more cardiac chambers (the same defects that were seen in young fetuses of alloxan-treated females). Both types of abnormalities were also present in controls (in the alloxan experiment, controls only had the neural tube condition), but only the frequency of the former was significantly greater in the test specimens than in the controls (10.0% versus 2.8%). In any case, neither of them was present in the 21st-day fetuses. Their transience means that they were not malformations, a vital component of which is persistence, but no doubt simply expressions of developmental delay. This subject will be fully explored below.

The older fetuses did have abnormalities, but these were entirely different in character from the conditions in the younger specimens. Present externally were omphalocele and micrognathia, and skeletal inspection detected incomplete ossification of sacral vertebrae. All abnormalities occurred in offspring of females with greatly elevated blood glucose, but only the ossification defect also in those of females with lesser levels.

The transitory phenomena in the fetuses and the absent skeletal ossification in the term offspring raise a question that has frequently bedeviled teratology. Deuchar (1977) claimed that there were no significant differences in length or weight between the experimental and control fetuses (no data were given, however); yet photographs presented at the same magnification of a control offspring and one with sacral vertebral defect clearly showed that the latter was substantially smaller than the former.

Small size for age cannot be taken as absolute evidence of developmental retardation, yet when coupled with "an increased rate of missing and incomplete ossification at a given time near term probably indicates nonspecific retardation of fetal growth" (Fritz and Hess 1970). Such facts invite the inference that delayed fetal skeletal maturation may proceed from toxic effects of a situation stressful to the pregnant female, which is an accepted concept in reproductive toxicology (Aliverti et al. 1979, Khera 1984).

It can therefore be reasoned that in Deuchar's experiment developmental delay occurred at embryonic and near-term stages, each presenting its own form of expression. So far as the later form is concerned, it would have been possible to demonstrate that the sacral condition was a persistent and therefore true defect by examining older prenatal offspring or allowing them to be born and following their skeletal development, as was done in a study previously described (Wilson et al. 1985).

The results of this study, and of similar ones examining younger fetuses of STZ-treated mice (Kawaguchi et al. 1994, Tatewaki et al. 1995), may be contrasted with those with follow-up to later stages. For example, offspring of females of a Hebrew University rat stock given STZ early in pregnancy were examined at several gestational stages (Zusman and Ornoy 1986). Younger ones (9th and 11th days) showed neural tube nonclosure or delayed development of various features; but older ones (15th and 17th days) had no such abnormalities. The authors, however, missed the opportunity of offering the obvious explanation of this discrepancy—that of transient retarded development—and held instead that the abnormalities were no longer found because many of the abnormal fetuses had died and been resorbed. But the facts contradicted this, since the resorption rates at the oldest stages examined were similar to those in the controls. Which can only leave the conclusion that whatever irregularities were present in the earliest stages had faded away with time, and quite a brief time at that.

INSULIN ADMINISTRATION

Malformation versus Developmental Delay

Among the studies in which insulin was administered to modify the prenatal effects of the diabetes are two of particular interest. Both experiments, by administering insulin during embryonic stages to pregnant diabetic rats, were directed at substantiating the belief that strict management of diabetic women from early pregnancy prevents fetal maldevelopment (Reece and Hobbins 1986). Furthermore, both sprang from the supposition that the lumbosacral abnormalities in offspring of diabetic animals were analogous to the human defects in that region, which were held to be "specifically linked to maternal diabetes mellitus" (Baker et al. 1981). In one study, Sprague-Dawley rats were given 40 mg/kg STZ iv on the 7th or 12th day of gestation, plus multi-day insulin to those given STZ on the former day (Baker et al. 1981). Defects of two types were noted in the lumbosacral area, but only in those of 7th-day STZ-treated animals: (1) failure of "neural tube fusion…(spina bifida occulta)" and (2) lack of ossification. Both very likely entailed no more than delayed skeletal maturation at different sites, a likelihood supported by the near-term offspring weighing 25% less than the controls. Defects of cartilage were not mentioned, although the method of skeletal preparation used stains both cartilage and ossified bone.

Insulin supplementation decreased the frequency of the defects, but did not abolish them. In fact even when the maternal blood glucose level was greatly reduced the defect frequency was not significantly different from that in the nonsupplemented group. Only when the mean level was further reduced did the frequency return to the control level. Though in neither case was the fetal weight restored to normal, weight was roughly related to defect frequency. The question thus comes down to the nature of the relation between maternal hyperglycemia, fetal weight impairment, and defect frequency. Whatever this may be—and only elaborate multifactorial analysis could have disentangled it—the point the authors were at pains to make, that it was "meticulous control of diabetes during organogenesis" that produced this mitigation, and hence that early control in diabetic women would prevent the sacral abnormality in their children, being predicated on the animal and human abnormalities being analogous, is clearly indefensible.

The second study, recognizing the difficulty presented by developmental delay in masking the occurrence of "true" malformations, attempted to distinguish these phenomena from each other (Eriksson et al. 1982). Sprague-Dawley female rats were given 45–50 mg/kg STZ iv before conception. Those with manifest diabetes (defined as a serum glucose concentration greater than 360 mg/dL) were used; and one-third also given 2–6 U/day insulin sc. Offspring of three late prenatal ages (19th, 21st, and 23rd days) were examined.

Skeletal abnormalities were divided into anomalies and malformations. Anomalies consisted of minor departures from normal patterns of ossification in various sites, and minor abnormalities such as extra ribs, and so on; malformations consisted of micrognathia and caudal dysgenesis. Caudal dysgenesis was defined as "lack of the tail" and "failing ossification of the caudal vertebrae." Only fetuses with micrognathia or both of the components of the caudal dysgenesis were classified as malformed. Strangely, micrognathia and caudal dysgenesis were rarely present in the same animal (U.J. Eriksson et al. 1989).

Several things raise the possibility that the expression "lack of the tail" did not mean absent tail. A photograph in the article captioned with this expression shows an Alizarin-stained skeleton in which the tail vertebrae are absent, but it is not clear that the tail is missing. It was noted in the text that calcified ossification centers (those stained by Alizarin) had not yet appeared in 19th-day fetuses—the youngest age examined—and hence caudal dysgenesis could not be detected in them. The apparent incongruity is presented, however, that older abnormal fetuses were said to lack the tail and by implication younger ones did not. The suspicion is thus reinforced that by this term only absence of tail vertebrae was intended. This is strengthened by the fact that imperforation of the anus was not reported in the offspring with the supposed absent tail, which is remarkable since in various experiments producing anal imperforation the latter was almost always part of the syndrome that included taillessness (eg, Gillman et al. 1948, Kalter and Warkany 1961, Grüneberg 1963). Incidentally, it is difficult to understand why in an earlier study routine inspection of several hundred live late fetuses and newborn offspring of diabetic females failed to disclose any with gross external malformations, presumably including lack of tail (Eriksson et al. 1980).

Turning to other findings in this study (Eriksson et al. 1982), diabetic females were severely hyperglycemic, which was correlated with an elevated fetal resorption rate and greatly retarded fetal growth. A sign of the latter was the significantly reduced mean number of ossification centers at many skeletal sites in the 19th-day fetuses. In older ones this was greatly improved, indicating that with further growth normality in this regard might have been reached.

Insulin supplementation improved all fetal conditions, not only largely preventing the malformations, but also ameliorating the anomalies. With respect to the latter, the improvement can be viewed as an augmentation of the effects of progressing skeletal maturation in association with the fetal weight gain that aging alone increasingly brings. Thus, it seems that one of the objects of the study was met, since the two sorts of abnormalities—anomalies and malformations—were dissevered, in the sense that one was remediable and the other not. Another goal—"To elucidate the teratogenic mechanisms in diabetic pregnancy" (whatever that means)—failed to be achieved, perhaps because the insulin was given throughout pregnancy.

Teratological Mechanism

As part of investigating teratological "mechanism," studies were made to learn when during pregnancy the maternal diabetic state exerted its teratological effects (R.S. Eriksson et al. 1989, U.J. Eriksson et al. 1989). This was done by administering insulin either by daily injection or implanted minipump to diabetic rats throughout pregnancy, except for successive 2- or 4-day periods from the 3rd through 12th days of gestation. Again, insulin reduced the frequency of the malformations, except when omitted on the 9th and succeeding days, indicating that the abnormalities were determined during the early to middle embryonic period.

It is not amiss, in considering malformation frequency to note that the definition of malformation underwent a change in this study (R.S. Eriksson et al. 1989). Whereas before, as already noted, an animal was considered malformed if it had micrognathia or caudal dysgenesis, in this one it was so defined if it had these or exencephaly, thus broadening the definition and making comparison with previous studies difficult. In addition, lumping these disparate malformations made it impossible to define susceptible periods for each of them. Finally, again, as elsewhere, the maternal glycemic state seemed irrelevant to the teratological outcome, since the serum glucose levels did not differ in rats with and without malformed offspring. And uninterpretable variations in beta-hydroxybutyrate concentrations in these two groups were of no help in understanding the etiology of the defects. Thus, understanding mechanism once more proved elusive.

STUDIES WITH DIFFERENT RAT STOCKS

The teratological findings in a study using two rat stocks differed in several respects from those previously described (Uriu-Hare at al. 1985). Sprague-Dawley and Wistar females were given 40–45 mg/kg STZ iv before conception and those meeting the criteria for diabetes were mated and late fetuses examined. Severe and approximately equal degrees of hyperglycemia were induced in females of both stocks, as were notable fetal weight and growth impairment, despite which external abnormalities occurred in only three Wistar and no Sprague-Dawley offspring. Significantly reduced numbers of ossification centers, indicative of growth retardation, as I have argued, did occur, however, at several sites including caudal vertebrae, in fetuses of both stocks, but in Wistar almost always to a greater extent than in Sprague-Dawley offspring. Thus, none of the external malformations were seen that occurred previously (Eriksson et al. 1982), and, on the contrary, various minor skeletal abnormalities occurred, but very infrequently, not seen previously.

In contrast, another study found surprising interstock variability (Eriksson et al. 1986). Although Sprague-Dawley rats long housed in Uppsala (the U line) and more recently imported Sprague-Dawley Hanover rats (the H line), both had similar degrees of STZ-induced hyperglycemia, micrognathia and caudal dysgenesis were entirely absent in offspring of the latter.

These differences are remarkable even though the stocks had been separated for about 20 years. For want of a better explanation, it can only be conjectured that the shift had its origin in a single gene mutation, as was likely the case for the difference in susceptibility to STZ-induced diabetes between two inbred mouse strains (Kaku et al. 1989). But this is doubtful, since a cross-breeding experiment found that both the maternal and fetal genotypes affected the malformation frequency (Eriksson 1988), a situation reminiscent of the findings in a study of the genetics of cortisone-induced cleft palate done long ago with inbred strains of mice (Kalter 1954).

Another study using the susceptible U and resistant H stocks (Styrud et al. 1995) had significance for much embryo culture work. Females of both lines were made diabetic by the usual procedure and early fetuses examined. Surprisingly, conditions such as those observed previously (Deuchar 1977)—malrotation, open neural tube, and heart hypertrophy—occurred in almost identical frequencies in both stocks. The explanation offered for this discrepant finding—that "embryonic changes are only barely detectable" in early gestation, "but become much more evident" later—is unconvincing. The authors were more realistic when they confessed that the "fundamental difference between the U and H strains that predisposes to the higher teratologic U vulnerability is not known...." What the authors failed to appreciate is that the apparent discrepancy clearly showed that the phenomena present in the early fetuses, demonstrative of developmental delay, were nonspecific in nature and unrelated to induction of major malformations.

In another largely negative study, CD rats were given 40–50 mg/kg STZ iv some days before conception or on the first day of pregnancy and near-term fetuses examined externally and skeletally (Giavini et al. 1986). As others often found, the rats seemed to be of two discrete populations, one showing moderate and the other severe degrees of hyperglycemia, with no overlap, regardless of the time of administration of the diabetogen. Nevertheless, there was very little difference in fetal consequence between them: those with the lower levels had offspring with no malformations, and those with the higher a very few abnormal offspring.

Great inconsistency between studies was again seen when in another one a wide variety of defects, but not taillessness, occurred (Padmanabhan and Al-Zuhair 1988). Wistar rats received single injections of 50 mg/kg STZ ip on the 3rd to 13th days of gestation. Many different kinds of external and internal defects were found, but mostly of unimpressive frequency. Furthermore, no specificity of type was discernible with respect to the time of treatment, whether on the days before implantation or during embryo formation and organogenesis. Among the many types were two (omphalocele and micrognathia) that have appeared in other such studies, and, on the contrary, one, cardiac septal defects, seldom reported in near-term fetuses. The latter, in fact, the most frequent defect seen, was seen after treatment on all days and also in an appreciable frequency in controls. The diagnosis of this condition was made by razor-blade sectioning of fixed specimens, which requires much experience and skill.

Skeletal defects noted consisted of lumbar ribs and deficiencies of ossification, including those of sacrococcygeal vertebrae. In light of the maternal toxicity and fetal growth impairment, this was not surprising. Interesting was the finding that insulin reduced all skeletal defects, contradicting a study in which insulin was barely successful in this respect (Eriksson et al. 1982). Giving rise to confusion was a study noting that insulin increased skeletal anomalies, perhaps through causing maternal hypoglycemia (Tanigawa et al. 1991). Insulin, it seems, in different hands, apparently has inconsistent effects.

NUTRITION AND STZ DIABETES

A new chapter was opened with the observation that trace element metabolism was disturbed in diabetic animals (Eriksson 1984, Uriu-Hare et al. 1989). Maternal nutritional status has been known to have a vital role in prenatal development since the 1930s and 1940s, when severe vitamin deficiency was discovered to cause fetal growth retardation and congenital malformations in domestic and laboratory animals (Kalter and Warkany 1959). It also later became established that maternal deficiency of mineral elements can be teratogenic (Hurley 1977).

This began with the discovery that fetuses of diabetic rats were deficient in zinc, despite the pregnant animals having elevated levels of several minerals. Coupled with the recognized teratological and growth-retarding effects of maternal zinc deficiency—among them abnormalities associated with maternal diabetes (Hurley and Swenerton 1966)—this led to attempts to prevent these abnormalities by adding large amounts of zinc to the drinking water of pregnant diabetic rats (Eriksson et al. 1984). The results were disappointing, since the fetal zinc level remained reduced, fetal growth was unimproved, and the malformation rate was unchanged.

Interesting results came from a study in which diabetic females were fed a marginal as well as a high level of zinc (Uriu-Hare et sl. 1989). The offspring of the former females had an intensified frequency of malformations, though of a similar variety. Thus, lack of zinc synergized some of the effects of diabetes, but zinc in excess could not abolish them.

These negative results did not discourage studies with other elements. Equally negative, however, was the evidence that deficiency of copper, magnesium, and protein had any part in the teratological effects of the maternal diabetes (Giavini et al. 1990, 1991, 1993, Jankowski et al. 1993). What the Giavini studies did accomplish—by documenting in great detail the defects, anomalies, and variants found—was, first, to reveal the limited ability of diabetes to cause major congenital malformations, at least in the animal stock used, next, to portray the qualitative variability the abnormalities could exhibit from one experiment to the next, and last, to affirm the nonspecificity of the teratological response to maternal diabetes.

A novel approach was used in an attempt to prevent diabetes-associated embryopathy (Hagay et al. 1995). Unfortunately, the confused and contradictory description of parts of the procedure hindered clear understanding of the outcome. But, as well as can be made out, the following is what was done and found. The subjects were mice homozygous for the human copper zinc superoxide dismutase transgene and others that did not possess the gene. Nontransgenic females were mated to transgenic or nontransgenic males and therefore carried embryos that were, respectively, transgenic, (ie, heterozygous for the gene) or nontransgenic (ie, did not possess the gene). Females were injected with 200 mg/kg STZ iv on each of the 7th and 8th days of pregnancy. Controls got citrate buffer.

Females were killed on the 11th day, an early developmental stage, and their embryos were examined for external morphological and other features. Compared with the transgenic embryos of diabetic females, the nontransgenic ones of such females were significantly smaller and more frequently dead and malformed. The malformations included exencephaly, cardiac hypertrophy, unnamed limb defects, and delayed anterior and posterior neuropore closure. The transgenic state thus was found to protect against the embryopathic changes. This protection was attributed to an excess of free oxygen radicals resulting from overexpression of the transgene, based on analogy to the improvement in the development of embryos subjected in vitro to teratogenic effects of hyperglycemic conditions afforded by the presence of such factors.

Certain facts argue against the malformation results and their interpretation. First, although the mice used in the study ordinarily, as it was stated, "have a low occurrence of fetal anomalies," appreciable frequencies of malformations occurred in the offspring, transgenic and nontransgenic, of nondiabetic females. Second, the malformation frequencies in the transgenic offspring of diabetic and nondiabetic females were not significantly different from each other. Unfortunately, detailed information of the sort that would have permitted a close analysis of the results—the types and frequencies of abnormalities in the offspring of the nondiabetic females and the individual frequencies of malformations in the offspring of the diabetic females—was not given, so that comparison and judgment were precluded. The same criticism is to be made of the results of administering insulin to diabetic females, which reduced the malformation frequency and simultaneously and probably not coincidentally improved embryonic size.

Many of the defects, it must be noted, were similar to those occurring in previous studies of embryos and young fetuses from diabetic animals, which did not persist to later stages and were no doubt expressions of delayed development. The significant size impairments noted in this study invite the conclusion that this was the case here as well.

18

DIABETIC PREGNANCY IN ANIMALS: II

SPONTANEOUS ANIMAL DIABETES

The importance of spontaneous diabetes in animals for examining effects on prenatal development, as it was pointed out (Funaki and Mikamo 1983), lies in the possibility that it may offer more valid models of the human condition than induced ones do. Diabetes occurs in several animal species (see Animal Resource Table in Salans and Graham, pp. 41–42), but pregnancy has been described in few of them.

Mouse Genes

A number of recessive genes in mice cause a diabetes syndrome, but most are maturity-onset states associated with obesity and sterility (Coleman 1982) and are not analogous to human type1 diabetes. One that does not lead to sterility, the semidominant yellow (A^y), when incorporated into the KK inbred mouse strain, which itself is prone to a polygenically determined diabetes, was reported in an abstract to cause external ear defects and various skeletal variations in offspring (Ooshima and Shiota 1991). The sparsity of details in this brief communication makes comment hazardous, but it seems that the effects of this noninsulin-dependent diabetes were associated with what sounded like a maternal stressful situation. Physical abnormalities apparently did not occur in offspring of KK mice without the yellow gene (Reddi et al. 1975). In a study of a congenic inbred mouse strain into which the yellow gene had been incorporated, there was no significant occurrence of congenital malformations in offspring of pregnant hyperglycemic females (Teramoto et al. 1991).

The NOD Mouse

Studies specifically directed to the prenatal effects of spontaneously developing mouse diabetes have been made only with the NOD (nonobese diabetic) mouse strain. As with the BB rat, discussed in the following section, its condition appears to simulate the human type 1 form of the disease, with the difference from the rat that the percent of affected female mice far exceeds that of males and permanent hyperglycemia is achieved in females far earlier than in males. Diabetic individuals require maintenance doses of 40–50 U/kg/day insulin for survival (Makino et al. 1980, Leiter et al. 1987, Tochino 1987).

In a teratology study of NOD mice, diabetic females were superovulated and 14th-day fetuses examined for malformations (Otani et al. 1991). Superovulation was used because NOD diabetic females do not ovulate "efficiently," and an early fetal stage was examined because a high resorption rate had previously been found in females allowed to continue to later pregnancy. But even by this early stage a high proportion of conceptuses of both diabetic and nondiabetic females—that is, with and without overt disease—were already dead. The live and examinable dead fetuses from diabetic females had various defects, two of which predominated: a relatively high frequency of exencephaly and a smaller one of spina bifida, a few with kinked or wavy vertebral column, and a case of "extreme delay in development [with] pathological umbilical herniation." (The last specimen will be discussed further in a later section in this chapter.) All of the defects, however, also occurred in offspring of nondiabetic NOD females, with only exencephaly greater in frequency in offspring of diabetic females. A morphological study also reported a relatively high frequency of neural tube defects, but no comparison was made with nondiabetic NOD mice (Ando et al. 1991).

A cross-transfer experiment attempted to clarify the maternal versus the conceptal source of the teratogenic response (Otani et al. 1991). Preimplantation embryos from diabetic females were implanted in pseudopregnant ICR nondiabetic females (a stock related to the one from which NOD were originally derived [Makino et al. 1980]), and those from ICR females were transferred to diabetic females. The two groups of offspring were examined on day 14. Considering only the exencephaly, since it was the only defect increased in the offspring of diabetic females, the two groups of offspring were not significantly different from each other (5.2% in the first group versus 11.1% in the second; $P<.05$).

Thus, while in the first experiment maternal diabetes was associated with an increased frequency of a malformation, in the second maternal diabetic and nondiabetic backgrounds did not lead to different teratological consequences. How can these seemingly discrepant results be interpreted? It might be that cross-transference itself was maldevelopmental and obscured different effects in the two groups, except that reciprocal cross-transference of ICR embryos was without this effect. It seems that the question remains unanswered.

Other experimenters studying a different colony of NOD mice reported a far greater diversity of malformations, after having no difficulty in obtaining and examining offspring at stages beyond the 14th day of pregnancy (Morishima et al. 1991). A large percentage of the offspring of females showing diabetic symptoms before the 9th day of pregnancy had abnormalities of the neural tube, face, tail, and ventral body wall, as well as complex viscerocardiac malformations; the last in fact were the focus of the experiment. Several of the abnormalities also occurred in offspring of nondiabetic NOD females, but in a far smaller overall frequency.

In none of the publications concerning NOD mice was insulin mentioned, which seems to contradict its reported need for survival in overt diabetic individuals (Makino et al. 1980, Leiter et al. 1987, Tochino 1987). A possible reason for this is that NOD mice can survive without insulin for some months after glycosuria is first detected (Leiter et al. 1987). Whether that was the case in the teratology studies is uncertain.

Other omissions directly bear on this one: the blood glucose levels in diabetic and nondiabetic females, with one exception (Morishima et al. 1991), were not reported, nor were differences in the glycemic state in females bearing and not bearing malformed offspring. Such data would have been useful in interpreting the results, since the age at which NOD female mice become permanently hyperglycemic apparently varies considerably. One article stated that the peak onset was at 16–20 weeks, another at an average age of 210 days, and a third that females as much as 52 weeks old had still not developed ketonuria and insulin dependency (Leiter et al. 1987, Tochino 1987, Formby et al. 1987). The absence of specific information regarding these variables adds another layer of uncertainty to the meaning of the results. More recent articles (Tatekawi et al. 1989a,b) reporting wide variations in blood glucose levels in NOD mice did not aid clarification.

Finally, the fact was also ignored that females of the NOD stock without overt diabetes also had offspring with malformations of the same sorts as occurred in the offspring of diabetic NOD females. What this fact might mean respecting the etiology of the malformations in the diabetic group was not alluded to. The passing remark that "there might be a genetic predisposition for external anomalies in NOD embryos" (Otani et al. 1991) seems to have referred to the stock's genetic composition that is associated with its diabetic tendencies, and not to the possibility that NOD mice have a tendency to malformation that is unrelated to diabetes, one that might be intensified by an additional maternal stressful situation. Examples of such potentiation are the exacerbated teratological consequences of administering triethylene thiophosphoramide (thio-TEPA) and alcohol to pregnant animals with alloxan- and STZ-induced diabetes, respectively (Takano et al. 1965, Lin et al. 1995).

The implied contention that various sorts of numerical and structural chromosomal anomalies, found in pre- and especially in postimplantation embryos from diabetic NOD females, were associated with the maternal disease state and fetal maldevelopment need not be taken seriously (Tatekawi et al. 1989a,b). No such anomalies were found in a study of offspring of hamsters with spontaneous diabetes (Funaki and Mikamo 1983).

The BB Rat

The study of spontaneous diabetes in rats began with the chance discovery of the condition in an outbred Wistar line, which was then given the name BB (Nakhooda et al. 1976). The condition entails clinical and pathological features similar to those of the human early-onset insulin-dependent form (Marliss et al. 1982). Signs of the disease appear abruptly at 2–6 months of age, in a percentage of animals and varies according to the degree and direction of selection the line has undergone. Soon after its onset diabetic animals require insulin daily for survival.

Despite the promise that the BB rat seemed to hold of enabling the investigation of the effects of a close mimic of human diabetes on fetal morphological development, and the opportunity it provided of testing the hypothesis that tight control of maternal diabetes before and during pregnancy would reduce fetal morbidity and maldevelopment, the model has been little exploited for these purposes.

In one of the few such studies, diabetic BB females, with plasma glucose levels of 300–700 mg/dL, receiving 0.8–4.8 U protamine zinc insulin daily, were bred to diabetic or nondiabetic males of the BB stock (Brownscheidle and Davis 1981). Many females proved to be sterile or resorbed entire litters, as was the case for the chemically induced disease. In pregnancies that continued, "gross malformations" occurred that included eye and central nervous system malformations and various undescribed sternebral, vertebral, and other skeletal defects. One of the latter was called an "anomaly of the pelvis and sacral spine, similar to that described in the caudal regression syndrome," obviously referring to the human diabetic outcome (Brownscheidle 1986). However, the illustration in the publication ostensibly supporting this opinion was wholly inappropriate for the purpose. Judging from the significant weight and size reduction of the offspring, some of the skeletal defects no doubt were instances of delayed ossification and can hardly be called malformations. The proportion of all the abnormalities that these formed was not divulged; hence the frequency of the undoubted malformations is unknown.

In another study, defects were seen in late fetal and newborn offspring all of which, without distinction, were considered malformations (Brownscheidle et al. 1983). True ones in the fetuses could be distinguished, since all the defects were named—malformations (anophthalmia, exencephaly, and gastroschisis), incomplete ossification of cranial elements and vertebral centra, and wavy and absent ribs—but not quantified; whereas in the newborn offspring the overall frequency of defects was recorded, but not that of each individually. Hence close analysis of the results was not possible. The statement that "lumbosacral dysgenesis was observed...specifically in dams with poor metabolic control" was uninterpretable, since the authors did not define what they meant by this term, but it probably referred to deficits in ossification.

The postnatal progress of the offspring was followed in those allowed to be delivered. In some cases, several developmental milestones were significantly delayed, but since the offspring were not fostered on nondiabetic females the meaning of these results is clouded.

So far as can be ascertained, only one other reproduction/teratology study has as yet been conducted with BB rats (U.J. Eriksson et al. 1989). Diabetic BB females from a colony maintained in Edinburgh bred to like males were given insulin daily throughout pregnancy or throughout except for interruption on 2 consecutive days from the 3rd through the 13th day. The fetal resorption rate, compared with that in a nondiabetic BB subline, was significantly increased to as high as about 30% after insulin interruption on the 9th–10th days, and the body weight was significantly reduced. The latter was no doubt the reason for the total number of ossification centers being less in the offspring of diabetic than nondiabetic females, regardless of continuous or interrupted insulin treatment. So far as congenital malformations are concerned, only two were seen in 47 surviving fetuses (an absent tail and caudal vertebrae, and a large omphalocele and exencephaly), the sparsity of which—in contrast with other findings (Brownscheidle et al. 1983)—was imputed to the resorption of malformed fetuses, for which, however, no evidence was presented.

Other Species

Reproduction studies apparently have been made only in one other species that develops diabetes spontaneously, Chinese hamsters. In one study except for slightly increased birth weight, no physical change was seen (Heisig and Schall 1971). In another preweaning mortality was increased, but its cause was not determined (Gerritsen et al. 1974).

The third was more extensive. Two related lines were used, one with a low and the other a high rate of diabetes, the latter produced by brother-sister inbreeding and selection (Funaki and Mikamo 1983). Near-term offspring of diabetic females of both lines had a low frequency of various gross malformations, including some seen in induced diabetes, such as agnathia and omphalocele, for a total of 4.0%. The occurrence of the latter in an offspring of a nondiabetic female of the low-rate line indicated that the instances of this malformation in the diabetic group may have been due to a synergistic situation.

Two important matters, the possible association of pregnancy outcome with maternal hyperglycemia and with fetal developmental retardation, were not taken into account by the authors. Since no glycemic data were given whether the blood glucose level in the diabetic females that bore offspring with major malformations was different from that of the others could not be examined.

The only information given, if only indirectly, about the second was that the proportion of underdeveloped fetuses of diabetic females was greatly increased; whether this growth retardation coincided with maldevelopment was not mentioned. The question is raised here because it may be as relevant to omphalocele—the most frequent malformation—as retarded development is to skeletal abnormalities previously discussed.

A photograph of an offspring presented in this publication (Funaki and Mikamo 1983) displays a malformation that is illustrated in no other article I have seen concerned with induced or spontaneous animal diabetes. This is a picture of a fetus labeled as having an "omphalocele," a defect seen often enough in offspring of diabetic animals to be suspected of constituting a characteristic abnormality. The photo affords insight into the possible nature of the defect that could not be guessed in its absence. This subject is dealt with in detail in the Critique section.

Postnatal Studies

A few studies have been made of the postnatal growth and development of offspring of female animals with STZ-induced diabetes. The findings of even this limited number have been inconsistent, however, owing in some measure to variations in levels of maternal hyperglycemia, but more likely to differences in procedure.

For example, postnatal weight gain was accelerated, perhaps only temporarily, in offspring of rats with STZ-induced hyperglycemia (Oh et al. 1988). But the soundness of this result was clouded by the offspring having been nursed by their own mothers. This also complicated a study in which the weight of 4-week-old offspring of STZ-treated mice was inconsistent (Linn et al. 1993) and another in which, although preweaning mortality was unaffected, the weight of older offspring and longevity of males (that of females was not mentioned) were significantly decreased (Iwase et al. 1995). The latter, the authors conjectured, may have been due to the combination of the diabetic intrauterine environment (postnatal diabetic influences were not considered) and the spontaneous hypertension afflicting the stock of rats used. It is obviously important to know whether the developmental detriments noted in these three studies were prenatal or postnatal in origin, but this matter was not addressed.

This uncertainty was removed by a study in which both experimental and control offspring were nursed on nondiabetic foster mothers (Vasilenko et al. 1989). Since delays in maturation—in linear growth and weight gain and in the developmental landmarks of pinna detachment and eye opening—occurred in offspring of diabetic as well as in those of nondiabetic animals fostered on diabetic ones, and the opposite, normality, when fostering was done in the other direction, the delays were attributed to maternal lactational inadequacy. The deleterious effects on postnatal growth of having a diabetic mother therefore obviously stemmed from conditions present after and not before birth.

Other studies supported this judgment. Although offspring of diabetic rats fostered on nondiabetic ones weighed significantly less than the controls at 30 days of age, the difference progressively diminished as they aged (Grill et al. 1991). Similarly, when female newborn of diabetic rats were fostered on nondiabetic ones, weight at weaning, time of vaginal opening, and proportion with normal estrous cycles were normal. Some of the offspring, nevertheless, were mildly carbohydrate intolerant at older ages (Foglia et al. 1987).

Preimplantation Studies

The impact of induced maternal diabetes on embryos in the period before implantation, in contrast with that after birth, was clear and consistent, retarded progress of blastocyst development being the sole and constant finding (Diamond et al. 1989, Vercheval et al. 1990, Moley et al. 1991, Hertogh et al. 1992); exceptional in this regard were embryos of spontaneously diabetic hamsters (Funaki and Mikamo 1983). This very early retardation, however, is just as irrelevant to furthering understanding of the supposed teratological repercussions of diabetes on the definitive embryo and fetus (as many of the authors of these articles thought it could do) as is the form of developmental retardation found in near-term fetuses. Regardless of anything else, however, these early-pregnancy studies complemented those of later stages in pointing to the noteworthy fact that maternal diabetes, at least the induced form, has the common effect of causing growth retardation at whatever prenatal stage it acts.

It is appropriate to note that an apparently identical inhibition of blastocyst development was caused by heat-shocking mice on the first day of pregnancy (Elliott and Ulberg 1971). The authors attempted to explain this as having a nutritional basis, which they themselves were not convinced by. Instead one may offer the interpretation that, whatever its proximate cause, the phenomenon may be a nonspecific consequence, due to whatever—heat, diabetes, and so on—of a systemic dislocation of maternal well-being.

EXPERIMENTALLY INDUCED DIABETES IN OTHER SPECIES

A limited number of studies have examined the effects of experimenally induced diabetes on reproduction and prenatal development in a few other species. An early study of female rabbits made diabetic by alloxan prior to conception was disappointing, since most of the pregnancies aborted, a few ended in premature delivery or stillbirth, and very few were considered full term. Congenital malformations were apparently not seen in any offspring (Miller 1947). A study of uterine glycogen in alloxanized pregnant rabbits at term failed to mention the consequences, if any, to the offspring (Vaes and Meyer 1957).

The only other such study of rabbits I am aware of had more positive results (Barashnev 1964). Females received alloxan before conception or at three times during pregnancy—before implantation, at an early embryonic stage, or at a late fetal stage—and were killed during the last week of pregnancy and their offspring examined grossly and histologically. The degree of ensuing diabetes was quite variable. Those treated prenatally and a few treated at the embryonic stage received insulin.

Most of the offspring were alive at examination, but were immature and growth-retarded. The brain was apparently the only internal structure studied. In most cases, it was reduced in size, but only in proportion to the decrease in overall body size. But in some others it was also malformed; the latter, it seems, judging from the diagrams, was particularly true of the cerebral hemispheres. In addition, a small percentage of offspring of females treated before conception or during the embryonic stage had external malformations, 2.8% and 0.9%, respectively. The abnormalities were not explicitly detailed, but may have been those of eyes and skull. The possible relation of the malformations to diabetes severity and whether those escaping maldevelopment were among the offspring of the females receiving insulin were not clarified.

In a study with dogs, three pregnancies of females of an unspecified breed given alloxan before conception ended at or near term with apparently morphologically normal offspring (Miller 1947). Studies with guinea pigs made diabetic by STZ injection before conception were similarly negative (Saintonge and Côté 1983, 1984). Studies of maternal diabetes in sheep and rhesus monkeys are of no relevance here since the diabetogens were administered after organogenesis (eg, Kohn and Bennett 1986, Lips et al. 1988, Miodovnik et al. 1989).

CRITIQUE

The Malformations: Direct versus Indirect Origin

The following remarks refer only to the minority of studies in which malformations were produced. A number of matters mentioned earlier in this chapter and the previous one must be dealt with further. The first, a question of fundamental importance, concerns the origin of the harm chemical-induced diabetes does to embryos and fetuses. When a substance is administered during pregnancy, as alloxan and STZ sometimes were, it can be unclear whether the fetal abnormalities that may ensue are due to the direct action of the substance on embryos or to an indirect action via some effect it may have on the pregnant animal, in this case, among others, hyperglycemia. This is an old problem in experimental teratology, and has often proved difficult to resolve (Khera 1984).

It was explicitly raised in a briefly reported early experiment (Ross and Spector 1952). Mice of an unnamed stock were injected with 100–150 mg/kg alloxan sc on 3 successive but undesignated days, probably during midpregnancy. The authors considered that the dose was subdiabetogenic since the maternal blood glucose level was in the normal range and because there were no changes in the pancreatic beta cells of examined pregnant animals. Nevertheless, several fetuses had a defect of the head, suggesting myeloencephalocele. In the discussion following this orally presenting paper, a listener proposed that the maldevelopment resulted from histotoxic effects of the alloxan rather than from its diabetogenic qualities, which the presenter of the paper agreed with.

It must therefore be seriously inquired whether, in the studies under discussion, diabetogenic chemicals, despite their brief presence, act directly on the conceptus, or indirectly by some intermediate instrument, that is, the maternal organism.

The argument that with chemicals like alloxan and STZ, which have extremely short half-lives (Patterson et al. 1949, Kerunanayake et al. 1976), their prenatal consequences must be of indirect origin modulated through the production of maternal diabetes, overlooks an important consideration. Which is, that if the brief moment of its potency is not too short to permit it to reach and destroy insulin-producing cells of the pancreas, why should it not also be able during such a short spell to reach embryos in sufficient quantities to harm them. Other chemicals, of established teratogenicity, share this attribute of brief existence (Nau 1987). What the question perhaps calls for is a comparison of the fetal consequences of alloxan administered before and at various times during pregnancy.

The Malformations: Pre- versus Postimplantation Origin

Various lines of reasoning may help answer the question whether diabetogenic chemicals harm conceptuses by impinging directly upon them or by acting via the maternal disease state. Although the action of these chemicals in destroying beta cells is rapid, the hyperglycemic consequences of this cytotoxicity take some time to be expressed. Therefore, when the chemical is administered during embryonic stages, some large proportion of its embryotoxic effects will be due to direct action, because diabetes may not yet have developed. It follows that the malformations thus caused, ceteris paribus, will be of specific types associated with the teratological vulnerability of the time of treatment.

When, on the other hand, a chemical is administered before or at the time of conception, sufficient time will usually have passed for diabetes to have been established when embryogenesis begins, and the anomalies induced will be due to the chronic maternal disease state. (Unfortunately, details were seldom provided about the severity of the latter prevailing during the vulnerable embryonic interval, which might have allowed something approximating a dose-response analysis.) With these matters in mind, it can be asked whether the *true* malformations induced by these different etiologic avenues were distinct from each other.

True malformations did occur, although usually of limited assortment and in relatively low frequencies. In mice, after alloxan, they were almost entirely of the neural tube, palate, and lower jaw. The same locations were also among the most common in rats after alloxan, but sometimes with a larger array. On the contrary, STZ in rats led to a narrow array of defects, with those of the neural tube, jaw, and ventral body wall predominating. The overall impression, with few exceptions, is of a patternless miscellany.

Nevertheless, there seem to be clear differences between the effects of direct and indirect action, despite the few overlaps that may blur the distinction. Strongly implicating direct action are the time-related malformation specificities following treatment on the 7th–14th days of gestation (Wilson et al. 1985, Watanabe and Ingalls 1963, Takano et al. 1965, Takano and Nishimura 1967, Padmanabhan and Al-Zuhair 1988). Some defects, in fact, occurred only after postimplantation treatment, such as digital and renal abnormalities.

In contrast, indirect action was indicated by agnathia and micrognathia occurring only after preconception treatment, and by neural tube defects and omphalocele after preconception and early postimplantation treatment. Other malformations, especially facial clefts, were shared by almost all the studies, regardless of treatment time.

Basis of the Fetal Growth Retardation

In the light of the discovery that maternal diabetes retards embryonic development in the blastocyst as well as the embryogenetic stage—perhaps throughout prenatal existence—the possibility is not to be disregarded that this feature is the common thread among many of the defects seen in offspring of diabetic animals. And indeed since it appears to be the most prevalent and pervasive of its effects, attention should be directed to attempts that were made to investigate and explain this phenomenon.

Several means were used to explore this question. The constant signs of embryonic growth and developmental retardation were significant reduction in crown-rump length and somite number (Eriksson et al. 1984). These were hypothesized to be due to disturbance in transfer of nutrients from mother to conceptus, stemming from reduced uteroplacental blood flow; a belief that was supported by measurements that found the total flow in the near-term placental circulation to be decreased by about half (Palacin et al. 1985, Eriksson and Jansson 1984, Chartrel et al. 1990). But this was cruelly negated by the contradictory finding that the flow in uterine and decidual tissue during midpregnancy was increased (Wentzel et al. 1995).

Attempts were made to reconcile these conflicting outcomes, in the quest to explain their connection to the occurrence of so-called malformations (explained in the text that follows). Decreased blood flow, it was reasoned, could be related to the fetal growth retardation, but not to the malformations in the near-term offspring, because the flow to malformed and nonmalformed fetuses was similar. The interpretation of the contrary findings was exactly the opposite; that is, increased flow to the embryos left their retarded growth unexplained, but for their defects "increased delivery of oxidative substrates" was called upon (Styrud et al. 1995).

Why so-called malformations? Altering a definition in midstream is unacceptable. In a preliminary study (Eriksson et al. 1994), the neural tube of growth-retarded embryos was not disproportionately changed, but instead the most conspicuous and constant "dysmorphogenetic" feature of the retardation was posterior neuropore nonclosure. This, as was admitted, is "a development that should take place" at an earlier stage of gestation than the one examined. In this paper, the authors thus wisely refrained from labeling the delayed closure a malformation. In a later article (Styrud et al. 1996), however, the same features that were earlier accepted as representing retardation—"neural tube closure abnormalities or rotational defects"—were called malformations. And the fanciful explanation of their supposed occurrence, as already stated, was then invoked.

Therefore, except for a vague "maternal nutritional inadequacy," the growth retardation caused by animal diabetes remains unexplained, as does its putative connection to malformations.

Missing Lower Vertebral Elements

The connection, however, between prenatal retardation and the anomalies of the lower vertebrae reported in several studies is not difficult to perceive. These anomalies are of particular interest because they are said to be the counterpart of the caudal dysplasia syndrome claimed to occur frequently in children of women with diabetes, a syndrome typically consisting of absent sacral vertebrae. The lower vertebral bodies missing in defective offspring of diabetic rats were different in an important respect from the human abnormality. The latter may be seen in newborn children, but is far more often detected in older ones. The rat condition, on the contrary, occurred in younger fetuses but not older ones. The "absence" in the rat is thus a phenomenon consequent upon a temporary retardation, which disappears with catch-up growth.

This conclusion is supported by a detailed analysis of the "order, time, and rate of ossification" of the Wistar rat skeleton made years ago (Strong 1925), which noted that ossification in the first sacral arch begins at 18 days and 10 hours of pregnancy, does not occur in more rostral arches until 22 days, that is, the time of birth, and in caudal bodies does not begin till 3 days postnatal. The implication therefore is that permitting catch-up growth of offspring of diabetic rats and examining their skeleton at postnatal ages, especially if they are allowed to be nursed by nondiabetic surrogate mothers, would reveal that the missing elements had appeared. The analogy to the human abnormality is thus entirely spurious.

Omphalocele

Prenatal growth retardation may also be associated with at least one of the malformations—omphalocele—that occurred in offspring in several studies of induced and spontaneous diabetes. (In all but two instances, the defect was labeled omphalocele; in the exceptions it was called gastroschisis. These are two distinctly different abnormalities, the latter the far more serious one, but they are often confused and misnamed. This was probably the case with the exceptions.)

Omphalocele consists of the presence at birth of intestine in the body stalk, due to partial or complete failure of the developing gut to return to the abdominal cavity during late first trimester, as it normally does. Although it is an abnormality when present at birth, in the embryo, in the form of a transient umbilical herniation, it is a normal phenomenon (deVries 1980).

Under certain conditions, such as growth disturbance, it may persist into later stages, and in some instances the omphalic sac may rupture before birth. Omphaloceles vary in size, and, as Warkany (1971, p. 759) has commented, "small and large omphaloceles should be distinguished because of their different nature and different prognosis." The photograph mentioned previously (Funaki and Mikamo 1983) of a fetus with what was labeled an omphalocele, shows a specimen with intestine, but no other abdominal organ, extruded, probably a relatively small ruptured omphalocele. It must, therefore, be considered a possibility, here and in other instances of the condition occurring in diabetic animal pregnancy, that the defect was another expression of the fetal growth-inhibiting influence of the maternal disease.

CONCLUSION

Animal models have been used to probe unresolved problems of human diabetic pregnancy, especially the one most regarded as still outstanding, the increased risk of congenital malformations in children of diabetic women. The current belief is that poor control of the maternal disease in early pregnancy is at its root, a belief that is supported by the beneficial fetal outcome apparently obtained by closely supervising the metabolic state of diabetic women from before or early in pregnancy (Steel et al. 1990). This salutary result seems to be complemented by findings of experimental studies in which insulin administration reduced the rate of malformations in offspring of diabetic animals. These and other outcomes, however, are not without difficulties of interpretation, and it is to these complications that attention will now turn.

First to be considered are the aberrant conditions found in the embryos and fetuses of diabetic animals. These were of two sorts, which differ qualitatively from each other in a crucial attribute, namely, whether they are permanent or not. Permanent aberrations are present at birth and continue to exist in postnatal life. Impermanent ones are those that are present at some time during prenatal life, but by the time birth approaches (or afterward in the case, eg, of many ventricular septal defects, as discussed elsewhere in this work) have disappeared. The first consist of congenital malformations, and the second are certain skeletal states, described earlier in this book.

The malformations made up a relatively small variety and could be almost completely divided into those caused by direct embryotoxic action of the chemical agents and those due indirectly to their diabetogenic repercussion. If any relation is to be sought between the human and animal effects of maternal diabetes and insight gained into the fundamentals of their occurrence, it is only those of indirect origin that can be relevant. In studies in which malformations of this origin were produced, the most often occurring, and which perhaps represented a "characteristic" cluster, were neural tube, ventral body wall, and mandible.

Many congenital malformations are said to be more common, some of them far more common, in the newborn children of women with diabetes than in those from normal pregnancies (eg, Greene 1989, Combs and Kitzmiller 1991). (These repeatedly cited statistics are largely based on a comparison of hospital series of diabetic pregnancies with wholly inappropriate and faulty control data [Kučera 1971a] and hence are untrustworthy, as often stated previously.) Of this large variety of malformations only a small number, however, are held to be part of the constellation—the so-called diabetic embryopathy—that denotes it as diabetes-specific, prominent among them holoprosencephaly and certain lower vertebral defects. The first of these, or any variety of this condition, was never reported in experimental studies of diabetic pregnancy. The second one occurred frequently.

The human malformation whose analogue the animal skeletal defects in question is assumed to be is absence of sacral vertebrae. It has the distinction of being considered the most common one; that is, the ratio of its occurrence in diabetic vis-à-vis nondiabetic pregnancies is greatest of any defect. This malformation, held to be foremost among the hallmarks of the embyropathic effects of human maternal diabetes, was the focus of many of the experimental studies already discussed, in their endeavor to reproduce it in the offspring of the diabetic animals. But as noted frequently, the analogy is false, since absence of lower vertebral elements in offspring of diabetic animals was invariably due to retarded fetal development, and where continued growth was permitted the supposedly missing ossification centers had appeared by the time birth approached.

Insulin was administered to diabetic animals in several studies (Horii et al. 1966, Baker et al. 1981, Eriksson et al. 1982, Wilson et al. 1985, Tanigawa et al. 1991). In one, in which diabetes was induced before conception (Eriksson et al. 1982), insulin almost entirely prevented the defects produced by the maternal diabetes: micrognathia and "caudal dysgenesis." The latter consisted of missing caudal vertebrae and "lack of the tail." But it is likely that it was absent only in the sense that no ossification sites were visible in it. That this defect was prevented by insulin was thus no doubt due to restored fetal growth. The prevention of the other defect, micrognathia, was apparently real. But its frequency in noninsulin-supplemented instances decreased with advancing fetal age, perhaps indicating that this defect also had some growth-retarded aspects. In the other preconception study (Tanigawa et al. 1991), skeletal defects were not prevented, but were induced, which was imputed to the hypoglycemic effects of the insulin.

In a study in which alloxan was given before implantation, insulin prevented the very low percentage of various axial skeletal ones and also all but prevented the neural tube and facial defects (Horii et al. 1966). STZ administered soon after implantation, that is, at an early embryonic stage, apparently caused only defects of the lower vetebral column, and insulin, not surprisingly, since it improved fetal growth, lowered the frequency of the defects (Baker et al. 1981). Finally, following treatment soon after implantation, a single day of insulin treatment reversed the retarded ossification and mitigated the teratogenic effects (Wilson et al. 1985). Because at least some of the teratological results of these studies probably had an indirect basis, their mitigation or prevention by insulin largely supports the separability of the direct and indirect effects of diabetogens.

Whether diabetes induced by cytotoxic chemicals in mice and rats is a suitable counterpart of human type 1 diabetes for studying and clarifying some of its outstanding problems is still not fully agreed upon. What seems indisputable is that the abnormalities of the vertebral column in offspring of animals with this diabetes are temporary by-products of fetal growth retardation and do not correspond at all to the sacral abnormality in children of diabetic women. With respect to the malformations in the animals, most of the relatively small variety they consist of are not among the ones occurring frequently in children. Even putting this fact aside, it is still to be proved whether these teratological experiments, indeed whether the diabetes induced, have any relevance for the investigation of human diabetic pregnancy.

So far as the experiments themselves are concerned, it is abundantly clear that the induction of diabetes by chemicals is often inefficient and that, when induced, the diabetes is frequently not teratogenic or only weakly teratogenic. Finally, facts such as the poor relation between maternal blood glucose level and teratogenesis, and that animal stocks made equally hyperglycemic by diabetogens nevertheless differ in teratologic susceptibility, throw profound doubt on the concept that puts the entire blame upon hyperglycemia for harming embryos and the belief that management of the human disease is the preventive formula.[13]

13 A version of this chapter appeared in *Reproductive Toxicology*, vol. 10, pp. 417–438, 1996.

19

IS DIABETES TERATOGENIC?

> It is of use, from time to time, to take stock, so to speak, of our knowledge of a particular disease, to see exactly where we stand in regard to it, to inquire to what conclusions the accumulated facts seem to point, and to ascertain in what direction we may look for fruitful investigations in the future (Osler 1885).

INTRODUCTION

The basis of the supposed cause of congenital malformations by maternal diabetes, as the orderly mind conceives it, must be either genetic or not genetic. Let us consider that the former is true. If so, the instrumentality may be construed as analogous to the hereditary pattern of insulin-dependent diabetes mellitus itself, which probably has a multifactorial mode of transmission (Neel 1970, Vadheim and Rotter 1989). But serious inquiry into whether genetic factors play some role in the occurrence of these phenomena has never been made, such as by familial studies of malformations in sibs of affected individuals born before the clear advent of maternal diabetes, or of like patterns of malformations in offspring of maternal nondiabetic sibs, and so on.

As it happens, a certain consistent finding overleaped the question and made speculation unnecessary, namely that the frequency of congenital malformations in the children of prediabetic women or, even more conclusively, in those of insulin-dependent diabetic men does not exceed that in the overall population (Koller 1953, Rubin 1958a, Hagbard 1959, Neave 1967, White 1971, Chung and Myrianthopoulos 1975b, Theile et al. 1985). So, the reasoning goes, it cannot be the diabetes-related genes diabetic mothers transmit to their children that are the reason for the increased risk of congenital malformations, because children also inherit such genes from diabetic fathers (El-Hashimy et al. 1995). The proneness to maldevelopment must therefore be due to nongenetic, that is, environmental, forces.

The knowledge that congenital malformations may be caused by environmental forces was only very recently acquired. Previously, it was largely taken for granted that human and other mammalian embryos were sheltered from external damage and that prenatal maldevelopment must be genetic in origin.

Observation of congenital malformations in human beings is as old as recorded history (Martin 1880, Ballantyne 1894, Warkany 1977), but extensive and detailed description and analysis of these phenomena, intermingled with inquiries into their origins, began only in the 19th century (Saint-Hilaire 1832, Ballantyne 1902, Schwalbe 1906, Mall 1908). Full realization that human maldevelopment can be caused extrinsically (aside from various superstitious notions [Glenister 1964]) only dawned with the discovery that therapeutic x-irradiation can be teratogenic (Goldstein and Murphy 1929, Murphy 1929). But this was little regarded, because that causative agency was felt to be unnatural and hence hardly physiologically relevant.

This attitude very soon greatly altered when it was announced just a few years later that rubella, or German measles, a common infectious disease, and a long-standing part of humankind's everyday surroundings, an epidemic of which had struck wartime Australia, caused congenital abnormalities in offspring of infected pregnant women in that country (Gregg 1941). The final stroke, forcing the most reluctant skeptic to accept that environmental factors were capable of gravely damaging human embryos, came with the revelation that what had been considered to be a relatively harmless sedative, thalidomide, had caused devastating malformations (Lenz 1961, McBride 1961). In addition, several other environmental agents and situations have been confirmed to be human teratogens, as noted in an authoritative summary of the contemporary understanding of the causation of congenital malformations in human beings (Kalter and Warkany 1983).

DIABETES AND MALFORMATIONS

Can type 1 diabetes mellitus be considered one such cause? Many authors have thought so; some, exposing their naiveté, have even written that "maternal diabetes is the only proven teratogen" (Kotzot et al. 1993). Some have provided a long list of defects so caused (eg, Reece and Hobbins 1986) and loftily expounded on their etiology, mechanisms, and metabolic basis (Hoet, 1986, Freinkel 1989, Cousins 1991b, Goto and Goldmann 1994, Sadler et al. 1995).

A small number of authors, especially from the past, were more circumspect, and expressed doubt. They did this especially by noting the wide range of malformation frequencies, some not varying from normal, which had been found by different studies of the outcomes of diabetic pregnancies (see early review by Kyle 1963). And in trying to explain the reasons for this great variability sounded their many weaknesses. Examples follow.

Some authors may have included every trivial abnormality found on clinical examination, whereas others used technical aids to diagnosis or recorded only the lethal malformations discovered at autopsy. Some have mentioned only those anomalies which are obvious only in the first week whereas others have followed their cases and have added those malformations which were discovered later (Farquhar 1959).

The [congenital malformation] figures vary with the source of information, the completeness of the clinical examination or autopsy, the age of the child at which the review is made, and the definition of a congenital abnormality (Breidahl 1966).

Ces [malformation] variations considérable tiennent aux moyens d'investigation mise en œuvre mais aussi et peut-être surtout à la définition des malformations congénitales, à l'âge du dépistage, à la possibilité de surveillance des infants (Mimouni 1972).

Physicians would be remiss if they failed to appreciate the methodologic shortcomings in available studies. All studies lacked proper controls. Studies usually compared prevalences of anomalies studied prospectively in offspring of mothers with DM to prevalences in controls gathered retrospectively at different times by different investigators who may or may not have utilized identical criteria...no infants were examined in "blind" fashion, i.e., by physicians unaware of whether their mother did or did not have DM. These represent quite serious objections and justify withholding definitive statements concerning the relationship between maternal diabetes and anomalies (Simpson 1978).

No recent findings have made it necessary to alter this declaration.

A further element, at least as capable as those noted above of prejudicing the findings of such inquiries, is nonrandom selection, or biased ascertainment as it is known, of diabetic subjects, as declared in the quotation of Fisher's cited in an earlier chapter. This is not a trivial matter, but the necessity and importance of "neutrality" in this regard have almost never been given due consideration by those dealing with pregnancy outcome of diabetic women. Unbiased ascertainment is the crux in the investigation of the etiology of congenital malformations (Little and Carr-Hill (1984).

THE PRINCIPLES OF TERATOLOGY

Of paramount importance in judging assertions regarding the teratogenicity of diabetes is determining whether this supposed etiological factor conforms with certain teratological principles (Wilson 1973). These were formulated over the years through experimental studies with laboratory animals, and within the limitations imposed by human situations apply as well to people.

These principles are as follows:

(1) Susceptibility to teratogens depends on the genotypes of the conceptus and the gravida.
(2) The nature of the adverse outcome varies with the prenatal stage exposed to the harmful agent and
(3) The nature of the agent,
(4) The latter because agents act in specific ways.
(5) The harmful effects are ultimately expressed as prenatal growth retardation, malformation, death, and functional impairment,
(6) Whose frequency and severity depend on the dosage of the agent.

Because they offer the most abundant and best documented material for analysis, it is the malformations alleged to be caused by maternal insulin-dependent diabetes, the excessive perinatal mortality rate in diabetic pregnancy, and the possible relation between the two, that will be the focus in this chapter.

Teratogens may be considered to be of two sorts, according to the manner pregnant subjects are exposed to them: those to which the subject is exposed once or intermittently, and those present chronically. Examples are therapeutic pharmaceutical agents and environmental pollutants, respectively. The principles just outlined are most clearly seen to apply to the former, but both conform to them.

Not all the principles are well illustrated by human teratogens. There are few explicit examples of the role played by genetics in determining susceptibility. The principle, well known from experimental teratology, that agents that cause maldevelopment at given dosages kill at larger ones (Kalter 1980), has not been able to be confirmed in humans, because dosages of human teratogens have rarely been experienced at levels that might be prenatally lethal. The principles of specificity of timing and response, however, are closely adhered to by teratogens as they act in humans, as illustrated by several examples.

Ionizing irradiation, whether of medical or military origin, displayed its target specificity by almost exclusively causing microcephaly. Its effects, in addition, were time-limited, since the abnormality occurred virtually entirely after exposure in the 6th–11th weeks of pregnancy; and dose-related, as calculated by the relation of offspring head circumference to maternal distance from the Hiroshima atomic-bomb hypocenter (Miller and Blot 1972, Miller and Mulvihill 1976).

Rubella viremia, different from radiation in having a protracted presence during pregnancy, also displayed defect and time specificity by causing a particular combination of congenital abnormalities and those in the majority of cases only when the infection was contracted in the first trimester (eg, Munro et al. 1987). But the nature of the disease did not allow a dose-response analysis of the variability of its consequences (Warkany and Kalter 1961, Warkany, 1971, p. 62 et seq.).

Although suspicion fell early on thalidomide as the cause of an epidemic of limb malformations that were seen in several countries (Lenz 1961, McBride 1961), it took an arduous epidemiological investigation to establish the connection firmly (Weicker 1963, 1969). Various systems were affected, but unusual abnormalities of the limbs were by far the most common (Smithells and Newman 1992). A most meticulous time specificity was discovered to have existed as well, exposure on only the 35th to 50th days after the last menstrual period (23rd to 38th days after conception) being teratogenic, with different parts being affected at different times during this interval (Nowack 1965, Kreipe 1967).

Children of pregnant women with epilepsy who took anticonvulsant drugs in the first trimester had an increased risk of being congenitally malformed, with certain malformations predominating. Risk factors of primary importance were gestation time of exposure, high drug dosage, and the particular anticonvulsant drug used (Janz 1982, Bossi 1983, Kaneko and Kondo 1995).

DOES DIABETES OBEY THE TERATOLOGICAL PRINCIPLES?

The Influence of Genotype

Type 1 diabetes is not always present during all of a woman's reproductive years. Yet seldom have the outcomes of the pregnancies of diabetic women preceding the onset of the disease been mentioned (neglecting the prediabetic misconception), so that it is difficult to say whether an untoward outcome is conditioned by genetic factors. Instances of several pregnancies of diabetic women producing malformed children follow.

Glasgow et al. (1979) saw two women who each twice delivered congenitally malformed children: one, first a baby with cardiovascular abnormalities and then a baby with an accessory auricle and tooth asymmetry (hardly major defects); and the other successively a child with anencephaly, a normal one, one with transposition of the great vessels, and finally another without defects. Coustan et al. (1980) noted one child with an absent tibia who had an older sibling with the same defect (it was unstated whether the mother was also diabetic in the previous pregnancy). Small et al. (1986) reported two sets of malformed siblings, a pair with pyloric stenosis and pulmonary valve disease, and three children with cleft palate, anencephaly, and hypoplastic heart, respectively. Stubbs et al. (1987) noted two women each with a malformed child who had each previously had a malformed baby, but the nature of the older children's defects and whether the mothers were diabetic during those pregnancies were not stated.

The possible intrinsic basis of some diabetes-associated malformations might have been examined by the simple matter of studying the family histories of diabetic women. But such studies have never been performed. Congenital malformations such as pulmonary stenosis, recorded several times as being due to diabetes, have long been known to have a significant familial rate of recurrence (eg, Warkany 1971, p. 549). Numerous other malformations share this propensity.

Specificity of Teratological Response

It has claimed by some, denied by others, and both claimed and denied successively by still others that maternal diabetes is especially associated with an increased frequency of specific congenital malformations, namely, cardiovascular malformations, particularly ventricular septal defect, anencephaly, and certain other malformations of the central nervous system, and abnormalities of the caudal spinal column.

The thoroughgoing review appearing on preceding pages of this work have nullified these claims. In its place is left the belief that there is a general increase in the malformation incidence without a preponderance of any one type of abnormality. The rationale for a nonspecific outcome, as one author put it, would be that "the diabetic state persists throughout pregnancy; thus one could reason that nonspecific anomalies of all organ systems would be expected, in contrast to the specific group of anomalies characteristic of drug- or virus-induced teratogenesis" (Simpson 1978).

This is specious reasoning. With respect first to viral teratogenesis, fetuses may be infected with rubella throughout gestation and be born infected, and yet the teratogenic effects will be related to the stage of gestation at the time of maternal infection (Ueda et al. 1979). Another example of a "chronic" or constitutional teratogenic maternal disease, thus present throughout pregnancy, yet whose embryopathic effects show organ and time specificity, is phenylketonuria (Koch et al. 1994).

Since, as shown in previous pages, diabetes is not associated with a specific constellation of congenital malformations whose analysis could assign particular ones to different susceptible periods of early gestation, it departs in this respect from other human teratogens. It thus does not adhere to the specificity tenet required for being considered a teratogen.

Dose-Response Relation

The dosage of teratogens determines the frequency, type, and severity of the response. Dosages below a threshold level are without apparent harm to embryos; above it the teratological effects are progressively more frequent and severe until prenatal death begins to occur. Death may be due to damage to vital fetal organs, to nonspecific effects of the agent on the conceptus, or to indirect effects of maternal toxicity. But in any particular instance, even in experimental studies, it may not be easy to say which of these avenues is responsible for death (Kalter 1980).

Very early in the study of the outcome of diabetic pregnancy, vigorous attempts were made to relate various features considered to indicate severity of the diabetic state to the high perinatal mortality rates of the day, such as maternal age at onset of the disease, the length of time the disease had endured, required insulin dosage, pathological complications, sex hormone imbalance, and so on. None of these was clearly tied to infant death. But later, closely supervised maternal care and its product, normal or nearly normal blood glucose levels, were noted to be related to improved survival.

The great decline in the death rate beginning about 1950 turned attention to the most prominent remaining lethal factor, malformations; here also attempts were made to find maternal correlates that would give insight to prevention. Taking a hint from the beneficial effects of maternal glycemic control, studies were made of the association of malformation frequency and glucose level in early in pregnancy.

If congenital malformations were caused by maternal diabetes, mediated by maternal carbohydrate imbalance, the degree (ie, "dosage") of this imbalance, gauged by level of glycosylated hemoglobin, should have been correlated with the intensity of the effect, perhaps logarithmically, at least above a threshold, as appears to be the case for adult diabetic complications (Viberti 1995). This proposition was tested by determining the frequency of congenital malformations in diabetic women with different mean levels of this component. But as noted, clear-cut, consistent findings supporting this contention have eluded investigators.

In experimental teratology, the interrelation of malformation frequency and fetal death rate as a response to teratogenic dosage is complex. In some studies the malformation frequency seen at term was reduced by the death and resorption of severely abnormal fetuses induced by larger dosages of the agent; in other studies the malformation frequency and death rate both increased with dosage, indicating nondifferential mortality (Kalter 1980). In diabetic pregnancy the perinatal mortality rate has greatly decreased over time, probably partly owing to improved metabolic management (ie, "lowered dosage"), but the malformation frequency, according to the results outlined in previous chapters, remained constant in surviving offspring. Conforming to the first paradigm, ceteris paribus, the malformation rate should have increased, according to the second it should have decreased. It did neither. This would seem to be further indication of the nonteratogenicity of maternal diabetes.

A SUMMARY OF SORTS

In the present work, evidence as to whether diabetes can cause malformations in the offspring of diabetic women was drawn separately from surviving and nonsurviving offspring. These were considered individually to avoid the confusion introduced by the fact that the frequency of congenital malformations in perinatal mortalities has increased significantly in the last 40 or so years—the consequence of the inverse relation between the rates of malformation and mortality due to the recalcitrance of malformations to prevention.

Congenital malformations in perinatal mortalities were looked into first. The record for all mortalities gave an unambiguous picture. In each decade since early in the insulin era, the frequency of congenital malformations in mortalities was not different from that in perinatal mortalities in the general population (see Table 10.1).

Supplementing this information was that from well-examined autopsy material. When 40 years ago Rubin and Murphy (1958) pointed to autopsies as a means of exploring the effects of maternal diabetes on pregnancy outcome, they were able to identify only three reports of such data, with a mean malformation frequency in the 93 specimens of 22.6%. Time has added many more such studies, but has not changed the outcome. As summarized in Table 10.3 the total number identified that have been autopsied stands at present at 815, with a malformation frequency of 20.2%. Unfortunately in only four of the studies was the vital ingredient of controls examined as well, but the frequency in them of 17.4% provided no evidence that maternal diabetes leads to an increased level of malformations.

It is unfortunate that the rate of autopsies of infants of diabetic pregnancies has greatly diminished in recent years. Of course, the number of diabetic perinatal mortalities is greatly reduced also. Still the scarcity of autopsies is to be deplored because of the possible loss it entails of further evidence regarding effects of diabetes on prenatal development. It may be wishful thinking, however, to expect clarification from this source, since the efficacy of autopsies for ferreting out the causes of death are, as always, so poor these days (Cartlidge et al. 1995).

An unusual matter concerning malformations in autopsied infants from diabetic pregnancies is that, contrary to mortalities in general, there was no temporal increase in their frequency; that in the earliest and in the latest were both about 20%, whereas malformations in general population mortalities showed a manyfold rise over the years (see Table 10.1). Thus, the malformation frequency in autopsies did not vary with the perinatal mortality rate, as it has in overall mortalities. But why it did not is hard to say, except to guess that those autopsied were not always a random sample.

It is also unfortunate (incredible, one should say) that, with rare exceptions, no spontaneous abortuses of diabetic women have been examined for structural abnormalities, despite the valuable indications the study of such material would surely yield of the question here pondered. One says this because of the abundance of abortuses, but especially because malformations in abortuses are far more common than in neonates (Shiota 1993).

Last comes the issue of malformations in surviving offspring. The final account that has emerged from combing through the many studies of every variety that were published in the last 75 or more years was also unmistakable in its meaning. This, too, has told us that congenital malformations are not and never were increased in the children of diabetic women, despite the dramatically lowered perinatal mortality rate in their pregnancies; thus the present "lowered" levels are not the outcome of the great improvements in care of these women.

I have used sources from as many sides of this question as exist. As Gibbon put it long ago, the serious historian "is obliged to consult a variety of testimonies, each of which taken separately is perhaps imperfect and partial." And in sum their testimonies have obliged me to come to this conclusion, done at great peril. Research, someone once said, involves the shedding not the confirmation of our preconceptions.

The overwhelming majority of workers in the field of diabetic pregnancy—obstetricians, diabetologists, metabolists, clinical and experimental teratologists, medical geneticists, epidemiologists, and so on—have never expressed the smallest doubt that type 1 maternal diabetes is teratogenic, that, on the contrary, as some have ventured and others parroted, it causes a two-, four-, sixfold, or even greater elevation in the rate of defects beyond that occurring generally in the population (eg, the very latest, Fraser 1994, Garner 1995, Coustan 1998). And I—an outsider, as they may say—have the impudence to gainsay them all. But I have worked long and diligently and with much circumspection reached this conclusion, and any who will attempt to dispute it must work as hard and long to do so.

APPENDIX. Major Congenital Malformations (MCM) in Liveborn Offspring Not Dying Neonatally, of Unselected, Conventionally Managed Pregestational Diabetic Women[a]

Reference	Years of Survey	Number Offspring	Number MCM	Excluded Abnormalities Named by Author(s)
	America			
1930–1949				
Lavietes et al. 1943	1921–43	19	0	
White and Hunt 1943	1936-42	108	4	2 each: syndactylism, dwarfism, pancreatic cysts, short tendon; 1 each: clubfoot, webbed toes, congenital hip, cretinism, feeblemindedness, angioma, cysts of the mouth, varices of the heart
Palmer and Barnes 1945	1930–44	33	0	Deafness
Randall 1947	1933–46	40	1	Down
Hall and Tillman 1951	1923–46	85	0	
Moss and Mulholland 1951	1929–48	13	0	
Gaspar 1945	1935–44	24	0	
Graham and Lowrey 1953	1947–52	10	0	
McCain and Lester 1950	1932–48	12	0	
Palumbo 1954	1944–53	37	0	
Pedowitz and Shlevin 1952	1932–50	124	2	
Reis et al. 1950	1935–49	66	0	Hypospadias
Whitely et al. 1953	1941–52	58	2	Partial rectal stricture, hypospadias, microcephaly
Total (%)		629	9 (1.4)	
1950–1969				
Dekaban 1959	–	79	2	
Whitehouse et al. 1956	1947–56	61	0	3 hypospadias, cerebral palsy
McLendon and Bottomy 1960	1949–57	121	1	
Moss and Connor 1965	1949–63	77	3	Unilateral polydactyly hand
Stephens et al. 1963	1951–61	100	2	Hypospadias, "inconspicuous fusion of maxilla," unilateral clubfoot
Horger et al. 1967	1955–65	89	1	
Warrner and Cornblath 1969	1966–68	17	0	
Lufkin et al. 1984	1950–79	187	6	4 microcephaly, 2 clubfoot, VSD, PDA, deafness, 7th nerve palsy, undescended testes, congenital cataracts
Total (%)		731	15 (2.0)	
1970 to mid 90s				
Eshai and Gutberlet 1975	1971–73	17	0	Hirschsprung disease
Goldstein et al. 1978	1974–76	29	1	Microcephaly, left colon syndrome, hydrocele, cyanotic CHD

APPENDIX. *continued*

Reference	Years of Survey	Number		Excluded Abnormalities Named by Author(s)
		Offspring	MCM	
Leveno et al. 1979	1974–79	116	1	2 hypospadias, 2 VSD, 4 unspecified limb defects
Martin et al. 1979	1971–77	43	0	2 VSD, PDA, clubfoot, hemangioma
O'Shaughnessy et al. 1979	1978	13	1	
Sehgal 1976	1968–73	18	0	Down
Whittle et al. 1979	–	70	1	Unspecified cardiac anomalies
Coustan et al. 1980	1975–79	56	3	VSD
Skyler et al. 1980	1975–79	18	0	
Lemons et al. 1981	1969–76	81	4	Down, 2 VSD
Tunçer and Tunçer 1981	1970–79	88	3	Urethral stricture, hypospadias, absent metacarpal, syndactyly foot
Bourgeois and Duffer 1990	1980–87	39	0	2 renal dysplasia
Budhraja and Danel 1986	1981–84	48	1	PDA
Johnson et al. 1988	1983–86	47	1	VSD, trisomy 18
Landon et al. 1987	1982–84	74	1	
Clarson et al. 1989	–	19	0	
Landon et al. 1989	1986–87	35	1	
McFarland and Hemaya 1985	1978–83	103	2	Ladd's bands, VSD
Aucott et al. 1994	1984–87	77	3	VSD, clubfoot
Coustan et al. 1986	–	22	0	
Rose et al. 1988	1981–85	71	5	VSD, hydrocephalus + clubfoot
Total (%)		1084	29 (2.7)	
	Europe			
1930–1949				
Barns 1941	1927–40	14	1	
Lawrence and Oakley 1942	1923–41	33	0	Transient congenital morbis cordis
Peel and Oakley 1949	1942–49	107	3	Clubfoot, 2 "CHD", unnamed defect
Andersson 1950	1940–49	27	1	
Koller 1953	1922–49	76	1	
Majewski 1953	1933–52	22	0	
Total (%)	279	6	(2.2)	
1950–1969				
Hagbard 1956	1948–54	308	9	2 ear "deformities"
Pedersen 1954b	1946–53	142	2	
Svanteson 1953	1947–52	14	0	
Constam et al. 1963	1941–63	77	2	Hypospadias, clubfoot, facial weakness + microcephaly, lens subluxation
Komrower and Langley 1961	1951–60	179	4	2 hypospadias, 3 hemangioma

APPENDIX. *continued*

Reference	Years of Survey	Number Offspring	Number MCM	Excluded Abnormalities Named by Author(s)
Sanctis 1969	1967–68	12	1	
Schwartz et al. 1960	–	15	0	Clubfoot
Aubertin et al. 1964	–	72	2	
Bass 1970	1964–69	25	0	Thrombosis renal vein, aneurysm left coronary artery, Down
Slot et al. 1967	1959–66	60	2	Hypospadias, 2 microcornea (sibs), VSD
Bernard and Delahaye–Plouvier 1971	1966–69	43	1	Systolic murmur
Brearley 1975	1961–73	92	2	Clubfoot, hypospadias, PDA, VSD
Degen et al. 1970	1953–65	38	1	2 polydactyly
François et al. 1974a	1958–74	91	1	Dermal sinus, PDA
Grenet et al. 1972	1961–72	130	3	VSD, hypospadias, coloboma, uveitis
Lübken 1970	1959–69	55	1	Clubfoot, brain damage
Manzke et al. 1977	1959–70	58	2	(? 1 diagnosed postneonatally)
Pardou et al. 1977	1964–74	56	1	
Salvioli et al. 1976	1963–72	38	1	
Smorenberg–School et al. 1970	1963–69	80	2	Trisomy 17-18
Steindel and Mohnike 1971	1963–70	97	2	3 VSD, PDA
Total (%)		1682	39 (2.3)	
1970 to mid-90s				
Auinger 1978	1962–77	65	1	Hip dysplasia
Cruveiller et al. 1977	1970-76	71	2	VSD
Goudé et al. 1975	1970–73	9	1	
Wald et al. 1979	–	25	1	
Peacock et al. 1979	–	25	1	Sacral sinus, syndactyly
Airaksinen et al. 1990	1983–97	92	2	Hydrocele, vertebral anomaly
Apeland et al. 1992	1982–90	74	2	2 VSD, PDA
Burkart et al. 1988	1979–86	110	4	Hermaphroditism, clubfoot, VSD
Carta et al. 1986	–	29	1	Patent foramen ovale
Cullimore et al. 1990	1981–85	84	3	Hypertrophic cardiomyopathy
Gregory et al. 1992	1984–90	78	2	
Hawthorne et al. 1994	1977–90	103	3	VSD, hemangioma, nonfunctioning kidney, hypospadias, pilonidal cyst, inguinal hernia + undescended testes, 2 clubfoot, 2 polydactyly, syndactyly, accessory aureoles, single umbilical artery, 2 undescended testes

APPENDIX. *continued*

Reference	Years of Survey	Number Offspring	Number MCM	Excluded Abnormalities Named by Author(s)
Heller et al. 1984	1977–83	58	1	PDA, sacral dimple
Kimmerle et al. 1992	1987–90	85	1	
Duffty and Lloyd 1989	1986–87	45	1	
Gillmer et al. 1984	1980–83	65	1	
Kühl and Møller-Jensen 1989	1982–85	42	0	Hypospadias
Schmid et al. 1984	1972–78	31	0	Dwarfism
Small et al. 1986	1971–84	123	5	2 hypospadias, pyloric stenosis, hydrocele, VSD
Smorenberg-School et al. 1983	1969–82	66	5	
Lizan et al. 1984	1980–83	12	0	VSD
Lloyd and Duffty 1984	1979–82	41	0	
Peck et al. 1991	1979–87	114	1	Thoracic dystrophy, hypospadias, 2 clubfoot
Zanardo et al. 1983	–	18	1	
Visser et al. 1985	–	8	0	
Nielsen and Nielsen 1994	1976–92	264	7	2 VSD, hypoplasia hand + clubfoot
Total (%)		1473	46 (3.1)	

CHD, congenital heart disease; PDA, patent ductus arteriosus; VSD, ventricular septal defect.

[a] Abnormalities excluded are those that author(s) called minor or did not name or specify; also excluded were reports in which results from mortalities and survivors were not given separately and studies of preconception or early-gestation glycemic control.

BIBLIOGRAPHY

Abell DA, Beischer NA. 1975. Evaluation of the three-hour glucose tolerance test in detection of significant hyperglycemia and hypoglycemia in pregnancy. Diabetes 24:874–80.

Abu-Harb M, Hey E, Wren C. 1994. Death in infancy from unrecognised congenital heart disease. Arch Dis Child 71:3–7.

Adashi EY, Pinto H, Tyson JE. 1979. Impact of maternal euglycemia on fetal outcome in diabetic pregnancy. Am J Obstet Gynecol 133:268–74.

Adler P, Fett KD, Bohatka L. 1977. The influence of maternal diabetes on dental development of the non-diabetic offspring in the stage of dental transition. Acta Paediatr Hung 18:181–95.

Airaksinen KEJ, Anttila LM, Linnaluoto MK, et al. 1990. Autonomic influence on pregnancy outcome in IDDM. Diab Care 13:756–61.

Alberman E, Blatchley N, Botting B, et al. 1997. Medical causes on stillbirth certificates in England and Wales: distribution and results of hierarchical classifications tested by the Office for National Statistics. Br J Obstet Gynecol 104:1043–9.

Albert TJ, Landon MB, Wheller JJ, et al. 1996. Prenatal detection of fetal anomalies in pregnancies complicated by insulin-dependent diabetes mellitus. Am J Obstet Gynecol 174:1424–8.

Ales KL, Santini DL. 1989. Should all pregnant women be screened for gestational glucose intolerance? Lancet 1:1187–91.

Algert S, Shragg P, Hollingsworth DR. 1985. Moderate caloric restriction in obese women with gestational diabetes. Obstet Gynecol 65:487–91.

Aliverti V, Bonanomi L, Giavini E, et al. 1979. The extent of fetal ossification as an index of delayed development in teratogenic studies on the rat. Teratology 20:237–42.

Allen, E. 1939. The glycosurias of pregnancy. Am J Obstet Gynecol 38:982–92.

Allen RD, Palumbo PJ. 1987. Respiratory distress and neonatal mortality in infants of diabetic and prediabetic mothers. Acta Diabetol Lat 18:101–6.

Alles AJ, Sulik KK. 1993. A review of caudal dysgenesis and its pathogenesis as illustrated in an animal model. In: Opitz JM, ed. Blastogenesis: normal and abnormal. Wiley-Liss, New York, pp. 83–102.

Altemus LA, Ferguson AD. 1965. Comparative incidence of birth defects in Negro and white children. Pediatrics 36:56–61.

Amendt P. 1975. Die somatisch-geistige Entwicklung von Kindern diabetischer Mütter: Ergebnisse Nachuntersuchung im Alter zwischen 4 bis 16 Jahren. Acta Paediatr Acad Sci Hung 16:299–315.

Amendt P, Gödel E, Amendt U, et al. 1974. Missbildungen bei mütterlichem Diabetes mellitus unter besonderer Berücksichtigung des kaudalen Fehlbildungssyndroms. Zentralbl Gynecol 96:950–8.

American Diabetes Association Workshop-Conference on Gestational Diabetes. 1980. Summary and recommendations. Diab Care 3:499–501.

Ananijevic-Pandey J, Jarebinski M, Kastratovic B, et al. 1992. Case-control study of congenital malformations. Eur J Epidemiol 8:871–4.

Anderson RH. 1984. The morphology of ventricular septal defects. Perspect Paediatr Pathol 8:235–68.

Anderson RH. 1991. Simplifying the understanding of congenital malformations of the heart. Int J Cardiol 32:131–42.

Anderson RH, Lenox CC, Zuberbuhler JE. 1984. The morphology of ventricular septal defects. Perspect Paediatr Pathol 8:235–68.

Andersson B. 1950. Diabetes and pregnancy. Acta Med Scand 138:259–78.

Ando S, Otani H, Tanaka O, et al. 1991. Morphological analysis of neural tube defects in non-obese diabetic (NOD) mouse embryos. Congenital Anom 31:23–32.

Angervall L. 1959. Alloxan diabetes and pregnancy in the rat: effects on the offspring. Acta Endocrinol 31 Suppl 44:1–86.

Angervall RA, Stevenson JA. 1960. Effects of alloxan-induced diabetes on the pregnancy of rats. Am J Obstet Gynecol 80:536–41.

Anon. 1954. Fetal salvage in patients with diabetes mellitus. Am J Obstet Gynecol 67:210-ll.

Anon. 1963. Advance report: final natality statistics, 1962. Mon Vit Stat Rep 12 (6) Suppl (Aug. 20, 1963):1–4.

Anon. 1980. Abnormal infants of diabetic mothers. Lancet 1:633–44.

Anon. 1988. Congenital abnormalities in infants of diabetic mothers. Lancet 1:1313–5.

Anon. 1989. Contribution of birth defects to infant mortality—United States, 1986. MMWR 38:633–5.

Anon. 1990. Cincinnati-Hamilton, OH. US census data. Database: C90STF3C1. Venus Lookup (1.4). http://venus.census.gov/cdrom

Anon. 1991. Maternal mortality surveillance, United States, 1979–1986. MMWR 40 (55–2):1–13.

Anon. 1992. Diagnosing congenital dislocation of the hip. Br Med J 305:435–6.

Anon. 1994. Stratification by size in the epidemiology of ventricular septal defects. EUROCAT 8:1–2.

Apeland T, Bergrem H, Berget M. 1992. Gravide diabetikere: en retrospektiv undersøkelse av svangerskap og fødsel hos type 1-diabetikere i Sør-Rogaland 1982–90. T Norske Laegeforen 112:2520–3.

Arey JB. 1949. Pathologic findings in the neonatal period. J Paediatr 34:44–8.

Armstrong D. 1986. The invention of infant mortality. Sociol Health Illness 8:211–32.

Artal R, Golde SH, Dorey F, et al. 1983. The effect of plasma glucose variability on neonatal outcome in the pregnant diabetic patient. Am J Obstet Gynecol 147:537–41.

Assemany SR, Muzzo S, Gardner LI. 1972. Syndrome of phocomelic diabetic embryopathy (caudal dysplasia). Am J Dis Child 123:489–91.

Aubertin E, Aubertin J, Gay J. 1964. Importance de la valeur du traitement antidiabétique chez les diabétiques enceintes. J Med Bord 141:333–60.

Aucott SW, Williams TG, Hertz RH, et al. 1994. Rigorous management of insulin-dependent diabetes mellitus during pregnancy. Acta Diabetol 31:126–9.

Auinger W. 1978. Diabetes und Schwangerschaft. 1. Mitteilung. Stoffwechselführung und Erfahrungen bei 90 manifest diabetischen Schwangerschaften. Wien Klin Wochenschr 90:109–16.

Ayromlooi J, Mann LI, Weiss RR, et al. 1977. Modern management of the diabetic pregnancy. Obstet Gynecol 49:137–43.

Bachman C. 1952. Diabetes mellitus and pregnancy with special reference to fetal and infantile loss. Am J Med 223:681–93.

Bacigalupa G, Langner K, Saling E. 1984. Glycosylated hemoglobin (HbA_1), glucose tolerance and neonatal outcome in gestational diabetic and non-diabetic mothers. J Perinat Med 12:137–45.

Baird D. 1942. Discussion on stillbirth and neonatal mortality. Proc R Soc Med 36:59–60.

Baird D, Walker J, Thomson AM. 1954. The causes and prevention of stillbirths and first week deaths. Part III. A classification of deaths by clinical cause: the effect of age, parity and length of gestation on death rates by cause. J Obstet Gynecol Br Emp 61:433–48.

Baker L, Egler JM, Klein SH, et al. 1981. Meticulous control of diabetes during organogenesis prevents congenital lumbosacral defects in rats. Diabetes 30:955–9.

Bakketeig LS, Hoffman HJ, Oakley AR. 1984. Perinatal mortality. In: Bracken, MB, ed. Perinatal Epidemiology. Oxford University, New York, pp. 99–151.

Balkau B, King H, Zimmet P, et al. 1985. Factors associated with the development of diabetes in the Micronesian population of Nauru. Am J Epidemiol 122:594–605.

Ballantyne JW. 1894. The teratological records of Chaldea. Teratologia 1:127–42.

Ballantyne JW. 1902. Manual of Antenatal Pathology and Hygiene: The Foetus. Green and Sons, Edinburgh.

Ballantyne JW. 1904. Manual of Antenatal Pathology: The Embryo. Green and Sons, Edinburgh.

Ballard JL, Holroyde J, Tsang RC, et al. 1984. High malformation rates and decreased mortality in infants of diabetic mothers managed after the first trimester of pregnancy (1956–1978). Am J Obstet Gynecol 148:1111–7.

Banta JV, Nichols O. 1969. Sacral agenesis. J Bone Joint Surg 51A:693–703.

Banting FG, Best CH. 1923. The discovery and preparation of insulin. U Toronto Med J 1:94–8.

Barach JH. 1928. Historical facts in diabetes. Ann Med Hist 10:387–401.

Barashnev YI. 1964. Malformations of the fetal brain resulting from alloxan diabetes in the mother. Ark Pat 26:T382–6.

Barlow TG. 1962. Early diagnosis and treatment of congenital dislocation of the hip. J Bone Joint Surg 44B:292–301.

Barnes PH. 1961. Prediabetes and pregnancy. Can Med Assoc J 85:681–8.

Barns HHF. 1941. Diabetes mellitus and pregnancy. J Obstet Gynecol Br Emp 48:707–25.

Barns HHF, Morgans ME. 1948. Prediabetic pregnancy. J Obstet Gynecol Br Emp 55:449–54.

Barns HHF, Morgans ME. 1949. Pregnancy complicated by diabetes mellitus. Br Med J 1:51–4.

Barr M, Burdi MM. 1978. Arhinencephaly and polysplenia syndrome associated with maternal diabetes mellitus. Teratology 17:20A.

Barr, M, Hanson JW, Currey K, et al. 1983. Holoprosencephaly in infants of diabetic mothers. J Paediatr 102:565–8.

Bartelheimer H, Kloos K. 1952 Die Auswirkung des experimentellen Diabetes auf Gravidität und Nachkommenschaft. Z Ges Exp Med 119:246–65.

Basil-Jones BJ. 1949. Diabetes in pregnancy: laboratory assistance. Med J Aust 2:558–64.

Bass G. 1970. Diabetes und Schwangerschaft. Schweiz Rundsch Med Prax 59:69–74.

Beard RW, Hoet JJ. 1982. Is gestational diabetes a clinical entity? Diabetologia 23:307–12.

Beard RW, Oakley NW. 1976. The fetus of the diabetic. In: Beard RW, Nathanielsz PW, eds. Fetal Physiology and Medicine: the basis of neonatology. Saunders, London, pp. 137–57.

Beaufils M. 1990. Prise en charge de l'hypertension chez la femme enceinte diabétique:arterial blood pressure, pregnancy and diabetes. Diab Metab 16:144–8.

Becerra JE, Khoury MJ, Cordero JF, et al. 1990. Diabetes mellitus during pregnancy and risks for specific birth defects: a population-based case-control study. Pediatrics 85:1–9.

Beischer NA, Oats JN, Henry OA, et al. 1991. Incidence and severity of gestational diabetes mellitus according to country of birth in women living in Australia. Diabetes 40:35–8.

Beláustegui A, Ruiz A, Omeñaca F, et al. 1980. Aspectos anatomoclínicos en el recién nacido hijo de madre diabética. An Esp Paediatr 13:101–10.

Bendon RW, Mimouni F, Khoury J, et al. 1990 Histopathology of spontaneous abortion in diabetic pregnancies. Am J Perinatol 7:207–10.

Benirschke K. 1987. You need a sympathetic pathologist: the borderline of embryology and pathology revisited. Teratology 36:389–93.

Benjamin E, Winters D, Mayfield J, et al. 1993. Diabetes in pregnancy in Zuni Indian women. Diab Care 16:1229–35.

Benjamin F, Wilson SJ, Deutsch S, et al. 1986. Effect of advancing pregnancy on the glucose tolerance test and on the 50-g oral glucose load screening test for gestational diabetes. Obstet Gynecol 68:362–5.

Bennett KA, Cheverud JM, Booth SN. 1981. Deciduous tooth dimensions in fetal rhesus monkeys from mothers with induced diabetes. Am J Phys Anthropol 55:411–7.

Bennett PH, Burch TA, Miller M. 1971. Diabetes mellitus in American (Pima) Indians. Lancet 2:125–8.

Bennett PH, Webner C, Miller M. 1978. Congenital anomalies and the diabetic and prediabetic pregnancy. Ciba Found Symp 63:207–25.

Bennewitz HG. 1824. De Diabete Mellito, Graviditatis Symptomate (Diabetes Mellitus: a symptom of pregnancy). Inaugural Dissertation in Medicine, Berlin.

Berdon WE, Slovis TL, Campbell JB, et al. 1977. Neonatal small left colon syndrome: its relationship to aganglionosis and meconium plug syndrome. Radiology 125:457–62.

Berendes HW, Weiss B. 1970. The NIH collaborative study—a progress report. In: Fraser FC, McKusick VA, eds. Congenital Malformations: Proceedings of the Third International Conference. Excerpta Medica, Amsterdam, pp. 293–8.

Berg AT. 1991. Menstrual cycle length and the calculation of gestational age. Am J Epidemiol 133:585–9.

Bergmann RL, Bergmann KE, Eisenberg A. 1984. Offspring of diabetic mothers have a higher risk for childhood overweight than offspring of diabetic fathers. Nutr Res 4:545–52.

Bergqvist N. 1954. The influence of pregnancy on diabetes. Acta Endocrinol 15:166–81.

Bergstein NAM. 1978. The influence of preconceptional glucose values on the outcome of pregnancy. Ciba Found Symp 63:255–64.

Berk MA, Mimouni F, Miodovnik M, et al. 1989. Macrosomia in infants of insulin-dependent diabetic mothers. Pediatrics 83:1029–34.

Berkeley C, Bonney V, MacLeod D. 1938. The Abnormal in Obstetrics. Wood & Co., Baltimore.

Berkowitz GS, Lapinski RH, Dolgin SE, et al. 1993. Prevalence and natural history of cryptorchidism. Pediatrics 92:44–9.

Berkowitz GS, Lapinski RH, Wein R, et al. 1992. Race/ethnicity and other risk factors for gestational diabetes. Am J Epidemiol 135:965–73.

Berkus MD, Langer O. 1993. Glucose tolerance test: degree of glucose abnormality correlates with neonatal outcome. Obstet Gynecol 81:344–8.

Bernard S, Delahaye-Plouvier G. 1971. Pronostic foetal et réanimation néo-natale des enfants nés en milieu opératoire de mères diabétiques: (à propos de 47 observations). Anesth Analg (Paris) 28:563–75.

Berry RJ, Buehler JW, Strauss LT, et al. 1987. Birth weight-specific infant mortality due to congenital anomalies, 1960 and 1980. Public Health Rep 102:169–81.

Bix H. 1933. Über Beziehungen zwischen mütterlichem Diabetes und Riesenkindern. Med Klin 29:50–2.

Blank A, Grave GD, Metzger BE. 1995. Effects of gestational diabetes on perinatal morbidity reassessed. Diab Care 18:127–9.

Bliss M. 1982. The Discovery of Insulin. University of Chicago, Chicago.

Blot H. 1856. De la glycosurie physiologique chez les femmes en couches, les nourrices, et un certain nombre de femmes enceintes. C R Acad Sci 43:676–8.

Blumel J, Evans B, Eggers GWN. 1959. Partial and complete agenesis or malformation of the sacrum with associated anomalies: etiologic and clinical study with special reference to heredity: a preliminary report. J Bone Joint Surg 41A:497–518.

Bone AJ. 1990 Animal models of insulin-dependent diabetes. In: Pickup JC, Williams G, eds. Textbook of Diabetes. Blackwell Scientific, London, pp. 151–63.

Böök J-A, Fraccaro M. 1956. Research on congenital malformations. Etud Neonat 5:39–54.

Borman B, Cryer C. 1990. Fallacies of international and national comparisons of disease occurrence in the epidemiology of neural tube defects. Teratology 42:405–12,

Borrelli M, Bruschin H, Nahas WC, et al. 1985. Sacral agenesis: why is it so frequently misdiagnosed? Urology 26:351–5.

Boscq G. 1979. Diabète et grossesse: réflexions sur la surveillance actuelle des grossesses des diabétiques. Rev Fr Gynecol 74:395–402.

Bossi L. 1983. Fetal effects of anticonvulsants. In: Morselli PL, Pippenger CE, Penry JK, eds. Antiepileptic Drug Therapy in Pediatrics. Raven Press, New York, pp. 37–64.

Bottazzo GF. Banting Lecture. On the honey disease. A dialogue with Socrates. Diabetes 1993;42:778–800.

Bouchardat A. 1875. De la Glycosurie ou Diabète Sucré. Baillière, Paris.

Boué J, Boué A, Lazar P. 1975. Retrospective and prospective epidemiological studies of 1500 karyotyped spontaneous human abortions. Teratology 12:11–26.

Boughton C, Perkins E. 1957. Pregnancy in diabetic women: an analysis of a series. J Obstet Gynecol Br Emp 64:105–12.

Bound JP, Logan WF. 1977. Incidence of congenital heart disease in Blackpool 1957–1971. Br Heart J 39:445–50.

Bourgeois FJ, Duffer J. 1990. Outpatient obstetric management of women with type-1 diabetes. Am J Obstet Gynecol 163:1065–73.

Boutte P, Valla J-S, Lambert J-C, et al. 1985. L'association vater chez un nouveau-né de mère diabétique. Pediatrie 40:219–22.

Bowen BD, Heilbrun N. 1932. Pregnancy and diabetes, with a report of 5 cases and a review of the literature. Am J Med Sci 32:780–811.

Bower C, Stanley F, Connell AF, et al. 1992. Birth defects in the infants of Aboriginal and non-Aboriginal mothers with diabetes in Western Australia. Med J Aust 156:520–4.

Boyd ME, Usher RH, McLean FH. 1983. Fetal macrosomia: prediction, risks, proposed management. Obstet Gynecol 61:715–22.

Brandstrup E, Okkels H. 1938. Pregnancy complicated with diabetes. Acta Obstet Gynecol Scand 18:136–63.

Brearley BF. 1975. The management of pregnancy in diabetes mellitus. Practitioner 215:644–52.

Breidahl HD. 1966. The growth and development of children born to mothers with diabetes. Med J Aust 1:268–70.

Brown ZA, Mills JL, Metzger BE, et al. 1992. Early sonographic evaluation for fetal growth delay and congenital malformations in pregnancies complicated by insulin-requiring diabetes. Diab Care 15:613–9.

Brownscheidle CM. 1986. The BB rat: type I diabetes and congenital malformations. In: Jovanovic L, Peterson CM, Fuhrmann K, eds. Diabetes and Pregnancy: teratology, toxicity and treatment. Praeger, New York, pp. 15–36.

Brownscheidle CM, Davis DL. 1981. Diabetes in pregnancy: a preliminary study of the pancreas, placenta and malformations in the BB Wistar rat. Placenta Suppl 3:203–16.

Brownscheidle CM, Wooten V, Mathieu MH, et al. 1983. The effects of maternal diabetes on fetal maturation and neonatal health. Metabolism 32:148–55.

Brudenell M. 1975. Care of the clinical diabetic woman in pregnancy and labour. In: Sutherland HW, Stowers JM, eds. Carbohydrate Metabolism in Pregnancy and the Newborn. Churchill Livingstone, Edinburgh, pp. 221–9.

Buchanan TA. 1991. Glucose metabolism during pregnancy: normal physiology and implications for diabetes mellitus. Isr J Med Sci 27:432–41.

Buck BJ, Day MB. 1955. Diabetic pregnancies at Hartford Hospital. Conn State Med J 19:458–61.

Budhraja M, Danel I. 1986. Control of overt maternal diabetes during pregnancy in a county hospital. Arch Intern Med 146:311–5.

Bunn HF, Haney DN, Kamin S, et al. 1976. The biosynthesis of human hemoglobin A1c: slow glycosylation of hemoglobin in vivo. J Clin Invest 57:1652–9.

Burck U, Riebel T, Held KR, et al. 1981. Bilateral femoral dysgenesis with micrognathia, cleft palate, anomalies of the spine and pelvis, and foot deformities. Helv Paediatr Acta 36:473–82.

Burkart W, Fischer-Guntenhöner E, Standl, E, et al. 1989. Menarche, Zyklus und Fertilität bei der Diabetikerin. Geburtsh Frauenh 49:149–54.

Burkart W, Hanker JP, Schneider HP. 1988. Complications and fetal outcome in diabetic pregnancy: intensified conventional versus insulin pump therapy. Gynecol Obstet Invest 26:104–12.

Burt RL. 1956. Peripheral utilization of glucose in pregnancy. III. Insulin tolerance. Obstet Gynecol 7:658–65.

Burt RL. 1960. Carbohydrate metabolism in pregnancy. Clin Obstet Gynecol 3:310–25.

Butler NR, Alberman ED, eds. 1969. Perinatal Problems: The Second Report of the 1958 British Perinatal Mortality Survey. Livingstone, Edinburgh.

Butler NR, Bonham DG. 1963. Perinatal Mortality: The First Report of the 1958 British Perinatal Mortality Survey. Livingstone, Edinburgh.

Buyse ML, ed. 1990. Birth Defects Encyclopedia. Center for Birth Defects Information Services, Dover, Massachusetts.

Bye A, Henderson-Smart DJ, Storey B, et al. 1980. Incidence of the respiratory distress syndrome in infants of diabetic mothers: perinatal influences. Aust NZ J Obstet Gynecol 20:99–102.

Calle EE, Khoury MJ. 1991. Completeness of the discharge diagnoses as a measure of birth defects recorded in the hospital birth record. Am J Epidemiol 134:69–77.

Calzolari E, Contiero MR, Roncarati E, et al. 1986. Aetiological factors in hypospadias. J Med Genet 23:333–7.

Camerini-Dávalos RA. 1964. Prediabetes. In: Danowski TS, ed. Diabetes Mellitus: diagnosis and treatment. American Diabetes Association, New York, pp. 195–9.

Campbell DM, Bewsher PD, Davidson JM, et al. 1974. Day-to-day variations in fasting plasma glucose and fasting plasma insulin levels in late normal pregnancy. J Obstet Gynecol Br Commonw 81:615–21.

Campbell LV, Ashwell SM, Borkman M, et al. 1992. White coat hyperglycaemia: disparity between diabetes clinic and home blood glucose concentrations. Br Med J 305:1194–6.

Campbell S, Pearce JM. 1983. Ultrasound visualization of congenital malformations. Br Med Bull 39:322–31.

Cardell BS. 1953. The infants of diabetic mothers: a morphological study. J Obstet Gynecol Br Emp 60:834–53.

Carlgren L-E. 1959. The incidence of congenital heart disease in children born in Gothenburg 1941–1950. Br Heart J 21:40–50.

Carpenter MW, Coustan DR. 1982. Criteria for screening tests for gestational diabetes. Am J Obstet Gynecol 144:768–73.

Carr DH. 1983. Cytogenetics of human reproductive wastage. In: Kalter H, ed. Issues and Reviews in Teratology. Vol. l. Plenum Press, New York, pp. 33–72.

Carrington ER. 1960. The effect of maternal prediabetes. Clin Obstet Gynecol 3:911–20.

Carta Q, Meriggi E, Trossarelli GF, et al. 1986. Continuous subcutaneous insulin infusion versus intensive conventional insulin therapy in type I and type II diabetic pregnancy. Diabete Metab 12:121–9.

Cartlidge PH, Dawson, AT, Stewart JH, et al. 1995. Value and quality of perinatal and infant postmortem examinations: cohort analysis of 400 consecutive deaths. Br Med J 310:155–7.

Casey BM, Lucas MJ, McIntire DD, et al. 1997. Pregnancy outcomes in women with gestational diabetes compared with the general obstetric population. Obstet Gynecol 90:869–73.

Chappard D, Lauras B, Fargier P, et al. 1983. Sirénomélie et dysplasie rénale multikystique. J Genet Hum 31:403–11.

Chappiet. 1907. Contribution à l'étude des rapports du diabéte sucré et de la puerpéralité. Thése de Paris.

Chartrel NC, Clabaut MT, Boismare FA, et al. 1990. Uteroplacental hemodynamic disturbances in establishment of fetal growth retardation in streptozotocin-induced diabetic rats. Diabetes 39:743–6.

Chase HC. 1967. International comparison of perinatal and infant mortality: the United States and six west European countries. U.S. Government Printing Office, Washington, DC.

Chauhan SP, Perry KG Jr, McLaughlin BN, et al. 1996. Diabetic ketoacidosis complicating pregnancy. J Perinatol 16:173–5.

Chávez GF, Cordero JF, Becerra JE. 1988. Leading congenital malformations among minority groups in the United States, 1981–1986. MMWR 37:17–24.

Christianson RE, van den Berg BJ, Milkovitch L, et al. 1981. Incidence of congenital anomalies among white and black live births with long-term follow-up. Am J Public Health 71:1333–41.

Chung CS, Myrianthopoulos NC. 1975a. Factors affecting risks of congenital malformations. I. Epidemiological analysis. Birth Defects 11(10):1–22.

Chung CS, Myrianthopoulos NC. 1975b. Factors affecting the risks of congenital malformations. II. Effect of maternal diabetes on congenital malformations. Birth Defects 11(10):23–37.

Churchill HA, Berendes HW, Nemore J. 1969. Neuropsychological deficits in children of diabetic mothers: a report from the Collaborative Study of Cerebral Palsy. Am J Obstet Gynecol 105:257–68.

Clarson C, Tevaarwerk GJ, Harding PG, et al. 1989. Placental weight in diabetic pregnancies. Placenta 10:275–82.

Claye AM, Craig WS. 1959. Pregnancy complicated by diabetes mellitus: a study in combined obstetric and paediatric management. Arch Dis Child 34:312–7.

Clayton SG. 1956. The pregnant diabetic: a report on 200 cases. J Obstet Gynecol Br Emp 63:532–41.

Cobley JF, Lancaster HO. 1955. Carbohydrate tolerance in pregnancy. Med J Aust 1:171–5.

Cocilovo G. 1989. Screening for gestational diabetes: an update. In: Morsiani, M, ed. Epidemiology and Screening of Diabetes. CRC, Boca Raton, Florida, pp. 69–75.

Coetzee EJ, Jackson WP. 1979. Metformin in management of pregnant insulin-dependent diabetics. Diabetologia 16:241–5.

Coffey VP. 1974. Twenty-one years' study of anencephaly in Dublin. Ir Med J 67:553–8.

Cohen MM. 1989. Perspectives on holoprosencephaly. III. Spectra, distinctions, continuities and discontinuities. Am J Med Genet 34:271–88.

Cohn JA, Cerami A. 1979. The influence of genetic background on the susceptibility of mice to diabetes induced by alloxan and on recovery from alloxan diabetes. Diabetologia 17:187–91.

Coleman DL. 1982. Diabetes-obesity syndromes in mice. Diabetes 31 Suppl 1:1–6.

Colwell KA, Baldwin VJ, Yong SL. 1991. Sirenomelia and caudal regression—two distinct entities? Teratology 43:420.

Combs CA, Kitzmiller JL. 1991. Spontaneous abortion and congenital malformations in diabetes. Baillière Clin Obstet Gynecol 5:315–31.

Comess LJ, Bennett PH, Burch TA, et al. 1969. Congenital anomalies and diabetes in the Pima Indians of Arizona. Diabetes 18:471–7.

Conn JW, Fajans SS. 1961. The prediabetic state: a concept of dynamic resistance to a genetic diabetogenic influence. Am J Med 31:839–50.

Connell FA, Vadheim C, Emanuel I. 1985. Diabetes in pregnancy: a population-based study of incidence, referral for care, and perinatal mortality. Am J Obstet Gynecol 151:598–603.

Connor EJ. 1967. Congenital malformations in offspring of diabetic mothers. Med Ann DC 36:465–7.

Constam GR, Jost L, Rust T, et al. 1963. Diabetes und Schwangerschaft. Schweiz Med Wochenschr 93:1611–5, 1647–53.

Contreras-Soto J, Forsbach G, Vazquez-Rosales J, et al. 1991. Noninsulin dependent diabetes mellitus and pregnancy in Mexico. Int J Gynecol Obstet 34:205–10.

Cooper MJ, Enderlein MA, Tarnoff H, et al. 1992. Asymmetric septal hypertrophy in infants of diabetic mothers: fetal echocardiography and the impact of maternal diabetic control. Am J Dis Child 146:226–9.

Cordero L, Landon MB. 1993. Infant of the diabetic mother. Clin Perinatol 20:635–48.

Corsello G, Buttita P, Cammarata M, et al. 1990. Holoprosencephaly: examples of clinical variability and etiologic heterogeneity. Am J Med Genet 37:244–9.

Corwin RS. 1979. Pregnancy complicated by diabetes mellitus in private practice: a review of ten years. Am J Obstet Gynecol 134:156–9.

Cossard F, Horovitz J, Mage, P, et al. 1982. La grossesse chez la diabétique. J Gynecol Obstet 11:495–504.

Cousins L. 1987. Pregnancy complications among diabetic women: review 1965–1985. Obstet Gynecol Surv 42:140–9.

Cousins L. 1988. Obstetric complications. In: Reece EA, Coustan, DR, eds. Diabetes Mellitus in Pregnancy: principles and practice. Churchill Livingstone, New York, pp. 455–68.

Cousins L. 1991a. Insulin sensitivity in pregnancy. Diabetes 40:39–43.

Cousins L. 1991b. Etiology and prevention of congenital anomalies among infants of overt diabetic women. Clin Obstet Gynecol 34:481–93.

Cousins L. 1991c. The California Diabetes and Pregnancy Programme: a statewide collaborative programme for the pre-conception and prenatal care of diabetic women. Baillière Clin Obstet Gynecol 5:443–59.

Cousins L, Dattel B, Hollingsworth D, et al. 1985. Screening for carbohydrate intolerance in pregnancy: a comparison of two tests and reassessment of a common approach. Am J Obstet Gynecol 153:381–5.

Cousins L, Key TC, Schorzman L, et al. 1988. Ultrasonic assessment of early fetal growth in insulin-treated diabetic pregnancies. Am J Obstet Gynecol 159:1186–90.

Coustan DR. 1991. Diagnosis of gestational diabetes: what are our objectives? Diabetes 40:14–7.

Coustan DR. 1998. Pre-conception planning: the relationship's the thing. Diab Care 21:887–8.

Coustan DR, Berkowitz R, Hobbins JC. 1980. Tight metabolic control of overt diabetes in pregnancy. Am J Med 68:845–52.

Coustan DR, Lewis SB. 1978. Insulin therapy for gestational diabetes. Obstet Gynecol 51:306–10.

Coustan DR, Nelson C, Carpenter MW, et al. 1989. Maternal age and screening for gestational diabetes: a population-based study. Obstet Gynecol 73:557–61.

Coustan DR, Reece EA, Sherwin RS, et al. 1986. A randomized clinical trial of the insulin pump vs intensive conventional therapy in diabetic pregnancies. JAMA 255:631–6.

Crampton JH, Palmer LJ, Steenrod WJ, et al. 1950. Pregnancy in the diabetic. Proc Am Diabetes Assoc 10:93–99.

Cretius K. 1957. Ist die Geburt eines Riesenkindes Symptom eines mütterlichen Prädiabetes? Gynaecologia 143:18–32.

Croen LA, Shaw GM, Lammer EJ. 1996. Holoprosencephaly: epidemiologic and clinical characteristics of a California population. Am J Med Genet 64:465–72.

Crook A. 1925. Incidence of glycosuria during pregnancy. Lancet 1:656–8.

Crosse VM, Mackintosh JM. 1954. Perinatal mortality. In: Recent Advances in Paediatrics. Little, Brown, Boston, pp. 63–86.

Cruveiller J, Véron P, Benichou J-E. 1977. Embryofoetopathie diabétique: à propos de cent observations. Sem Hop 53:3217–26.

Cullimore J, Roland J, Turner G. 1990. The mangement of diabetic pregnancy in a regional centre: a five year review. J Obstet Gynecol 10:171–5.

Cummins M, Norrish M. 1980. Follow-up of children of diabetic mothers. Arch Dis Child 55:259–64.

Cunningham GF, MacDonald PC, Leveno K.J, et al. 1993. William Obstetrics. Appleton & Lange, Norwalk, Connecticut.

Cunningham MD, McKean HE, Gillispie DH, et al. 1982. Improved prediction of fetal lung maturity in diabetic pregnancies: a comparison of chromatographic methods. Am J Obstet Gynecol 142:197–204.

Curet LB, Izquierdo L, Gilson G, et al. 1992. Perinatal outcome and diabetes mellitus. Am J Obstet Gynecol 166:307.

Czeizel A, Keller S, Bod M. 1983. An etiological evaluation of increased occurrence of congenital limb reduction abnormalities in Hungary, 1975–1978. Int J Epidemiol 12:445–9.

D'Esopo DA, Marchetti AA. 1942. The causes of fetal and neonatal mortality. Am J Obstet Gynecol 44:1–22.

Daentl DL, Smith, DW, Scott CI, et al. 1975. Femoral hypoplasia-unusual facies syndrome. J Paediatr 86:107–11.

Damm P, Mølsted-Pedersen L. 1989. Significant decrease in congenital malformations in newborn infants of an unselected population of diabetic women. Am J Obstet Gynecol 161:1163–7.

Dampeer TK. 1958. Diabetes and pregnancy. J La State Med Soc 110:350–4.

Dandona P, Boag F, Fonseca V, et al. 1986. Diabetes mellitus and pregnancy. N Engl J Med 314:58.

Dandrow RV, O'Sullivan JB. 1966. Obstetric hazards of gestational diabetes. Am J Obstet Gynecol 96:1144–7.

David MP, Fein A. 1974. Sirenomelia: report of a case with thoughts on the teratogenic mechanism. Obstet Gynecol 44:91–8.

Davis WS, Allen RP, Favara BE, et al. 1974. Neonatal small left colon syndrome. Am J Roentgenal 120:322–9.

Davis WS, Campbell JB. 1975. Neonatal small left colon syndrome: occurrence in asymptomatic infants of diabetic mothers. Am J Dis Child 129:1024–7.

Davison JM, Lovedale C. 1974. The excretion of glucose during normal pregnancy and after delivery. J Obstet Gynecol 81:30–4.

Day RE, Insley J. 1976. Maternal diabetes mellitus and congenital malformation: survey of 205 cases. Arch Dis Child 51:935–8.

Degen R, Scholz G, Kunze C. 1970. Die Früh- und Spätprognose von Kindern diabetischer Mütter. Pädiatrie 9:265–76.

Dekaban AS. 1959. The outcome of pregnancy in diabetic women. II. Analysis of clinical abnormalities and pathologic lesions in offspring of diabetic mothers. J Paediatr 55:767–76.

Delaney JJ, Ptacek J. 1970. Three decades of experience with diabetic pregnancies. Am J Obstet Gynecol 106:550–6.

DeMyer W, Zeman W. 1963. Alobar holoprosencephaly (arhinencephaly) with median cleft lip and palate: clinical, electroencephalographic and nosologic considerations. Conf Neurol 23:1–36.

DeMyer W, Zeman W, Palmer CG. 1964. The face predicts the brain: diagnostic significance of median facial anomalies for holoprosencephaly (arhinencephaly). Pediatrics 34:256–63.

Deuchar EM. 1977. Embryonic malformations in rats, resulting from maternal diabetes: preliminary observations. J Embryol Exp Morphol 41:93–9.

deVries PA. 1980. The pathogenesis of gastroschisis and omphalocele. J Paediatr Pathol 15:245–51.

Diabetes Control and Complications Trial Research Group. 1996. Pregnancy outcomes in the Diabetes Control and Complications Trial. Am J Obstet Gynecol 174:1343–53.

Diabetic Pregnancy Study Group of the European Association for the Study of Diabetes. 1989. A prospective multicentre study to determine the influence of pregnancy upon the 75-g oral glucose tolerance test (OGTT). In: Sutherland HW, Stowers JM, Pearson DW, eds. Carbohydrate Metabolism in Pregnancy and the Newborn. V. Springer, New York, pp. 209–26.

Diamond MP, Moley KH, Pellicer A, et al. 1989. Effects of streptozotocin- and alloxan-induced diabetes mellitus on mouse follicular and early embryo development. J Reprod Fertil 86:1–10.

Dicker D, Feldberg D, Karp M, et al. 1987. Preconceptional diabetes control in insulin-dependent diabetes mellitus patients with continuous subcutaneous insulin infusion therapy. J Perinat Med 15:161–7.

Dicker D, Feldberg D, Samuel N, et al. 1988. Spontaneous abortion in patients with insulin-dependent diabetes mellitus: the effect of preconceptional diabetic control. Am J Obstet Gynecol 158:1161–4.

DiGeorge AM. 1968. Congenital absence of the thymus and its immunological consequences: concurrence with congenital hypoparathyroidism. Birth Defects 4(1):116–21.

Dippel AL. 1934. Death of foetus in utero. Bull Johns Hopkins Hosp 54:24–47.

Doery JC, Edis K, Healy, D, et al. 1989. Very high prevalence of gestational diabetes in Vietnamese and Cambodian women. Med J Aust 151:11.

Dolger H, Bookman JJ, Nechemias C, et al. 1966. The need for modification of the classification of diabetes in pregnancy. Diabetes 15:532.

Dolk H, De Wals P, Gillerot Y, et al. 1991. Heterogeneity of neural tube defects in Europe: the significance of site of defects and presence of other major anomalies in relation to geographic differences in prevalence. Teratology 44:547–59.

Dooley SL, Metzger BE, Cho NH. 1991. Gestational diabetes mellitus: influence of race on disease prevalence and perinatal outcome in a U.S. population. Diabetes 40:25–9.

Downing DF, Goldberg H. 1956a. Cardiac septal defects. I. Ventricular septal defect: analysis of one hundred cases studied during life. Dis Chest 29:475–91.

Downing, DF, Goldberg H. 1956b. Cardiac septal defects. II. Atrial septal defect: analysis of one hundred cases studied during life. Dis Chest 29:492–507.

Dowse GK, Spark RA, Mavo B, et al. 1994. Extraordinary prevalence of non-insulin-dependent diabetes mellitus and bimodal plasma glucose in the Wanigela people of Papua New Guinea. Med J Aust 160:767–74.

Drexel H, Bichler A, Sailer S, et al. 1988. Prevention of perinatal morbidity by tight metabolic control in gestational diabetes mellitus. Diab Care 11:761–8.

Driscoll SG. 1965. The pathology of pregnancy complicated by diabetes mellitus. Med Clin North Am 49:1053–67.

Driscoll SG, Benirschke K, Curtis GW. 1960. Neonatal deaths among infants of diabetic mothers: postmortem findings in ninety-five infants. Am J Dis Child 100:818–35.

Drury MI. 1961. Diabetes mellitus complicating pregnancy. Ir J Med Sci 6th ser, No. 430:425–33.

Drury MI. 1966. Pregnancy in the diabetic. Diabetes 15:830–5.

Drury MI. 1979. Pregnancy in the clinical diabetic: a personal experience of 739 cases. Ir J Med Sci 148:75–9.

Drury MI. 1986. Management of the pregnant diabetic patient: are the pundits right? Diabetologia 29:10–2.

Drury MI. 1989. "They give birth astride of a grave." Diab Med 6:291–8.

Drury MI, Greene AT, Stronge JM. 1977. Pregnancy complicated by clinical diabetes mellitus: a study of 600 pregnancies. Obstet Gynecol 49:519–22.

Drury MI, Stronge JM, Foley ME, et al. 1983. Pregnancy in the diabetic patient: timing and mode of delivery. Obstet Gynecol 62:279–82.

Drury TF, Powell AL. 1987. Prevalence of known diabetes among black Americans. U.S. Public Health Service, Hyattsville, Maryland.

Duffty P, Lloyd DJ. 1989. The infant of the diabetic mother: recent experience. In: Sutherland HW, Stower JM, Pearson DW, eds. Carbohydrate Metabolism in Pregnancy in the Newborn. IV. Springer, London, pp. 327–32.

Duhamel B. 1959. Malformations ano-rectales et anomalies vertébrales. Arch Fr Paediatr 16:534–40.

Duhamel B. 1961. From the mermaid to anal imperforation: the syndrome of caudal regression. Arch Dis Child 36:152–5.

Duncan EH, Baird D, Thomson AM. 1952. The causes and prevention of stillbirths and first week deaths. I. The evidence of vital statistics. J Obstet Gynecol Br Emp 59:183–96.

Duncan JM. 1882. On puerperal diabetes. Trans Obstet Soc Lond 24:256–85.

Dundan S, Murphy A, Rafferty J, et al. 1974. Infants of diabetic mothers. J Ir Med Ass 67:371–5.

Dunn JS, McLetchie NGB. 1943. Experimental alloxan diabetes in the rat. Lancet 2:384–7.

Dunn PM. 1964. Congenital malformations and maternal diabetes. Lancet 2:644–5.

Dunn PM. 1989. Baron Dupuytren (1777–1835) and congenital dislocation of the hip. Arch Dis Child 64:969–70.

Eastman JR, Escobar V. 1978. Femoral hypoplasia-unusual facies syndrome: a genetic syndrome? Clin Genet 13:72–6.

Eastman NJ. 1946. Diabetes mellitus and pregnancy: a review. Obstet Gynecol Surv 1:3–31.

Edmonds LD, Layde PM, James LM, et al. 1981. Congenital malformations surveillance: two American systems. Int J Epidemiol 10:247–52.

Edouard L, Alberman E. 1980. National trends in the certified causes of perinatal mortality, 1968 to 1978. Br J Obstet Gynecol 87:833–8.

Edwards JH, Leck I, Record RG. 1964. A classsification of malformations. Act Genet 14:76–90.

Ehrenfest H. 1924. Carbohydrate metabolism during pregnancy and the value of insulin to the obstetrician. Am J Obstet Gynecol 8:685–709.

Ekelund H, Kullander, S, Källén B. 1970. Major and minor malformations in newborns and infants up to one year of age. Acta Paediatr Scand 59:297–302.

El-Hashimy M, Angelico MC, Martin BC, et al. 1995. Factors modifying the risk of IDDM in offspring of an IDDM parent. Diabetes 44:295–9.

Elliott DS, Ulberg LC. 1971 Early embryo development in the mammal. I. Effects of experimental alterations during first cell division in the mouse zygote. J Anim Sci 33:86–95.

Ellison AC, Maren TH. 1972 The effects of metabolic alterations on teratogenesis. Johns Hopkins Med J 130:87–94.

Elwood JH. 1975. Secular trends in the incidence of anencephalus and spina bifida in Belfast and Dublin 1953–1973. Ir J Med Sci 144:388–94.

Elwood JH, Elwood JM. 1984. Investigation of area differences in the prevalence at birth of anencephalus in Belfast. Int J Epidemiol 13:45–52.

Elwood JH, MacKenzie G. 1971. Comparison of secular and seasonal variations in the incidence of anencephalus in Belfast and four Scottish cities 1956–66. Br J Prev Soc Med 25:17–25.

Elwood JM, Elwood JH. 1980. Epidemiology of Anencephalus and Spina Bifida. Oxford University, Oxford, England.

Emanuel I. 1993. Intergenerational factors in pregnancy outcome: implications for teratology? In: Kalter H, ed. Issues and Reviews in Teratology. Vol. 6. Plenum Press, New York, pp. 47–84.

Endo A. 1966 Teratogenesis in diabetic mice treated with alloxan prior to conception. Arch Environ Health 12:492–500.

Endo A, Ingalls TH. 1968 Chromosomal anomalies in embryos of diabetic mice. Arch Environ Health 16:316–25.

Engelhardt W, Schrieber MA, Elser H. 1976. Beobachtungen zum Entbindungszeitpunkt bei 144 Gestations-Diabetikerinnen. Geburts Frauenheilk 36:603–9.

Engleson G, Lindberg T. 1962. Detection of prediabetes by modified Exton-Rose glucose tolerance test sensitised by cortisone. Acta Obstet Gynecol Scand 41:321–7.

Erhardt CL, Nelson FG. 1964. Reported congenital malformations in New York City, 1958–1959. Am J Public Health 54:1489–1506.

Erickson JD. 1976. Racial variations in the incidences of congenital malformations. Ann Hum Genet 39:315–20.

Erickson JD. 1991. Risk factors for birth defects: data from the Atlanta Birth Defects Case-Control Study. Teratology 43:41–51.

Erickson JD, Mulinare J, McClain PW, et al. 1984a. Vietnam veterans' risk for fathering babies with birth defects. JAMA 252:903–12.

Erickson JD, Mulinare JD, McClain, PW, et al. 1984b. Vietnam Veterans' Risk of Fathering Babies with Birth Defects. U.S. Department of Health and Human Services, Atlanta.

Eriksson RS, Thunberg L, Eriksson UJ. 1989. Effects of interrupted insulin treatment on fetal outcome of pregnant diabetic rats. Diabetes 38:764–72.

Eriksson UJ. 1984. Diabetes in pregnancy: retarded fetal growth, congenital malformations and feto-maternal concentrations of zinc, copper and manganese in the rat. J Nutr 114:477–84.

Eriksson UJ. 1988. Importance of genetic predispostion and maternal environment for the occurrence of congenital malformations in offspring of diabetic rats. Teratology 37:365–74.

Eriksson UJ, Andersson A, Effendic S, et al. 1980. Diabetes in pregnancy: effects on the foetal and new-born rat with particular regard to body weight, serum insulin concentration and pancreatic contents of insulin, glucagon and somatostatin. Acta Endocrinol 94:354–64.

Eriksson UJ, Bone AJ, Turnbull DM, et al. 1989. Timed interruption of insulin therapy in diabetic BB/E rat pregnancy: effect on maternal metabolism and fetal outcome. Acta Endocrinol 120:800–10.

Eriksson UJ, Dahlström E, Hellerström C. 1983. Diabetes in pregnancy: skeletal malformations in the offspring of diabetic rats after intermittent withdrawal of insulin in early pregnancy. Diabetes 32:1141–5.

Eriksson UJ, Dahlström E, Larsson KS, et al. 1982 Increased incidence of congenital malformations in the offspring of diabetic rats and their prevention by maternal insulin therapy. Diabetes 31:1–6.

Eriksson UJ, Dahlström VE, Lithell HO. 1986. Diabetes in pregnancy: influence of genetic background and maternal diabetic state on the incidence of skeletal malformations in the fetal rat. Acta Endocrinol Suppl 277:66–73.

Eriksson UJ, Jansson L. 1984. Diabetes in pregnancy: decreased placental blood flow and disturbed fetal development in the rat. Paediatr Res 18:735–8.

Eriksson UJ, Lewis NJ, Freinkel N. 1984. Growth retardation during early organogenesis in embryos of experimentally diabetic rats. Diabetes 33:281–4.

Eriksson UJ, Styrud J, Eriksson RS. 1989. Diabetes in pregnancy: genetic and temporal relationships of maldevelopment in the offspring of diabetic rats. In: Sutherland HW, Stowers DW, eds. Carbohydrate Metabolism in Pregnancy and the Newborn. IV. Springer, New York, pp. 51–63.

Eshai R, Gutberlet RL. 1975. The infant of the diabetic mother. Paediatr Ann 4:318–22.

Eshner AA. 1907. The relations between diabetes and pregnancy: with the report of a case of diabetes in which the glycosuria disappeared with the inception of pregnancy and reappeared after delivery. Am J Med Sci 134:375–90.

Essex NL. 1976. Diabetes and pregnancy. Br J Hosp Med 15:333–44.

Essex NL, Pyke DA. 1979. Management of maternal diabetes in pregnancy. In: Sutherland HW, Stowers JM, eds. Carbohydrate Metabolism in Pregnancy and the Newborn. Springer, Berlin, pp. 357–68.

Essex NL, Pyke DA, Watkins PJ, et al. 1973. Diabetic pregnancy. Br Med J 4:89–93.

Eunpu DL, Zackai EH, Mennuti MT. 1983. Neural tube defects, diabetes, and serum α-fetoprotein screening. Am J Obstet Gynecol 147:729–30.

EUROCAT Working Group. 1991. Prevalence of neural tube defects in 20 regions of Europe and the impact of prenatal diagnosis, 1980–1986. J Epidemiol Comm Health 45:52–8.

Evans JR, Rowe RD, Keith JD. 1960. Spontaneous closure of ventricular septal defects. Circulation 22:1044–54.

Fadel HE, Hammond SD, Huff TA, et al. 1979. Glycosylated hemoglobins in normal pregnancy and gestational diabetes mellitus. Obstet Gynecol 54:322–6.

Farmer G, Russell G. 1984. Indices of fetal growth and neonatal morbidity in relation to glucose tolerance during pregnancy. In: Sutherland HW, Stowers JM, eds. Carbohdrate Metabolism in Pregnancy and the Newborn. Churchill Livingstone, Edinburgh, pp. 190–4.

Farmer G, Russell G, Hamilton-Nicoli DR, et al. 1988. The influence of maternal glucose metabolism on fetal growth, development and morbidity in 917 singleton pregnancies in nondiabetic women. Diabetologia 31:134–41.

Farquhar JW. 1959. The child of the diabetic woman. Arch Dis Child 34:76–96.

Farquhar JW. 1965. The influence of maternal diabetes on foetus and child. In: Gairdner D, ed. Recent Advances in Paediatrics, vol. 3. Little, Brown, Boston, pp. 121–53.

Farquhar JW. 1969a. The infant of the diabetic mother. Postgrad Med J Suppl 45:806–11.

Farquhar JW. 1969b. Prognosis for babies born to diabetic mothers in Edinburgh. Arch Dis Child 44:36–47.

Feigenbaum A, Chitayat D, Robinson B, et al. 1996. The expanding clinical phenotype of the tRNA$^{Leu(UUR)}$ A→G mutation at np 3243 of mitochondrial DNA: diabetic embryopathy associated with mitochondrial cytopathy. Am J Med Genet 62:404–9.

Feldt RH, Avasthey P, Yoshimasu F, et al. 1971. Incidence of congenital heart disease in children born to residents of Olmsted County, Minnesota, 1959–1969. Mayo Clin Proc 46:794–9.

Feller A, Sternberg H. 1931. Zur Kenntnis der Fehlbildungen der Wirbelsäule. III. Mitteilung. Über den vollständigen Mangel der unteren Wirbelsäulenabschnitte und seine Bedeutung für die formale Genese der Defektbildungen des hinteren Körperendes. Virchow Arch Pathol 280:649–92.

Fenichel P, Hieronimus S, Bourlon F, et al. 1990. Macrosomie du foetus de mère diabétique. Presse Méd 19:255–8.

Ferencz C, Rubin JD, McCarter RJ, et al. 1985. Congenital heart disease: prevalence at livebirth: the Baltimore-Washington Infant Study. Am J Epidemiol 121:31–3.

Ferencz C, Rubin JD, McCarter RJ, et al. 1987. Cardiac and noncardiac malformations: observations in a population-based study. Teratology 35:367–78.

Ferencz C, Rubin JD, McCarter RL, et al. 1990. Maternal diabetes and cardiovascular malformations: predominance of double outlet right ventricle and truncus arteriosus. Teratology 41:319–26.

Ferret P, Lindan O, Morgans ME. 1950 Pregnancy in insulin-treated alloxan diabetic rats. J Endocrinol 7:100–2.

Fink A. 1955. Die perinatale Sterblichkeit (eine Übersicht über 55 300 Geburten der letzten 20 Jahre). Zentralbl Gynecol 77:1094–1104.

Fischer L. 1935. Riesenkinder bei mütterlichem Diabetes. Zentralbl Gynecol 59:249–60.

Fisher RA. 1934. The effect of methods of ascertainment upon the estimation of frequencies. Ann Eugenics 6:13–25.

FitzGerald MG, Malins JM, O'Sullivan DJ. 1961. Prevalence of diabetes in women thirteen years after bearing a big baby. Lancet 1:1250–2.

Fixler DE, Paster P, Chamberlin M, et al. 1989. Trends in congenital heart disease in Dallas County births 1971–1984. Circulation 81:137–42.

Flynn FV, Harper C, de Mayo P. 1953. Lactosuria and glycosuria in pregnancy and the puerperium. Lancet 2:698–704.

Foglia VG, Heller CL, Becu-Villalobos D, et al. 1987. Neuroendocrine changes in female rats born from streptozotocin-diabetic mothers. Horm Metab Res 19:545–8.

Formby B, Schmid-Formby F, Jovanovic L, et al. 1987. The offspring of the female diabetic "nonobese diabetic" (NOD) mouse are large for gestational age and have elevated pancreatic insulin content: a new animal model of human diabetic pregnancy. Proc Soc Exp Biol Med 184:291–4.

Forsbach G, Contreras-Soto JJ, Fong G, et al. 1988. Prevalence of gestational diabetes and macrosomic newborns in a Mexican population. Diab Care 11:235–8.

François R, Picaud J-J, Ruitton-Ugliengo A, et al. 1974a. The newborn of diabetic mothers: observations on 154 cases, 1958–1972. Biol Neonat 24:1–31.

François R, Picaud J-J, Ruitton-Ugliengo A, et al. 1974b. Le nouveau-né de mère diabétique (expérience de 168 cas 1958–1974). Diabete 22:69–91.

Frankel AN. 1950. Pregnancy complicated by diabetes. NY State J Med 50:1233–6.

Frantz GH, Aitken GT. 1967. Complete absence of the lumbar spine and sacrum. J Bone Joint Surg 49A:1531–40.

Fraser FC. 1960. Discussion. In: Wolstenholme GE, O'Connor CM, eds. Ciba Foundation Symposium on Congenital Malformations. Little, Brown, Boston, p. 236.

Fraser FC. 1976. The multifactorial/threshold concept—uses and misuses. Teratology 14:267–80.

Fraser R. 1994. Diabetes in pregnancy. Arch Dis Child 71:F224–30.

Fredrikson H, Hagbard L, Olow I, et al. 1957. Efterundersökning av barn till diabetiska Mödrar. Nord Med 57:669–71.

Freinkel N. 1989. The metabolic basis for birth defects in pregnancies complicated by diabetes mellitus. In: Sutherland HW, Stowers JM, Pearson DW, eds. Carbohydrate Metabolism in Pregnancy and the Newborn. IV. Springer, New York, pp. 39–49.

Freinkel N, Gabbe SG, Hadden DR, et al. 1985. Summary and recommendations of the Second International Workshop-Conference on Gestational Diabetes Mellitus. Diabetes 34:123–6.

Freinkel N, Metzger BE, Phelps RL, et al. 1986. Gestational diabetes mellitus: a syndrome with phenotypic and genotypic heterogeneity. Horm Metab Res 18:427–30.

Fritz H, Hess R. 1970. Ossification of the rat and mouse skeleton in the perinatal period. Teratology 3:331–8.

Froehlich LA, Fujikura T. 1969. Congenital malformations in perinatal, infant and child deaths. In: Nishimura H, Miller JR, eds. Methods for Teratological Studies in Experimental Animals and Man. Igaku Shoin, Tokyo, pp. 167–94.

Froewis J, Rogovits N. 1969. Diabetische Schwangerschaft und Geburt. Wien Klin Wochenschr 81:129–35.

Fuhrmann K. 1982. Diabetic control and outcome in the pregnant patient. In: Peterson CM, ed. Diabetes Management in the '80s. Praeger, New York, pp. 66–79.

Fuhrmann K, Reiher H, Semmler K, et al. 1983. Prevention of congenital malformations in infants of insulin-diabetic mothers. Diab Care 6:219–23.

Fuhrmann K, Reiher H, Semmler K, et al. 1986. Congenital anomalies: etiology, prevention, and prenatal diagnosis. In: Jovanovic L, Peterson,CM, Fuhrmann K, eds. Diabetes and Pregnancy: teratology, toxicology and treatment. Praeger, New York, pp. 168–84.

Funaki K, Mikamo K. 1983. Developmental-stage-dependent teratogenic effects in the Chinese hamster. Diabetes 32:637–43.

Futcher PH, Long NW. 1954. Hospital data on the birth of large infants to "prediabetic" women. Bull Johns Hopkins Hosp 94:128–38.

Gabbe SG. 1977. Congenital malformations in infants of diabetic mothers. Obstet Gynecol Surv 32:125–32.

Gabbe SG. 1986. Diabetes mellitus. In: Danforth DN, Scott JR, eds. Obstetrics and Gynecology. Lippincott, Philadelphia, pp. 546–51.

Gabbe SG, Landon MB. 1989. Management of diabetes mellitus in pregnancy: survey of maternal-fetal medicine subspecialists in the United States. In: Sutherland HW, Stowers JM, Pearson DW, eds. Carbohydrate Metabolism in Pregnancy and the Newborn. IV. Springer, London, pp. 309–17.

Gabbe SG, Lowensohn RI, Wu PY, et al. 1978. Current patterns of neonatal morbidity and mortality in infants of diabetic mothers. Diab Care 1:335–9.

Gabbe SG, Mestman JH, Freeman RK, et al. 1977. Management and outcome of class A diabetes mellitus. Am J Obstet Gynecol 127:465–9.

Gamsu HR. 1978. Neonatal morbidity in infants of diabetic mothers. J Roy Soc Med 71:211–22.

Gandhi JA, Zhang XY, Maidman JE. 1995. Fetal cardiac hypertrophy and cardiac function in diabetic pregnancies. Am J Obstet Gynecol 173:1132–6.

Gardner RJ, Veale, AM, Parslow MI, et al. A survey of 972 cytogenetically examined cases of Down's syndrome. NZ Med J 78:403–8.

Garner P. 1995. Type I diabetes mellitus and pregnancy. Lancet 346:157–61.

Garner P, Okun N, Keely E, et al. 1997. A randomized control trial of strict glycemic control and tertiary level obstetric care versus routine obstetric care in the management of gestational diabetes: a pilot study. Am J Obstet Gynecol 177:190–5.

Garner PR, D'Alton ME, Dudley DK, et al. 1990. Preeclamplsia in diabetic pregnancies. Am J Obstet Gynecol 163:505–8.

Gaspar JL. 1945. Diabetes mellitus and pregnancy: a survey of 49 deliveries. West J Surg 53:21–7.

Gaspart E. 1985. Glucose. In: Siest G, Henny J, Schiele F, et al., eds. Interpretation of Clinical Laboratory Tests. Biomedical Publications, Foster City, California, pp. 253–69.

Gellis SS, Hsia DY 1959. The infant of the diabetic mother. Am J Dis Child 97:1–41.

Gendell M, Hellegers AE. 1973. The influence of the changes in maternal age, birth order, and color on the changing perinatal mortality, Baltimore, 1961–66. Health Serv Rep 88:733–42.

Gens E, Michaelis D. 1990. The frequency of disturbances of somatic development in young people with type I diabetes in dependence on duration and age at onset of the disease. Exp Clin Endocrinol 95:97–104.

Gerritsen GC, Johnson MA, Soret MG, et al. 1974. Epidemiology of Chinese hamsters and preliminary evidence for genetic heterogeneity of diabetes. Diabetologia 10:581–8.

Gestation and Diabetes in France Study Group. 1991. Multicenter survey of diabetic pregnancy in France. Diab Care 14:994–1000.

Giavini E, Airoldi L, Broccia ML, et al. 1993. Effect of diets with different content in protein and fiber on embryotoxicity induced by experimental diabetes in rats. Biol Neonat 63:353–9.

Giavini E, Broccia ML, Prati M, et al. 1986. Effects of streptozotocin-induced diabetes on fetal development of the rat. Teratology 34:81–8.

Giavini E, Broccia ML, Pratti M, et al. 1991. Diet composition modifies embryotoxic effects induced by experimental diabetes in rats. Biol Neonat 59:278–86.

Giavini E, Pratti M. 1990. Morphogenesis of diabetes-induced congenital cataract in the rat. Acta Anat 137:132–6.

Giavini E, Prati M, Roversi G. 1990. Congenital malformations in offspring of diabetic rats: experimental study on the influence of the diet composition and magnesium intake. Biol Neonat 57:207–17.

Gilbert JA 1949. The association of maternal obesity, large babies, and diabetes. Br Med J 1:702–4.

Gilbert JA, Dunlop DM. 1949. Diabetic fertility, maternal mortality, and foetal loss rate. Br Med J 1:48–51.

Gillman J, Gilbert C, Gillman T, et al. 1948. A preliminary report on hydrocephalus, spina bifida, and other congenital anomalies in the rat produced by trypan blue. S Afr J Med Sci 13:47–90.

Gillmer MD, Holmes SM, Moore MP, et al. 1984. Diabetes in pregnancy: obstetric management 1983. In: Carbohydrate Metabolism in Pregnancy and the Newborn. Sutherland HW, Stowers JM, Pearson DW, eds. Churchill, London, pp. 102–18.

Gillmer MD, Oakley NW, Beard RW, et al. 1980. Screening for diabetes during pregnancy. J Obstet Gynecol 87:377–82.

Gittelsohn AM, Milham S. 1965. Vital record incidence of congenital malformations in New York State. In: Neel JV, Shaw MW, Schull WJ, eds. Genetics and Epidemiology of Chronic Disease. U.S. Department of Health, Education and Welfare, Washington, DC, pp. 305–20.

Given WP, Douglas RG, Tolstoi E. 1950. Pregnancy and diabetes. Am J Obstet Gynecol 59:729–47.

Given WP, Douglas RG, Tolstoi E. 1951. Pregnancy and diabetes. Med Clin North Am 35:659–65.

Given WP, Tolstoi E. 1957. Present day management of the pregnant diabetic: success or failure? Surg Clin North Am 37:369–78.

Gladman G, McCrindle BW, Boutin C, et al. 1997. Fetal echocardiographic screening of diabetic pregnancies for congenital heart disease. Am J Perinatol 14:59–62.

Glasgow AC, Harley JM, Montgomery DA 1979. Congenital malformations in infants of diabetic mothers. Ulster Med J 48:109–17.

Glenister TW. 1964. Fantasies, facts and foetuses: the interplay of fancy and reason in teratology. Med Hist 8:18–30.

Golde SH, Montoro M, Good-Anderson B, et al. 1984. The rate of nonstress tests, fetal biophysical profile, and contraction stress tests in the outpatient management of insulin-requiring diabetic pregnancies. Am J Obstet Gynecol 148:269–73,

Goldenberg RL, Humphrey JL, Hal CB, et al. 1983. Lethal congenital anomalies as a cause of birthweight-specific neonatal mortality. JAMA 250:513–5.

Golding J. 1987. Epidemiology of fetal and neonatal death. In: Keeling JW, ed. Fetal and Neonatal Pathology. Springer, London, pp. 151–65.

Golding J. 1991. The epidemiology of perinatal death. In: Kiely M, ed. Reproductive and Perinatal Epidemiology. CRC, Boca Raton, FL, pp. 401–36.

Goldman JA. 1976. Glucose tolerance in mothers of offspring with congenital malformations. Isr J Med Sci 10:1434–7.

Goldman JA, Dicker D, Feldberg D, et al. 1986. Pregnancy outcome in patients with insulin-dependent diabetes mellitus with preconceptional control: a comparative study. Am J Obstet Gynecol 155:293–7.

Goldstein AI, Cronk DA, Garite T, et al. 1978. Perinatal outcome in the diabetic pregnancy: a retrospecive analysis. J Reprod Med 20:61–6.

Goldstein E, Porter B, Galil A. 1991. Neurodevelopmental outcome of offspring of the diabetic mother: need for further research. Am J Dis Child 145:602–3.

Goldstein L, Murphy D. 1929. Microcephalic idiocy following radium therapy for uterine cancer during pregnancy. Am J Obstet Gynecol 18:189–95.

Gomez KJ, Dowdy K, Allen, G, et al. 1988. Evaluation of ultrasound diagnosis of fetal anomalies in women with pregestational diabetes: University of Florida experience. Am J Obstet Gynecol 159:584–6.

Goodman MJ. 1976. Maternal diabetes and congenital malformations among live births in Hawaii. Acta Diab Lat 13:99–106.

Goto MP, Goldman AS. 1994. Diabetic embryopathy. Curr Opin Paediatr 6:486–91.

Goudé H, Cozic A, Franck JB, et al. 1975. La grossesse chez la femme diabétique: à propos de neuf grossesses: conduite à tenir. J Gynecol Obstet Biol Reprod 4:541–50.

Gould GM, Pyle WL. 1898. Anomalies and Curiosities of Medicine. Saunders, Philadelphia.

Graefe. 1898. Über die Einwirkung des Diabetes mellitus auf die weiblichen Sexualorgane und ihre Functionen. Munch Med Wochenschr 14:127–8.

Graham BD, Lowrey GH. 1953. Chemical findings in infants born of diabetic mothers: a preliminary report. Univ Mich Med Bull 19:267–72.

Graham G. 1924. Pregnancy complicating diabetes treated with insulin. Lancet 206:953.

Graham TP Jr, Gutgesell HP. 1995. Ventricular septal defects. In: Emmanouilides GC, Riemenschneider, TA, Allen HD, et al., eds. Moss and Adams Heart Disease in Children and Adolescents including the Fetus and Young Adult, 5th ed. Williams & Wilkins, Baltimore, pp. 724–46.

Granat M, Sharf M, Cooper A. 1979. Glucose intolerance during pregnancy. Obstet Gynecol 53:157–61.

Granroth G. 1978. Defects of the central nervous system in Finland. III. Diseases and drugs in pregnancy. Early Hum Dev 2:147–62.

Granroth G, Hakama M, Saxén L. 1977. Defects of the central nervous system in Finland. I. Variations in time and space, sex distribution, and parental age. Br J Prev Soc Med 31:164–70.

Graves WK, Neff R, Mark P. 1967. Altered glucose metabolism in pregnancy: its determination and fetal outcome. Am J Obstet Gynecol 98:602–8.

Graviss ER, Monteleone PA, Wampler LR, et al. 1980. Proximal femoral focal deficiency associated with the Robin anomalad. J Med Genet 17:390–2.

Gray SH, Feemster LC. 1926. Compensatory hypertrophy and hyperplasia of the islands of Langerhans in the pancreas of a child born of a diabetic mother. Arch Pathol Lab Med 1:348–55.

Greb AE, Pauli RM, Kirby RS. 1987. Accuracy of fetal death reports: comparison with data from an independent stillbirth assessment program. Am J Public Health 77:1202–6.

Greco P, Loverro G, Selvaggi L. 1994. Does gestational diabetes represent an obstetrical risk? Gynecol Obstet Invest 37:242–45.

Greene MF. 1989. Congenital malformations. In: Hare JW, ed. Diabetes Complicating Pregnancy: the Joslin Clinic method. Liss, New York, pp. 147–61.

Greene MF, Allred EN, Leviton A. 1995. Maternal metabolic control and risk of microcephaly among infants of diabetic mothers. Diab Care 18:166–9.

Greene MF, Benacerraf BR. 1991. Prenatal diagnosis in diabetic gravidas: utility of ultrasound and maternal serum alpha-fetoprotein screening. Obstet Gynecol 77:520–4.

Greene MF, Hare JW, Cloherty JP, et al. 1989. First-trimester hemoglobin A_1 and risk for major malformation and spontaneous abortion in diabetic pregnancy. Teratology 39:225–32.

Gregg MB. 1979. Temporal trends in the incidence of birth defects—United States. MMWR 28:401–3.

Gregg NM. 1941. Congenital cataract following German measles in the mother. Trans Ophth Soc Aust 3:35–46.

Gregory R, Scott AR, Mohajer M, et al. 1992. Diabetic pregnancy 1977–1990: have we reached a plateau? J Roy Coll Phys 26:162–6

Grenet P, Paillerets FD, Badoual J, et al. 1972. Le nouveau-né de mère diabétique. Arch Fr Paediatr 29:925–33.

Grill V, Johansson B, Jalkanen P, 1991. Influence of severe diabetes-mellitus early in pregnancy in the rat: effects of insulin sensitivity and insulin secretion in the offspring. Diabetologia 34:373–8.

Grimaldi RD. 1968 Significance and management of abnormal oral glucose tolerance tests during pregnancy. Obstet Gynecol 32:713–20.

Gruenwald P. 1947. Mechanisms of abnormal development. I. Causes of abnormal development in the embryo. II. Embryonic development of malformations. Arch Pathol 44:398–436, 495–559.

Gruenwald P. 1966. Growth of the human fetus. II. Abnormal growth in twins and infants of mothers with diabetes, hypertension or isoimmunization. Am J Obstet Gynecol 94:1120–32.

Grüneberg H. 1963. The Pathology of Animals: a study of inherited skeletal disorders in animals. Wiley, New York.

Guivarc'h-Levêque A, Poulain P, Levêque J, et al. 1992. La grossesse de la femme diabétique: incidence des malformations, de la macrosomie, mise à jour sur la conduite obstétricale. J Gynecol Obstet Biol Reprod 21:697–700.

Gürakan B, Karaaslan E, Balci S. 1996. Sirenomelia in an infant of a diabetic mother. Turk J Pediatr 38:393–7.

Gutgesell HP, Mullins CE, Gillette PC, et al. 1976. Transient hypertrophic subaortic stenosis in infants of diabetic mothers. J Pediatr 89:120–5.

Gutgesell HP, Speer ME, Rosenberg HS. 1980. Characterization of the cardiomyopathy in infants of diabetic mothers. Circulation 61:441–50.

Gyves MT, Rodman HM, Little AB, et al. 1977. A modern approach to management of pregnant diabetics: a two-year analysis of perinatal outcomes. Am J Obstet Gynecol 128:606–12.

Hadden DR. 1975. Glucose tolerance tests in pregnancy. In: Sutherland HW, Stowers JM, eds. Carbohydrate Metabolism in Pregnancy and the Newborn. Livingstone, Edinburgh, pp. 19–41.

Hadden DR. 1979. Asymptomatic diabetes in pregnancy. In: Sutherland HW, Stowers JM, eds. Carbohydrate Metabolism in Pregnancy and the Newborn 1978. Springer, Berlin, pp. 407–24.

Hadden DR. 1980. Screening for abnormalities of carbohydrate metabolism in pregnancy 1966–1977: the Belfast experience Diab Care 3:440–6

Hadden DR. 1985. Geographic, ethnic, and racial variations in the incidence of gestational diabetes mellitus. Diabetes 34 Suppl 2:8–12.

Hadden DR. 1986. Diabetes in pregnancy 1985. Diabetologia 29:1–9.

Hadden DR. 1989. The development of diabetes and its relation to pregnancy: the long-term and short-term historical viewpoint. In: Sutherland HW, Stowers JM, Pearson DW, eds. Carbohydrate Metabolism in Pregnancy and the Newborn. V. Springer, New York, pp. 1–8.

Hadden DR, Byrne E, Trotter I, et al. 1984. Physical and psychological health of children of type 1 (insulin-dependent) diabetic mothers. Diabetologia 26:250–4.

Hadden DR, Harley JM 1967. Potential diabetes and the foetus: a prospective study of the relation between maternal oral glucose tolerance and the foetal result. J Obstet Gynecol Br Commonw 74:669–74.

Hadden DR, Hillebrand B. 1989. The first recorded case of diabetic pregnancy (Bennewitz HG, 1824, University of Berlin). Diabetologia 32:625.

Hadden DR, Traub, AI, Harley JM 1988. Diabetes-related perinatal mortality and congenital fetal abnormality: a problem of audit. Diab Med 5:321–3.

Hagay ZJ, Weiss Y, Zusman I, et al. 1995. Prevention of diabetes-associated embryopathy by overexpression of the free radical scavenger copper zinc superoxide dismutase in transgenic mouse embryos. Am J Obstet Gynecol 173:1036–41.

Hagbard L. 1956. Pregnancy and diabetes mellitus: a clinical study. Acta Obstet Gynecol Scand 35 Suppl 1:1–180.

Hagbard L. 1958. The "pre-diabetic" period from an obstetric point of view. Acta Obstet Gynecol Scand 37:497–518.

Hagbard L. 1961. Pregnancy and Diabetes Mellitus. Thomas, Springfield, Illinois.

Hagbard L, Olow I, Reinand T. 1959. A follow-up study of 514 children of diabetic mothers. Acta Paediatr 48:184–97.

Hagbard L, Svanborg A. 1960. Prognosis of diabetes mellitus with onset during pregnancy: a clinical study of seventy-one cases. Diabetes 9:296–302.

Hakosalo JK. 1973. Cumulative detection rates of congenital malformations in a ten-year follow-up study. Acta Pathol Microbiol Scand Sec A Suppl 242:7–58.

Hall RE, Tillman AJ 1951. Diabetes in pregnancy. Am J Obstet Gynecol 61:1107–15.

Hamanishi C. 1980. Congenital short femur: clinical, genetic and epidemiological comparison of the naturally occurring condition with that caused by thalidomide. J Bone Joint Surg 62B:307–20.

Hamburger V. 1988. The Heritage of Experimental Embryology: Hans Spemann and the organizer. Oxford University, New York.

Hamman L, Hirschman II. 1917. Studies on blood sugar. Arch Intern Med 20:761–808.

Hansen JP. 1986. Older maternal age and pregnancy outcome: a review of the literature. Obstet Gynecol Surv 41:726–42.

Hanson U, Persson B. 1993. Outcome of pregnancies complicated by type 1 insulin-dependent diabetes in Sweden: acute pregnancy complications, neonatal mortality and morbidity. Am J Perinatol 10:330–3.

Hanson U, Persson B, Enochsson E, et al. 1984. Self-monitoring of blood glucose by diabetic women during the third trimester of pregnancy. Am J Obstet Gynecol 150:817–21.

Hanson U, Persson B, Thunell S. 1990. Relationship between haemoglobin A_{1c} in early type 1 (insulin-dependent) diabetic pregnancy and the occurrence of spontaneous abortion and fetal malformation in Sweden. Diabetologia 33:100–4.

Hardy JB, Drage JS, Jackson EC. 1979. The First Year of Life. Johns Hopkins University, Baltimore.

Hare JW. 1985. Pregnancy and diabetes. In: Marble A, Krall LP, Bradley RF, eds. Joslin's Diabetes Mellitus. Lea & Febiger, Philadelphia, pp. 698–711.

Hare JW. 1989. Medical management. In: Hare JW, ed. Diabetes Complicating Pregnancy: the Joslin Clinic method. Liss, New York, pp. 3–51.

Hare JW. 1991. Insulin management of type I and type II diabetes in pregnancy. Clin Obstet Gynecol 34:494–506.

Hare JW. 1994. Diabetes and pregnancy. In: Kahn CR, Weir GC, eds. Joslin's Diabetes Mellitus. Lea & Febiger, Philadelphia, pp. 889–99.

Hare JW, White P. 1980. Gestational diabetes and the White classification. Diab Care 3:394.

Harlap S, Shiono PH, Ramcharan S, et al. 1979. A prospective study of spontaneous fetal losses after induced abortion. N Engl J Med 301:677–81.

Harlap S, Shiono PH, Ramcharan S. 1980. A life table of spontaneous abortions and the effects of age, parity, and other variables. In: Porter IH, Hook EB, eds. Human Embryonic and Fetal Death. Academic Press, New York, pp. 145–58.

Harlass FE, Brady K, Read JA. 1991. Reproducibility of the oral glucose tolerance test in pregnancy. Am J Obstet Gynecol 164:564–8.

Harley JM, Montgomery DA. 1965. Management of pregnancy complicated by diabetes. Br Med J 1:14–8.

Harris BA, Fisichella RA. 1950. Diabetes complicated by pregnancy. NY State J Med 50:1097–102.

Harris EL. 1990. Genetic epidemiology of hypospadias. Epidemiol Rev 12:29–40.

Harris JS, Woomer DF, Bruggers L. 1963. Diabetes in pregnancy: experience in three general hospitals in Saginaw. J Mich Med Soc 62:769–74.

Harris LE, Steinberg AG. 1954. Abnormalities observed during the first six days of life in 8,716 live-born infants. Pediatrics 14:314–26.

Harris MI. 1988. Gestational diabetes may represent discovery of preexisting glucose intolerance. Diab Care 11:403–11.

Harris MI, Hadden, WC, Knowler WC, et al. 1987. Prevalence of diabetes and impaired glucose tolerance and plasma glucose levels in U.S. population aged 20–74 years. Diabetes 36:523–34.

Hass J. 1951. Congenital Dislocation of the Hip. Thomas, Springfield, Illinois.

Haust MD. 1981. Maternal diabetes mellitus—effects on the fetus and placenta. In: Naeye RL, Kissane JM, Kaufman N, eds. Perinatal Diseases. Williams and Wilkins, Baltimore, pp. 201–85.

Haworth JC, McRae KN, Dilling LA. 1976. Prognosis of infants of diabetic mothers to neonatal hypoglycaemia. Dev Med Child Neurol 18:471–9.

Hawthorne G, Snodgrass A, Tunbridge M. 1994. Outcome of diabetic pregnancy and glucose intolerance in pregnancy: an audit of fetal loss in Newcastle General Hospital 1977–1990. Diab Res Clin Pract 25:183–90.

Hegge FN, Franklin RW, Watson PT, et al. 1990. Fetal malformations commonly detectable on obstetric ultrasound. J Reprod Med 35:391–8.

Heinonen OP, Slone D, Shapiro S. 1977. Birth Defects and Drugs in Pregnancy. Publishing Sciences Group, Littleton, Massachusetts.

Heisig N, Schall J. 1971. Untersuchungen über die Gravidität und Nachkommenschaft des spontandiabetischen chinesischen Zwerghamsters. Arch Gynäk 210:2–28.

Heller SR, Lowe JM, Johnson IR, et al. 1984. Seven years experience of home management in pregnancy in women with insulin-dependent diabetes. Diab Med 1:199–204.

Helwig EB. 1940. Hypertrophy and hyperplasia of islands of Langerhans in infants born of diabetic mothers. Arch Intern Med 65:221–39.

Henley WE. 1947. Diabetes and pregnancy. NZ Med J 46:386–91.

Henriques CU, Damm P, Tabor A, et al. 1991. Incidence of fetal chromosome abnormalities in insulin dependent diabetic women. Acta Obstet Gynecol Scand 70:295–7.

Henriques CU, Damm P, Tabor A, et al. 1993. Decreased alpha-fetoprotein in amniotic fluid and maternal serum in diabetic pregnancy. Obstet Gynecol 82:960–4.

Herman GH. 1902. Diabetes and pregnancy. Edinb Med J 11:119–23.

Herrick,WW, Tillman AJ. 1938. Diabetes and pregnancy. Surg Gynecol Obstet 66:37–43.

Hertogh R de, Vanderheyden I, Pampfer S, et al 1992. Maternal insulin treatment improves pre-implantation embryo development in diabetic rats. Diabetologia 35:406–8.

Hertz-Picciotto I, Samuels SJ. 1988. Incidence of early loss of pregnancy. N Engl J Med 319:1483–4.

Herzstein J, Dolger H. 1946. The fetal mortality in women during the prediabetic period. Am J Obstet Gynecol 51:420–2.

Hexter AC, Harris JA. 1991. Bias in congenital malformations information from the birth certificate. Teratology 44:177–80.

Hiekkala H, Koskenoja M. 1961. A follow-up study of children of diabetic mothers. I. General findings. Ann Paediatr Fenn 7:17–31.

Hirst KM, Butler NR, Dawkins MJ. 1968. Infant and Perinatal Mortality in England and Wales. PHS Publ. No. 1000, Ser. 3, No. 12. U.S. Government Printing Office, Washington, DC.

Hitti IF, Glasberg SS, Huggins-Jones D, et al. 1994. Bilateral femoral hypoplasia and maternal diabetes: case report and review of the literature. Paediatr Pathol 14:567–74.

Hod M, Merlob P, Friedman S, et al. 1992. Prevalence of minor congenital anomalies in newborns of diabetic mothers. Eur J Obstet Gynecol Reprod Biol 44:111–6.

Hod M, Rabinerson D, Kaplan B, et al. 1996. Perinatal complications following gestational diabetes mellitus: how "sweet" is ill? Acta Obstet Gynecol Scand 75:809–15.

Hoet JJ. 1954. Carbohydrate metabolism during pregnancy. Diabetes 3:1–12.

Hoet JJ. 1986. The etiology of congenital malformations in infants of diabetic mothers: environmental and genetic interaction. In: Jovanovic L, Peterson CM, Fuhrmann K, eds. Diabetes and Pregnancy: teratology, toxicology and treatment. Praeger, New York, pp. 72–81.

Hoet JP, Gommers A, Hoet JJ. 1960. Causes of congenital malformations: role of prediabetes and hypothyroidism. In: Wolstenholme GE, O'Connor CM, eds. CIBA Foundation Symposium on Congenital Malformations. Little, Brown, Boston, pp. 219–35.

Hoffman JI. 1968. Natural history of congenital heart disease: problems in its assessment with special reference to ventricular septal defects. Circulation 37:97–105.

Hoffman JI. 1987. Incidence, mortality and natural history. In: Anderson RH, Shinbourne EA, Macartney FJ, et al., eds. Paediatric Cardiology. Churchill Livingstone, Edinburgh, pp. 3–14.

Hoffman JI. 1990. Congenital heart disease: incidence and inheritance. Paediatr Clin North Am 37:25–43.

Hoffman JI, Christianson R. 1978. Congenital heart disease in a cohort of 19,502 births with long-term follow-up. Am J Cardiol 42:641–7.

Holing EV, Brown ZZ, Beyer CS, et al. 1998. Why don't women with diabetes plan their pregnancies? Diab Care 21:889–95.

Hollingsworth DR, Moore TR. 1987. Postprandial walking exercise in pregnant insulin-dependent (type I) diabetic women: reduction of plasma lipid levels but absence of a significant effect on glycemic control. Am J Obstet Gynecol 157:1359–63.

Hollingsworth DR, Vaucher Y, Yamamoto TR. 1991. Diabetes in pregnancy in Mexican Americans. Diab Care 14 Suppl 3:695–705.

Holmes LB. 1976. Current concepts in genetics: congenital malformations. N Engl J Med 295:204–7.

Holmes LB. 1992. Fetal environmental toxins. Paediatr Rev 13:364–3.

Holmes LB. 1994. Spina bifida: anticonvulsants and other maternal influences. In: Bock G, Marsh J, eds. Neural Tube Defects. Wiley, Chichester, pp. 232–9.

Holmes LB, Cann, C, Cook C. 1985. Examination of infants for both minor and major malformations to evaluate for possible teratogenic exposures. Prog Clin Biol Res 163B:59–63.

Holmes LB, Driscoll SG, Atkins L. 1976. Etiologic heterogeneity of neural-tube defects. N Engl J Med 294:365–9.

Holmes LB, Kleiner, BC, Leppig KA, et al. 1987. Predictive value of minor anomalies. III. Use in cohort studies to identify teratogens. Teratology 36:291–8.

Holthusen W. 1972. The Pierre Robin syndrome: unusual associated developmental defects. Ann Radiol 15:253–62.

Hook EB, Porter IH. 1980. Terminological conventions, methodological considerations, temporal trends, specific genes, environmental hazards, and some other factors pertaining to embryonic and fetal death. In: Porter IH, Hook EB, eds. Human Embryonic and Fetal Death. Academic Press, New York, pp. 1–18.

Horger EO, Kellett WW, Williamson HO. 1967. Diabetes in pregnancy: a review of 143 cases. Obstet Gynecol 30:46–53.

Horger EO, Miller C, Conner ED. 1975. Relation of large birthweight to maternal diabetes mellitus. Obstet Gynecol 45:150–4.

Horii K, Watanabe G, Ingalls TH. 1966. Experimental diabetes in pregnant mice: prevention of congenital malformations in offspring by insulin. Diabetes 15:194–204.

Hosemann H. 1950. Kindliche Masse und Neugeborenensterblichkeit. Naturwissenschaften 37:409–16.

Höst HF. 1925. Carbohydrate tolerance in pregnancy. Lancet 1:1022–5.

Hreidarsson AB, Geirsson RT, Helgason T. 1993. Diabetes mellitus in Iceland: prevalence, organization of services, pregnancy outcome and long-term complications. Diab Nutr Metab 6:333–4.

Hsia DY, Gellis SS. 1957. Birth weight in infants of diabetic mothers. Ann Hum Genet 22:80–92.

Hubbell JP, Muirhead DH, Drorbaugh JE. 1965. The newborn infant of the diabetic mother. Med Clin North Am 49:1035–52.

Huber J, Reinold E. 1985. Die perinatal verstorbenen Kinder in der I. Universitäts-Frauenklinik Wien zwischen 1981 und 1983. Wien Med Wochenschr 135:197–200.

Hultquist GT. 1950. Diabetes and pregnancy: an animal study. Acta Pathol Microbiol Scand 27:695–719.

Hunter DJ, Burrows RF, Mohide PT, et al. 1993. Influence of maternal insulin-dependent diabetes mellitus on neonatal morbidity. Can Med Ass J 149:47–52.

Hurley LS. 1977. Nutritional deficiencies and excesses. In: Wilson JG, Fraser FC, eds. Handbook of Teratology. Vol. 1. Plenum Press, New York, pp. 261–308.

Hurley LS, Swenerton H. 1966. Congenital malformations resulting fron zinc deficiency in rats. Proc Soc Exp Biol Med 123:692–6.

Hurst D, Johnson DF. 1980. Brief clinical report: femoral hypoplasia-unusual facies syndrome. Am J Med Genet 5:255–8.

Hurwitz D, Higano N. 1952. Diabetes and pregnancy. N Engl J Med 247:305–9.

Hurwitz D, Irving FC. 1937. Diabetes and pregnancy. Am J Med Sci 194:85–92.

Hurwitz D, Jensen D. 1946. Carbohydrate metabolism in normal pregnancy. N Engl J Med 234:327–9.

Hyett JA, Moscoso G, Nicolaides KH. 1995. First-trimester nuchal translucency and cardiac septal defects in fetuses with trisomy 21. Am J Obstet Gynecol 172:1411–3.

Hyett JA, Perdu M, Sharland G, et al. 1999. Using fetal nuchal translucency to screen for major congenital cardiac defectrs at 10–14 weeks of gestation: population based cohort study. Br Med J 318:81–5.

Imerslund O. 1948. Den føtale og neonatale dødelighet og fødselsvekten hos barn født av prediabetiske mødre. Sartryck Nord Med 40:1880–2.

Incerpi MH, Miller DA, Samadi R, et al. 1998. Stillbirth evaluation: what tests are needed? Am J Obstet Gynecol 178:1121–5.

Irsigler K, Leodolter S, Rosenkranz A, et al. 1986. Different approaches toward normoglycemia in pregnancy: the Vienna experience. In: Jovanovic L, Peterson CM, Fuhrmann K, eds. Diabetes and Pregnancy: teratology, toxicology and treatment. Praeger, New York, pp. 263–90.

Iwase M, Wada M, Shinohara N, et al. 1995. Effect of maternal diabetes on longevity in offspring of spontaneously hypertensive rats. Gerontology 41:181–6.

Jackson WP. 1952. Studies in pre-diabetes. Br Med J 2:690–6.

Jackson WP. 1959. Prediabetes: a synthesis. Postgrad Med J 35:287–96.

Jackson WP. 1961. Is pregnancy diabetogenic? Lancet 2:1369–72.

Jacobs HR. 1937. Hypoglycemic action of alloxan. Proc Soc Exp Biol Med 37:407–9.

Jacobson JD, Cousins L. 1989. A population-based study of maternal and perinatal outcome in patients with gestational diabetes. Am J Obstet Gynecol 161:981–6.

Jährig D, Stiete S, Jonas C. 1993. Offspring of diabetic mothers: problems of morbidity. Diab Metab 19:207–12.

Janerich DT, Polednak AP. 1983. Epidemiology of birth defects. Epidemiol Rev 5:16–37.

Jankowski MA, Uriu-Hare JY, Rucker RB, et al. 1993. Effect of maternal diabetes and dietary copper on fetal development in rats. Reprod Toxic 7:589–98.

Jansen RP. 1982. Spontaneous abortion incidence in the treatment of infertility. Am J Obstet Gynecol 143:451–73.

Janssen PA, Rothman I, Schwartz SM. 1996. Congenital malformations in newborns of women with established and gestational diabetes in Washington State, 1984–91. Paediatr Perinat Epidemiol 10:52–63.

Janz D. 1982. On major malformations and minor anomalies in the offspring of parents with epilepsy. In: Janz D, Bossi, L, Dam M, et al., eds. Epilepsy, Pregnancy, and the Child. Raven Press, New York, pp. 211–22.

Janz NK, Herman WH, Becker M.P, et al. 1995. Diabetes and pregnancy: factors associated with seeking pre-conception care. Diab Care 18:157–65.

Jarrett RJ. 1981. Reflections on gestational diabetes mellitus. Lancet 2:1220–2.

Jarrett RJ. 1993. Gestational diabetes: a non-entity? Br Med J 306:37–8.

Jarrett RJ. 1997. Should we screen for gestational diabetes? Br Med J 315:736–7.

Jervell J, Bjerkedal T, Moe N. 1980. Outcome of pregnancies in diabetic mothers in Norway, 1967–1976. Diabetologia 18:131–4.

Johnson JM, Lange IR, Harman CR, et al. 1988. Biophysical profile scoring in the management of the diabetic pregnancy. Obstet Gynecol 72:841–6.

Johnson JP, Carey JC, Gooch WM, et al. 1983. Femoral hypoplasia-unusual facies syndrome in infants of diabetic mothers. J Paediatr 102:866–72.

Jokipii SG. 1955. Diabetes and pregnancy. Ann Med Intern Fenn 44:185–205.

Jones KL, ed. 1988. Smith's Recognizable Patterns of Human Malformations. Saunders, Philadelphia.

Jones WS. 1952. Diabetes in pregnancy: a preliminary report. Rhode Island Med J 35:662–4, 666, 668.

Jones WS. 1953. Diabetes in pregnancy. Am J Obstet Gynecol 66:322–34.

Jones WS. 1956. The severity of diabetes in pregnancy. Am J Obstet Gynecol 71:319–25.

Jones WS. 1958. Management of the pregnant diabetic. Diabetes 7:439–45.

Joslin EP. 1915. Pregnancy and diabetes mellitus. Boston Med Surg J 23:841–9.

Joslin EP. 1923. Pregnancy and diabetes. In: Joslin EP, ed. The Treatment of Diabetes Mellitus. Lea & Febiger, Philadelphia, pp. 649–65.

Joslin EP. 1928. The Treatment of Diabetes Mellitus, 4th ed. Lea & Febiger, Philadelphia.

Jovanovic L, Druzin M, Peterson CM. 1981. Effect of euglycemia on the outcome of pregnancy in insulin-dependent women as compared with normal control subjects. Am J Med 71:921–7.

Jovanovic L, Peterson CM. 1982. Optimal insulin delivery for the pregnant diabetic patient. Diab Care 5:24–37.

Jovanovic L, Peterson CM. 1985. Screening for gestational diabetes: optimum timing and criteria for retesting. Diabetes 34 Suppl 2:21–3.

Joyce J. 1986. Ulysses (corrected text). Vintage, New York.

Julian-Reynier C, Philip N, Scheiner C, et al. 1994. Impact of prenatal diagnosis by ultrasound on the prevalence of congenital anomalies at birth in southern France. J Epidemiol Comm Health 48:290–6.

Junod A, Lambert AE, Orci L, et al. 1967. Studies of the diabetogenic action of streptozotocin. Proc Soc Exp Biol Med 126:201–5.

Kade H, Dietel H. 1952. Die Prognose der Schwangerschaft bei prädiabetischen und diabetischen Frauen. Deut Med Wochenschr 77:673–5.

Kaku K, McGill J, Province M, et al. 1989. A single major gene controls most of the difference in susceptibility to streptozotocin-induced diabetes between C57BL/6J and C3H/HeJ mice. Diabetologia 32:716–23.

Kalamchi A, Cowell GH, Kim KI. 1985. Congenital deficiency of the femur. J Paediatr Orthop 5:129–34.

Kalitzki M. 1965. Congenital malformations and diabetes. Lancet 2:641–2.

Kalkhoff RK. 1985. Therapeutic results of insulin therapy in gestational diabetes mellitus. Diabetes 34 (Suppl 2):97–100.

Källén B. 1985. Analysis of deliveries among diabetic women in Sweden: 1978–1981. Personal communication.

Källén B. 1987a. Search for teratogenic risks with the aid of malformation registries. Teratology 35:47–52.

Källén B. 1987b. Caudal aplasia. In: Vinker PJ, Bruyn G, Klawans HL, et al., eds. Handbook of Clinical Neurology. Vol. 50. Malformations. Elsevier, Amsterdam, pp. 509–18.

Källén B. 1989a. Population surveillance of congenital malformations: possibilities and limitations. Acta Paediatr Scand 78:657–63.

Källén B. 1989b. A prospective study of some aetiological factors in limb reduction defects in Sweden. J Epidemiol Comm Health 43:86–96.

Källén B, Castilla EE, Lancaster PA, et al. 1992. The cyclops and the mermaid: an epidemiological study of two types of rare malformation. J Med Genet 29:30–5.

Källén B, Hay S, Klingberg M. 1984. Birth defects monitoring systems: accomplishments and goals. In: Kalter H, ed. Issues and Reviews in Teratology. Vol. 2. Plenum Press, New York, pp. 1–22.

Källén B, Winberg J. 1968. A Swedish register of congenital malformations: experience with continuous registration during 2 years with special reference to multiple malformations. Pediatrics 41:765–76.

Källén B, Winberg J. 1974. Caudal mesoderm pattern of anomalies: from renal agenesis to sirenomelia. Teratology 9:99–111.

Kalter H. 1954. The inheritance of susceptibility to the teratogenic effects of cortisone in mice. Genetics 39:185–96.

Kalter H. 1968. Teratology of the Central Nervous System: induced and spontaneous malformations of laboratory, agricultural, and domestic animals. University of Chicago, Chicago.

Kalter H. 1980. The relation between congenital malformations and prenatal mortality in experimental animals. In: Porter IH, Hook EB, eds. Human Embryonic and Fetal Death. Academic Press, New York, pp. 29–44.

Kalter H. 1987. Diabetes and spontaneous abortion: a historical review. Am J Obstet Gynecol 156:1243–53.

Kalter H. 1990. Perinatal mortality and congenital malformations in infants born to women with insulin-dependent diabetes mellitus—United States, Canada, and Europe, 1940–1988. MMWR 39:363–5.

Kalter H. 1991. Five-decade international trends in the relation of perinatal mortality and congenital malformations: stillbirth and neonatal death compared. Int J Epidemiol 20:173–9.

Kalter H. 1993. Case reports of malformations associated with maternal diabetes: history and critique. Clin Genet 43:174–9.

Kalter H. 1996. Reproductive toxicology in animals with induced and spontaneous diabetes. Reprod Toxicol 10:417–38.

Kalter H. 1997. Flawed study alleging prevention of diabetic embryopathy. Am J Obstet Gynecol 177:1273 (letter).

Kalter H. 1998. The non-teratogenicity of gestational diabetes. Paediatr Perinat Epidemiol 12:456–8.

Kalter H, Warkany J. 1959. Experimental production of congenital malformations in mammals by metabolic procedure. Physiol Rev 39:69–115.

Kalter H, Warkany J. 1961. Experimental production of congenital malformations in strains of inbred mice by maternal treatment with hypervitaminosis A. Am J Pathol 38:1–20.

Kalter H, Warkany J. 1983. Congenital malformations: etiologic factors and their role in prevention. N Engl J Med 308:424–31, 491–7.

Kampmeier OF. 1927. On sireniform monsters, with a consideration of the causation and the predominance of the male sex among them. Anat Rec 34:365–89.

Kaneko S, Kondo T. 1995. Antiepileptic drugs and birth defects: incidence, mechanisms and prevention. CNS Drug 3:41–55.

Kaplan S. 1979. A mechanistic approach to teratogenesis: analysis of caudal dysplasia syndrome (sacral agenesis). In: Persaud T, ed. Advances in the Study of Birth Defects. Vol. 1. MTP Press, Lancaster, Pennsylvania, pp. 177–97.

Karlsson K, Kjellmer I. 1972. The outcome of diabetic pregnancies in relation to the mother's blood sugar level. Am J Obstet Gynecol 112:213–20.

Kast A. 1994. "Wavy ribs"—a reversible pathologic finding in rat fetuses. Exp Toxic Pathol 6:203–10.

Kawaguchi M, Tanigawa K, Tanaka O, et al. 1994. Embryonic growth impaired by maternal hypoglycemia during early organogenesis in normal and diabetic rats. Acta Diabetol 31:141–6.

Keeling, JW. 1987. Macerated stillbirth. In: Keeling JW, ed. Fetal and Neonatal Pathology. Springer, London, pp. 167–77.

Keen H. 1991. Gestational diabetes: can epidemiology help? Diabetes 40:3–7.

Kenna AP, Smithells RW, Fielding DW. 1975. Congenital heart disease in Liverpool: 1960–69. Q J Med 44:17–44.

Kennedy WP. 1967. Epidemiologic aspects of the problem of congenital malformations. Birth Defects 3:1–18.

Kerunanayake EH, Hearse DJ, Mellows G. 1976. Streptozotocin: its excretion and metabolism in the rat. Diabetologia 12:483–8.

Key TC, Giuffrida,R, Moore TR. 1987. Predictive value of early pregnancy glycohemoglobin in the insulin-treated diabetic patient. Am J Obstet Gynecol 156:1096–1100.

Khera KS. 1984. Maternal toxicity: a possible etiological factor in embryo-fetal deaths and fetal malformations of rodent-rabbit species. Teratology 31:129–53.

Khoury MJ. 1989. Epidemiology of birth defects. Epidemiol Rev 11:244–8.

Khoury MJ, Becerra, JE, Cordero J, et al. 1989. Clinical-epidemiological assessment of patterns of birth defects associated with human teratogens: application to diabetic embryopathy. Pediatrics 84:658–65.

Kilpatrick ES, Rumley AG, Dominiczak MH, et al. 1994. Glycated haemoglobin values: problems in assessing blood glucose control in diabetes mellitus. Br Med J 309:983–5.

Kimmerle R, Heinemann L, Delecki A, et al. 1992. Severe hypoglycemia incidence and predisposing factors in 85 pregnancies of type I diabetic women. Diab Care 15:1034–7.

Kimmerle R, Zass RP, Cupisti S, et al. 1995. Pregnancies in women with diabetic nephropathy: long-term outcome for mother and child. Diabetologia 38:227–35.

Kinch RA. 1958. Fetal hazards in the diabetic pregnancy. Can Med Ass J 79:713–8.

Kirk JS, Comstock H, Lee W, et al. 1997. Sonographic screening to detect fetal cardiac anomalies: a 5-year experience with 111 abnormal cases. Obstet Gynecol 89:227–32.

Kirk RL, Serjeantson SW, King H, et al. 1985. The genetic epidemiology of diabetes mellitus. In: Chakraborty R, Szathmary EJ, eds. Diseases of Complex Etiology in Small Populations. Liss, New York, pp. 119–46.

Kitzmiller JL. 1986. Macrosomia in infants of diabetic mothers: characteristics, causes, prevention. In: Jovanovic L, Peterson CM, Fuhrmann K, eds. Diabetes and Pregnancy: teratology, toxicology and treatment. Praeger, New York, pp. 85–119.

Kitzmiller JL. 1993. Sweet success with diabetes: the development of insulin therapy and glycemic control for pregnancy. Diab Care 16:107–21.

Kitzmiller JL, Aiello LM, Kaldany A, et al. 1981. Diabetic vascular disease complicating pregnancy. Clin Obstet Gynecol 24:107–23.

Kitzmiller JL, Buchanan TA, Kjos S, et al. 1996. Pre-conception care of diabetes, congenital malformations, and spontaneous abortions. Diab Care 19:514–41.

Kitzmiller JL, Cloherty JP, Graham CA. 1982. Management of diabetes and pregnancy. In: Kozak GP, ed. Clinical Diabetes Mellitus. Saunders, Philadelphia, pp. 203–14.

Kitzmiller JL, Cloherty JP, Younger MD, et al. 1978. Diabetic pregnancy and perinatal mortality. Am J Obstet Gynecol 131:560–80.

Kitzmiller JL, Combs CA. 1993. Maternal and perinatal implications of diabetic nephropathy. Clin Perinatol 20:561–70.

Kitzmiller JL, Gavin LA, Gin GD, et al. 1991. Preconception care of diabetes: glycemic control prevents congenital anomalies. JAMA 265:731–6.

Kitzmiller JL, Hoedt LA, Gunderson EP, et al. 1988. Macrosomia and birth trauma in infants of diet treated gestational diabetic women. In: Weiss PA, Coustan DR, eds. Gestational Diabetes. Springer, New York, pp. 160–6.

Kjaer K, Hagen C, Sandø SH, et al. 1992a. Epidemiology of menarche and menstrual disturbances in an unselected group of women with insulin-dependent diabetes mellitus compared to controls. J Clin Endocrinol Metab 75:524–9.

Kjaer K, Hagen C, Sandø SH, et al. 1992b. Inferility and pregnancy outcome in an unselected group of women with insulin-dependent diabetes mellitus. Am J Obstet Gynecol 166:1412–8.

Klemetti A. 1978. Congenital defects in a cohort followed for seven years. Acta Paediatr Scand 67:601–6.

Klingberg MA, Papier CM. 1979. Teratoepidemiology. J Biosoc Sci 11:233–58.

Kloos K. 1952. Zur Pathologie der Feten und Neugeborenen diabetischer Mütter. Virchow Arch 321:177–227.

Knight G, Worth RC, Ward JD. 1983. Macrosomy despite a well-controlled diabetic pregnancy. Lancet 2:1431.

Knowler WC, Bennett PH, Hamman RF, et al. 1978. Diabetes incidence and prevalence in Pima Indians: a 19-fold greater difference than in Rochester, Minnesota. Am J Epidemiol 108:497–505.

Knowler WC, Pettitt DJ, Bennett PH, et al. 1983. Diabetes mellitus in the Pima Indians: genetic and evolutionary considerations. Am J Phys Anthropol 62:107–14.

Knox EG, Armstrong, EH, Lancashire R. 1984. The quality of notification of congenital malformations. J Epidemiol Comm Health 38:296–305.

Koch R, Levy HL, Matalon R, et al. 1994. The international collaborative study of maternal phenylketonuria: status report 1994. Acta Paediatr Suppl 407:111–9.

Koch S, Lösche G, Jager-Röman E, et al. 1992. Major and minor birth malformations and antiepileptic drugs. Neurology 42:83–8.

Koenig RJ, Peterson CM, Jones RL, et al. 1976a. Correlation of glucose regulation and hemoglobin A_{1c} in diabetes mellitus. N Engl J Med 295:417–20.

Koenig RJ, Peterson CM, Kilo C et al. 1976b. Hemoglobin A_{1c} as an indicator of the degree of glucose intolerance in diabetes. Diabetes 25:230–2.

Kohn LA, Bennett KA. 1986. Fluctuating asymmetry in fetuses of diabetic rhesus macaques. Am J Phys Anthropol 71:477–84.

Koller O. 1953. Diabetes and pregnancy. Acta Obstet Gynecol Scand 32:80–103.

Koman LA, Meyer LC, Warren FH. 1982. Proximal femoral focal deficiency: a 50-year experience. Dev Med Child Neurol 24:344–55.

Komrower GM, Langley FA. 1961. The fate of the diabetic woman's child. Manchester Med Gaz 40:166–71.

Koskenoja M. 1961. Alloxan diabetes in the pregnant mouse. Acta Ophthalmol Suppl 68:1–92.

Kotzot D, Weigi J, Huk W, et al. 1993. Hydantoin syndrome with holoprosencephaly: a possible rare teratogenic effect. Teratology 48:15–9.

Krall LP. 1965. When is diabetes? Med Clin North Am 49:893–904.

Kramer W. 1936. Diabetes and pregnancy: a survey of 665 cases. Penn Med 39:702–7.

Kreipe U. 1967. Missbildungen innerer Organe bei Thalidomidembryopathie. Ein Beitrag zur Bestimmung der sensiblen Phase bei Thalidomideinnahme in der Frühschwangerschaft. Arch Kinderheilk 176:33–61.

Kreshover SJ, Clough OW, Bear DM. 1953. Prenatal influences on tooth development. I. Alloxan diabetes in rats. J Dent Res 32:246–61.

Kriss JP, Futcher PH. 1948. The relation between infant birthweight and subsequent development of maternal diabetes mellitus. J Clin Endocrinol 8:380–9.

Kritzer MD. 1952. The significance of the birth of a large baby. Med Clin North Am 36:1151–5.

Kubryk N, Schmatko M, Borde M, et al. 1981. Le syndrome de régression caudale: à propos d'une observation. Ann Paediatr 28:597–600.

Kučera J. 1971a. Rate and type of congenital anomalies among offspring of diabetic women. J Reprod Med 7:61–70.

Kučera J. 1971b. Movement of the frequencies of congenital malformations in time and space. Soc Biol 18:422–30.

Kučera J, Lenz W. 1967. Caudale Regression mit Oesophagusatresie und Nierenagenesie—ein Syndrom. Z Kinderheilk 98:326–9.

Kučera J, Lenz W, Maier W. 1965. Missbildungen der Beine und der kaudalen Wirbelsäule bei Kindern diabetischer Mutter. Deut Med Wochenschr 90:901–5.

Kühl C, Møller-Jensen B. 1989. Intensified insulin treatment in diabetic pregnancy. In: Sutherland HW, Stowers JM, Pearson DW, eds. Carbohydrate Metabolism in Pregnancy and the Newborn. IV. Springer, London, pp. 161–71.

Kyle GC. 1963. Diabetes and pregnancy. Ann Intern Med 59:1–82.

Labarrere CA, Faulk WP. 1991. Diabetic placentae: studies of the battlefield after the war. Diabetes Metab Rev 7:253–63.

Labate JS. 1947. A study of the causes of fetal and neonatal mortality on the obstetric service of Bellevue Hospital. Am J Obstet Gynecol 54:188–200.

Lage JM, Driscoll SG, Bieber FR. 1987. Transposition of the external genitalia associated with caudal regression. J Urol 138:387–9.

Lambie CG. 1926. Diabetes and pregnancy. J Obstet Gynecol 33:563–606.

Lammer EJ, Opitz JM. 1986. The DiGeorge anomaly as a developmental field defect. Am J Med Genet Suppl 2:113–27.

Landon MB, Gabbe SG. 1993. Fetal surveillance in the pregnancy complicated by diabetes mellitus. Clin Perinatol 20:549–60.

Landon MB, Gabbe SG. 1995. Diabetes mellitus. In: Barron WM, Lindheimer MD, Davison JM, eds. Medical Disorders During Pregnancy, 2nd ed. Mosby, St. Louis, pp. 63–88.

Landon MB, Gabbe SG, Piana R, et al. 1987. Neonatal morbidity in pregnancy complicated by diabetes mellitus: predictive value of maternal glycemic profiles. Am J Obstet Gynecol 156:1089–95.

Landon MB, Mintz MC, Gabbe SG. 1989. Sonographic evaluation of fetal abdominal growth: predictor of the large-for-gestational-age infant in pregnancies complicated by diabetes mellitus. Am J Obstet Gynecol 160:115–21.

Lang U, Künzel W. 1989. Diabetes mellitus in pregnancy: management and outcome of diabetic pregnancies in the state of Hesse, F.R.G.: a five-year-survey. Eur J Obstet Gynecol Reprod Biol 33:115–29

Langer O, Mazze R. 1988. The relationship between large-for-gestational-age infants and glycemic control in women with gestational diabetes. Am J Obstet Gynecol 159:1478–83.

Larsson G, Spjuth J, Ranstam J, et al. 1986. Prognostic significance of birth of large infant for subsequent development of maternal non-insulin-dependent diabetes mellitus: a prospective study over 20–27 years. Diab Care 9:359–64.

Laursen HB. 1980. Some epidemiological aspects of congenital heart disease in Denmark. Acta Paediatr Scand 69:619–24.

Lavietes PH, Leary DC, Winkler AW, et al. 1943. Diabetes mellitus and pregnancy. Yale J Biol Med 16:151–66.

Lavin JP, Lovelace DR, Miodovnik M, et al. 1983. Clinical experience with one hundred seven diabetic pregnancies. Am J Obstet Gynecol 147:742–51.

Law SW, Gibbons W, Poindexter AN. 1980. Patient cooperation: a determinant of perinatal outcome in the pregnant diabetic. J Reprod Med 24:197–201.

Lawrence AM, Contopoulos AN. 1960. Reproductive performance in the alloxan diabetic rat. Acta Endocrinol 33:175–84.

Lawrence RD, Oakley W. 1942. Pregnancy and diabetes. Q J Med 11:45–75.

Layde PM, Dooley K, Erickson JD, et al. 1980. Is there an epidemic of ventricular septal defects in the U.S.A.? Lancet 1:407–8.

Lazarow A, Heggestad CB. 1970. Offspring of animals with experimental diabetes. In: Camerini-Dávalos RA, Cole HS, eds. Early Diabetes. Academic Press, New York, pp. 229–37.

Leck I. 1972. The etiology of human malformations: insights from epidemiology. Teratology 5:303–14.

Leck I. 1984. Fetal malformations. In: Barron SL, Thomson AM, eds. Obstetrical Epidemiology. Academic Press, London, pp. 263–317.

Leck I. 1993. The contribution of epidemiologic studies to understanding human malformations. In: Stevenson RE, Hall JG, Goodan RM, eds. Human Malformations and Related Anomalies. Oxford University, New York, pp. 65–93.

Leck I, Record RG, McKeown T, et al. 1968. The incidence of malformations in Birmingham, England, 1950–1959. Teratology 1:263–80.

Lecorché E. 1885. Du diabète: dans ses rapports avec la vie utérine la menstruation et la grossesse. Ann Gynecol 24:257–73.

Leikin E, Jenkins JH, Graves WL. 1987. Prophylactic insulin in gestational diabetes. Obstet Gynecol 70:587–92.

Leiter EH, Prochazka M, Coleman DL. 1987. Animal model of human disease: the non-obese diabetic (NOD) mouse. Am J Pathol 128:380–3.

Leiva A, de, Lefebvre PJ, Nerup J. 1996. European dimensions of diabetes research. Diabetologia 39: Suppl 5–11.

Lejeune J, Turpin R, Goutier M. 1959. Le mongolisme: premier example d'aberration autosomique humaine. Ann Génét 1:s41–9.

Lemire RJ, Beckwith JB, Warkany J. 1978. Anencephaly. Raven Press, New York.

Lemons JA, Vargas P, Delaney JJ. 1981. Infants of the diabetic mother: a review of 225 cases. Obstet Gynecol 57:187–92.

Leng-Lévy J, Aubertin J, Le Gall F, et al. 1972. Pronostic de la grossesse chez les diabétiques en fonction de la correction du diabète pendant la gestation. Bord Med 5:887–96.

Lenz W. 1961. Discussionsbemerkung zu dem Vortrag von R.A. Pfeiffer und K. Kosenow: Zur Frage der exogenen Entstehung schwerer Extremitätenmissbildungen. In: Tagung der Rheinisch-Westfälischen Kinderärztevereinigung in Düsseldorf 19.11.

Lenz W, Knapp K. 1962. Die Thalidomid-Embryopathie. Deut Med Wochenschr 87:1232–42.

Lenz W, Kučera J. 1967. L'étiologie de la régression caudale (agénésie du sacrum). Med Hyg 25:241–3.

Lenz W, Maier W. 1964. Congenital malformations and maternal diabetes. Lancet 2:1124–5.

Lenz W, Passarge E. 1965. Syndrome of caudal regression in infants of diabetic mothers. In: Abstracts of the 5th Annual Meeting of the Teratology Society, San Francisco, May 26–28, p. 16.

Leonhardt T, Samuelson G, Spetz S. 1978. Erfarenheter av skötsel av gravida diabetiker vid ett länssjukhus. Lakartidningen 75:2709–11.

Leppig KA, Werler MM, Cann CI, et al. 1987. Predictive value of minor anomalies. 1. Association with major malformations. J Paediatr 110:531–7.

Leridon H. 1976. Facts and artifacts in the study of intrauterine mortality: a reconsideration from pregnancy histories. Popul Stud 30:319–36.

Leridon H. 1977. Human Fertility: the basic components. University of Chicago, Chicago.

Leslie RDG, Pyke DA, John PN, et al. 1978. Haemoglobin A_1 in diabetic pregnancy. Lancet 2:958–9.

Leveno KL, Jauth JC, Gilstrap LC, et al. 1979. Appraisal of "rigid" blood glucose during pregnancy of the overtly diabetic woman. Am J Obstet Gynecol 135:853–9.

Levy-Marchal C, Czernichow P, eds. 1992. Epidemiology and Etiology of Insulin-Dependent Diabetes in the Young. Karger, Basel.

Limb CJ, Holmes LB. 1994. Anencephaly: changes in prenatal detection and birth status, 1972–1990. Am J Obstet Gynecol 170:1333–8.

Lin Y, Lee M, Leichter J. 1995. Interactive effects of alcohol and diabetes during pregnancy on the rat fetus. Teratog Carcinog Mutagen 15:147–53.

Lind T. 1984. Reflections on the 1983 workshop on gestational diabetes. In: Sutherland HW, Stowers JM, eds. Carbohydrate Metabolism in Pregnancy and the Newborn. Livingstone, Edinburgh, pp. 220–5.

Lind T, Billewicz WZ, Brown G. 1973. A serial study of changes occurring in the oral glucose tolerance test during pregnancy. J Obstet Gynecol Br Commw 80:1033–39.

Lind T, Phillips PR, and the Diabetic Pregnancy Study Group of the European Association for the Study of diabetes. 1991. Influence of pregnancy on the 75-g OTGT: a prospective multicenter study. Diabetes 40:8–13.

Linn T, Lowek E, Schneider K, et al. 1993. Spontaneous glucose intolerance in the progeny of low dose streptozotocin-induced diabetic mice. Diabetologia 36:1245–51.

Lips JP, Jongsma HW, Eskes TK. 1988. Alloxan-induced diabetes mellitus in pregnant sheep and chronic fetal catheterization. Lab Anim 22:16–22.

Little DJ, Stubbs SM, Brudenell M, et al. 1979. Early growth retardation in diabetic pregnancy. Br Med J 1:488.

Little J, Carr-Hill RA. 1984. Problems of ascertainment of congenital anomalies. Acta Genet Med Gemell 33:97–105.

Little J, Elwood JM. 1991. Epidemiology of neural tube defects. In: Kiely M, ed. Reproductive and Perinatal Epidemiology. CRC, Boca Raton, pp. 251–336.

Little RR, McKenzie EM, Shyken JM, et al. 1990. Lack of relationship between glucose tolerance and complications of pregnancy in nondiabetic women. Diab Care 13:483–7.

Lizan G, Lucas P, Muller G. 1985. Diabète et grossesse: notre expérience de la pompe à insuline. Rev Fr Gynecol Obstet 80:451–7.

Lloyd DJ, Duffty P. 1984. Management of the infant of the diabetic mother: recent experience. In: Sutherland HW, Stowers JM, eds. Carbohydrate Metabolism in Pregnancy and the Newborn. Churchill, Edinburgh, pp. 144–9.

Loh KJ. 1988. Diabetes und Schwangerschaft: gynäkologische Aspekte. Arch Gynecol Obstet 245:266–72.

Long WN, Freeman MG. 1969. Diabetes and pregnancy. Johns Hopkins Med J 125:258–61.

Long WN, Hartmann WL, Futcher PH, et al. 1954. Diabetes mellitus and pregnancy. Obstet Gynecol 3:160–8.

López-Quijada C, Carrion LC. 1974. Maternal disorders of carbohydrate metabolism in cases of cardiac embryopathy. Acta Diabetol Lat 11:140–8.

Lord J, Beighton P. 1981. The femoral hypoplasia-unusual facies syndrome: a genetic entity? Clin Genet 20:267–75.

Lowy C, Beard RW, Goldschmidt J. 1986a. Congenital malformations in babies of diabetic mothers. Diab Med 3:458–62.

Lowy C, Beard RW, Goldschmidt J. 1986b. The UK diabetic pregnancy survey. Acta Endocrinol Suppl 277:86–9.

Lubetzki J, Duprey J, Sambourg C. 1973. Influence of mother's age, parity, obesity, and diabetes upon birth weight. Diabetologia 9:79.

Lübken W. 1970. Schwangerschaft und Diabetes mellitus. Munch Med Wochenschr 112:684–9.

Lucas MJ, Leveno, KJ, Williams ML, et al. 1989. Early pregnancy glycosylated hemoglobin, severity of diabetes, and fetal malformations. Am J Obstet Gynecol 161:426–31.

Lufkin EG, Nelson RL, Hill LM, et al. 1984. An analysis of diabetic pregnancies at Mayo Clinic, 1950–79. Diab Care 7:539–47.

Lukens FD. 1948. Alloxan diabetes. Physiol Rev 28:304–30.

Lund CJ, Weese WH. 1953. Glucose tolerance and excessively large babies in nondiabetic mothers. Am J Obstet Gynecol 65:815–9.

Lundbaek K. 1962. Intravenous glucose tolerance as a tool in definition and diagnosis of diabetes mellitus. Br Med J 1:1507–13.

Lunell N-O, Persson B. 1972. Potential diabetes in women with large babies. Acta Obstet Gynecol Scand 51:293–6.

Lurie S, Matzkel A, Weissman A, et al. 1992. Outcome of pregnancy in class A1 and A2 gestational diabetic patients delivered beyond 40 weeks' gestation. Am J Perinatol 9:484–8.

Macafee CA, Beischer NA. 1974. The relative value of the standard indications for performing a glucose tolerance test in pregnancy. Med J Aust 1:911–4.

Mackeprang M, Hay S, Lunde S. 1972. Completeness and accuracy of reporting of malformations on birth certificates. Public Health Rep 87:43–9.

Magnus R, Rogers JG, Haan EA 1983. Does sacral agenesis predispose to spina bifida? J Med Genet 20:313.

Maher JE, Colvin, EV, Samdarshi TE, et al. 1994. Fetal echocardiography in gravidas with historic risk factors for congenital heart diaeasse. Am J Perinatol 11:334–6.

Maisels DO, Stilwell JH. 1980. The Pierre Robin syndrome associated with femoral dysgenesis. Br J Plast Surg 33:237–41.

Majewski A. 1953. Beobachtungen an Neugeborenen diabetischer Mütter. Geburts Frauenheilk 13:25–34.

Majewski F, Nothjunge J, Bierich JR. 1979. Alcohol embryopathy and diabetic fetopathy in the same newborn. Helv Paediatr Acta 34:135–40.

Makino S, Kunimoto K, Muraoka Y, et al. 1980. Breeding of a non-obese, diabetic strain of mice. Exp Anim 29:1–13.

Malins J. 1968. Clinical Diabetes Mellitus. Eyre & Spottiswoode, London.

Malins J. 1979. Fetal anomalies related to carbohydrate metabolism: the epidemiological approach. In: Sutherland HW, Stowers JM, eds. Carbohydrate Metabolism in Pregnancy and the Newborn. Springer, Berlin, pp. 229–46.

Malins JM, FitzGerald MG. 1965. Childbearing prior to recognition of diabetes: recollected birth weights and stillbirth rate in babies born to parents who developed diabetes. Diabetes 14:175–8.

Mall FR. 1908. A Study of the Causes Underlying the Origin of Human Monsters. Wistar, Philadelphia.

Malpas P. 1937. The incidence of human malformations and the significance of changes in the environment in their causation. J Obstet Gynecol Br Emp 44:434–54.

Manning FA, Morrison I, Lange IR, et al. 1985. Fetal assessment based on fetal biophysical profile scoring: experince in 12,620 referred high-risk pregnancies. I. Perinatal mortality by frequency and etiology. Am J Obstet Gynecol 151:343–50.

Manzke H, Cromme E, Gutezeit G. 1977. Entwicklung von Kindern diabetischer Mütter. Med Welt 28:1409–14.

Marble, A. 1985. Insulin in the treatment of diabetes. In: Marble A, Krall LP, Bradley RF, et al. eds. Joslin's Diabetes Mellitus. Lea & Febiger, Philadelphia, pp. 380–405.

Marden PM, Smith DW, McDonald J. 1964. Congenital anomalies in the newborn infant, including minor variations. J Paediatr 64:357–71.

Maresh M, Beard RW, Bray CS, et al. 1989. Factors predisposing to and outcome of gestational diabetes. Obstet Gynecol 74:324–6.

Mariani AJ, Stern J, Khan AU, et al. 1979. Sacral agenesis: an analysis of 11 cases and review of the literature. J Urol 122:684–6.

Marks HH, Krall LP, White P. 1971. Epidemiology and detection of diabetes. In: Marble A, White P, Bradley RF, et al., eds. Joslin's Diabetes Mellitus. Lea & Febiger, Philadelphia, pp. 10–34.

Marliss EB, Nakhooda AF, Poussier P, et al. 1982. The diabetic syndrome of the "BB" Wistar rat: possible relevance to type 1 (insulin-dependent) diabetes in man. Diabetologia 22:225–32.

Marquardsen G. 1952. Fertilitäts- und Graviditätskatamnese von 100 Diabetikerinnen. Arzt Wochenschr 7:700–4.

Marquette GP, Klein VR, Niebyl JR. 1985. Efficacy of screening for gestational diabetes. Am J Perinatol 2:7–9.

Martin AA, Barrio AML, Guerrero GC, et al. 1990. Sirenomelia: presentacíon de tres casos. An Esp Pediatr 33:87–9.

Martin E. 1880. Histoire des Monstres depuis l'Antiquité jusqu'a nos Jours. Reinwald, Paris.

Martin GR, Perry LW, Ferencz C. 1989. Increased prevalence of ventricular septal defects: epidemic or improved diagnosis. Pediatrics 83:200–3.

Martin RA, Fineman RM, Jorde LB. 1983. Phenotypic heterogeneity in neural tube defects: a clue to causal heterogeneity. Am J Med Genet 16:519–26.

Martin TR, Allen AC, Stinson D. 1979. Overt diabetes in pregnancy. Am J Obstet Gynecol 133:275–80.

Martinez C, Grande F, Bittner JJ. 1954. Alloxan diabetes in different strain of mice. Proc Soc Exp Biol Med 87:236–7.

Martínez-Frías ML. 1994. Epidemiological analysis of outcomes of pregnancy in diabetic mothers: identification of the most characteristic and most frequent congenital anomalies. Am J Med Genet 51:108–13.

Martínez-Frías ML, Bermejo E, Cereijo A. 1992. Preaxial polydactyly of feet in infants of diabetic mothers: epidemiological test of a clinical hypothesis. Am J Med Genet 42:643–6.

Martínez-Frías ML, Bermejo E, García A, et al. 1994. Holoprosencephaly associated with caudal dysgenesis: a clincal epidemiological analysis. Am J Med Genet 53:46–51.

Martínez-Frías ML, Bermejo E, Rodriguez-Pinilla L, et al. 1998. Epidemiological analysis of outcomes of pregnancy in gestational diabetic mothers. Am J Med Genet 78:140–5.

Martínez-Frías ML, Frías JL, Salvador J. 1989. Clinical/epidemiological analysis of malformations. Am J Med Genet 35:121–5.

Mathers CD, Field B. 1983. Some international trends in the incidence of neural tube defects. Comm Health Stud 7:60–6.

Matsunaga E, Shiota K. 1977. Holoprosencephaly in human embryos: epidemiologic studies of 150 cases. Teratology 16:261–72.

Matsunaga E, Shiota K. 1980. Search for maternal factors associated with malformed human embryos: a prospective study. Teratology 21:323–31.

Matthiessen PC, Trolle D, Zachau-Christiansen B. 1967. Infant and perinatal mortality in Denmark. PHS Publ. No. 1000, Ser. 3, No. 9, U.S. Government Printing Office, Washington, DC.

Mattingly G. 1941. Catherine of Aragon. Little, Brown, Boston.

Mayer JB. 1952. Die Embryopathia diabetica. Z Kinderheilk 71:183–201.

Mayer JB. 1964. Der Einfluss des mütterlichen Diabetes auf das werdende Kind: die diabetogenen Embryopathien. Bull Schweiz Akad Med Wiss 20:470–86.

Mayer TK, Freedman ZR. 1983. Protein glycosylation in diabetes mellitus: a review of laboratory measurements and of their clinical utility. Clin Chim Acta 127:147–84.

Mazze RS, Krogh CL. 1992. Gestational diabetes-mellitus: now is the time for detection and treatment. Mayo Clin Proc 67:995–1003.

McBride WG. 1961. Thalidomide and congenital abnormalities. Lancet 2:1358.

McCain JR, Lester WM. 1950. Diabetes in pregnancy. J Med Ass Ga 39:57–63.

McCain DR, Hadden DR. 1989. Are all infants of diabetic mothers "macrosomic?" Br Med J 298:524–5.

McCracken JS. 1965. Absence of foetal femur and maternal prediabetes. Lancet 1:1274–5.

McDonald AD. 1961. Maternal health in early pregnancy and congenital defect: final report on a prospective inquiry. Br J Prev Soc Med 15:154–66.

McDonald GW, Fisher GF, Burnham C. 1965. Reproducibility of the oral glucose tolerance test. Diabetes 14:473–80.

McFarland KF, Case CA. 1985. The relationship of maternal age on gestational diabetes. Diab Care 8:598–600.

McFarland KF, Hemaya E. 1985. Neonatal mortality in infants of diabetic mothers. Diab Care 8:333–6.

McIntosh R, Merritt KK, Richards MR, et al. 1954. The incidence of congenital malformations: a study of 5,964 pregnancies. Pediatrics 14:505–21.

McKeown T. 1988. The Origins of Human Disease. Blackwell, London.

McKeown T, Record RG. 1960. Malformations in a population observed for five years after birth. In: Wolstenholme GE, O'Connor CM, eds. Ciba Foundation Symposium on Congenital Malformations. Little, Brown, Boston, pp. 2–16.

McKusick VA, ed. 1992. Mendelian Inheritance in Man: catalogs of autosomal dominant, autosomal recessive, and x-linked phenotypes. Johns Hopkins Univ, Baltimore.

McLendon H, Bottomy JR. 1960. A critical analysis of the management of pregnancy in diabetic women. Am J Obstet Gynecol 80:641–52.

McNeil C. 1943. The first month of life: general survey. Edinb Med J 50:491–9.

Meberg A, Otterstad JE, Frøland G, et al. 1994. Increased incidence of ventricular septal defects caused by improved detection rate. Acta Paediatr 83:653–7.

Medical Research Council. 1955. The use of hormones in the management of pregnancy in diabetics. Lancet 2:833–6.

Méhes K. 1983. Minor Malformations in the Neonate. Akadémiai Kiadó, Budapest.

Méhes K. 1988. Informative Morphogenetic Variants in the Newborm Infant. Akadémiai Kiadó, Budapest.

Meinert CL. 1972. Standardization of the oral glucose tolerance test: criticisms and suggestions invited. Diabetes 21:1197–8.

Meirik O, Smedby B, Ericson A. 1979. Impact of changing age and parity distributions of mothers on perinatal mortality in Sweden, 1953–1975. Int J Epidemiol 8:361–4.

Mellin GW. 1963. The frequency of birth defects. In: Fishbein M, ed. Birth Defects. Lippincott, Philadelphia, pp. 1–17.

Mello G, Parretti E, Mecacci F, et al. 1997. Livelli glicemi [soglia] e aborto spontaneo nel I trimestre nelle gestani affette da diabete mellito insulino-dipendente. Min Gin 49:365–70.

Mengert WF, Laughlin KA. 1939. Thirty-three pregnancies in diabetic women. Surg Gynecol Obstet 69:615–7.

Merkatz IR, Duchon MA, Yamashita TS, et al. 1980. A pilot community-based screening program for gestational diabetes. Diab Care 3:453–7.

Merlob P. 1994. Mild errors of morphogenesis: one of the most controversial subjects in dysmorphology. In: Kalter H, ed. Issues and Reviews in Teratology. Vol. 7. Plenum Press, New York, pp. 57–102.

Merlob P, Papier CM, Klingberg MA, et al. 1985. Incidence of congenital malformations in the newborn, particularly minor abnormalities. In: Marois, M, ed. Prevention of Physical and Mental Congenital Defects. Liss, New York, pp. 51–6.

Mestman LH. 1980. Oucome of diabetes screening in pregnancy and perinatal morbidity in infants of mothers with mild impairment in glucose tolerance. Diab Care 3:447–52.

Metzger BE, and the Organizing Committee. 1991. Summary and recommendations of the third international workshop-conference on gestational diabetes mellitus. Diabetes 40:197–201.

Meyer-Wittkopf M, Simpson JM, Sharland GK. 1996. Incidence of congenital heart defects in fetuses of diabetic mothers: a retrospective study of 326 cases. Ultrasound Obstet Gynecol 8:8–10.

Mickal A, Begneaud WP, Weese WH. 1966. Glucose tolerance and excessively large infants: a twelve year follow-up study. Am J Obstet Gynecol 94:62–4.

Miller E, Hare JW, Cloherty JP, et al. 1981. Elevated maternal hemoglobin A_{1c} in early pregnancy and major congenital anomalies in infants of diabetic mothers. N Engl J Med 304:1331–4.

Miller HC. 1945. The effect of the prediabetic state on the survival of the fetus and the birth weight of the newborn infant. N Engl J Med 233:376–8.

Miller HC. 1946. The effect of diabetic and prediabetic pregnancies on the fetus and newborn infant. J Pediatr 29:455–61.

Miller HC. 1947. The effect of pregnancy complicated by alloxan diabetes on the fetuses of dogs, rabbits and rats. Endocrinology 40:251–8.

Miller HC. 1956. Offspring of diabetic and prediabetic mothers. In: Levine SZ, ed. Advances in Pediatrics. Vol. 8. YearBook, Chicago, pp. 137–63.

Miller HC, Hurwitz D, Kuder K. 1944. Neonatal mortality in pregnancies complicated by diabetes mellitus. JAMA 124:271–5.

Miller HC, Wilson HM. 1943. Macrosomia, cardiac hypertrophy, erythroblastosis, and hyperplasia of the islands of Langerhans in infants born to diabetic mothers. J Pediatr 23:251–66.

Miller M. 1965. Diabetic pregnancy and foetal survival in a large metropolitan area. In: Leibel BS, Wrenshall GA, eds. On the Nature and Treatment of Diabetes. Excerpta Medica, Amsterdam, pp. 714–7.

Miller RW, Blot WJ. 1972. Small head size after in-utero exposure to atomic radiation. Lancet 2:784–7.

Miller RW, Mulvihill JJ. 1976. Small head size after atomic radiation. Teratology 16:355–7.

Miller SF. 1972. Transposition of the external genitalia associated with the syndrome of caudal regression. J Urol 108:818–22.

Mills JL. 1982. Malformations in infants of diabetic mothers. Teratology 25:385–94.

Mills JL, Baker L, Goldman AS. 1979. Malformations in infants of diabetic mothers occur before the seventh gestational week: implications for treatment. Diabetes 28:292–3.

Mills JL, Fishl AR, Knopp RH, et al. 1983. Malformations in infants of diabetic mothers: problems in study design. Prev Med 12:274–86.

Mills JL, Knopp RH, Simpson JL, et al. 1988b. Lack of relation of increased malformation rates in infants of diabetic mothers to glycemic control during organogenesis. N Engl J Med 318:671–6.

Mills JL, Simpson JL, Driscoll SG, et al. 1988a. Incidence of spontaneous abortion among normal women and insulin-dependent diabetic women whose pregnancies were identified within 21 days of conception. N Engl J Med 319:1617–23.

Mills JL, Withiam MJ. 1986. Diabetes, pregnancy, and malformations: an epidemiologic perspective. In: Jovanovic L, Peterson CM, Fuhrmann K, eds. Diabetes and Pregnancy: teratology, toxicity and treatment. Praeger, New York, pp. 3–14.

Milunsky A, Alpert E, Kitzmiller JL, et al. 1982. Prenatal diagnosis of neural tube defects. VIII. The importance of serum alpha-fetoprotein screening in diabetic pregnant women. Am J Obstet Gynecol 142:1030–2.

Mimouni F, Miodovnik M, Rosenn B, et al. 1992. Birth trauma in insulin-dependent diabetic pregnancies. Am J Perinat 9:205–8.

Mimouni F, Miodovnik M, Tsang R.C, et al. 1987. Decreased maternal serum magnesium concentration and adverse fetal outcome in insulin-dependent diabetic women. Obstet Gynecol 70:85–8.

Mimouni M. 1972. Les malformations congénitales des enfants nés de mères diabétiques traitées par l'insuline. J Paediatr 53:579–85.

Miodovnik M, Lavin JP, Knowles HC, et al. 1984. Spontaneous abortion among insulin-dependent diabetic women. Am J Obstet Gynecol 150:372–5.

Miodovnik M, Mimouni F, Berk M, et al. 1989. Alloxan-induced diabetes mellitus in the pregnant ewe: metabolic and cardiovascular effects on the mother and her fetus. Am J Obstet Gynecol 160:1239–44.

Miodovnik M, Mimouni F, Dignan PSJ, et al. 1988. Major malformations in infants of IDDM women: vasculopathy and early trimester poor glycemic control. Diab Care 11:713–8.

Miodovnik M, Mimouni F, Tsang RC, et al. 1986. Glycemic control and spontaneous abortion in insulin-dependent diabetic women. Obstet Gynecol 68:366–9.

Miodovnik M, Rosenn B, Siddiqi T, et al. 1998. Increased rate of congenital malformations (CM) and perinatal mortality (PM) in infants of mothers with insulin dependent diabetes (IDDM): myth or reality. Am J Obstet Gynecol 178:S52.

Miodovnik M, Skillman C, Holroyde JC, et al. 1985. Elevated maternal glycohemoglobin in early pregnancy and spontaneous abortion among insulin-dependent diabetic women. Am J Obstet Gynecol 153:439–42.

Mitchell SC, Berendres HW, Clark WM Jr. 1967. The normal closure of the ventricular septum. Am Heart J 83:334–8.

Mitchell SC, Korones SB, Berendes HW. 1971a. Congenital heart disease in 56,109 births: incidence and natural history. Circulation 43:323–32.

Mitchell SC, Sellman AH, Westphal MC, et al. 1971b. Etiologic correlates in a study of congenital heart diaease in 56,109 births. Am J Cardiol 28:653–7.

Modanlou HD, Dorchester WL, Thorosian A, et al. 1980. Macrosomia—maternal, fetal, and neonatal implications. Obstet Gynecol 55:420–4.

Modvig J, Schmidt L, Damsgaard MT. 1990. Measurement of total risk of spontaneous abortion: the virtue of conditional risk estimation. Am J Epidemiol 132:1021–38.

Moe DG, Guntheroth WG. 1987. Spontaneous closure of uncomplicated ventricular septal defect. Am J Cardiol 60:674–8.

Moe N, Paul P, Jervell J, et al. 1987. Diabetes mellitus og graviditet. T Norske Laegeforen 107:1746–50.

Moley KH, Vaughn WK, DeCherney AH, et al.1991. Effect of diabetes mellitus on mouse pre-implantation embryo development. J Reprod Fertil 93:325–32.

Möllerström J. 1950. Graviditetsförloppet vid diabetes. Nord Med 44:1570–1.

Mølsted-Pedersen, L. 1980. Congenital malformations in the offspring of diabetic women. In: Waldhaüsl WK, ed. Diabetes 1979. Proceedings of the 10th Congress of IDF, Vienna, Austria. Excerpta Medica, Amsterdam, pp. 758–62.

Mølsted-Pedersen, L. 1984. Detection of gestational diabetes. In: Sutherland HW, Stowers M, eds. Carbohydrate Metabolism in Pregnancy and the Newborn. Livingstone, Edinburgh, pp. 209–14.

Mølsted-Pedersen L, Pedersen J. 1967. Causes of perinatal death in diabetic pregnancy: a clinico-pathological analysis. Acta Med Scand Suppl 476:175–81.

Mølsted-Pedersen L, Tygstrup I, Pedersen J. 1964. Congenital malformations in newborn infants of diabetic women: correlation with maternal diabetic vascular complications. Lancet 1:1124–6.

Moore WM 1991. Naegele's rule. Lancet 337:910.

Moreau R, Deuil R, Hadjissotiriou, G, et al. 1955. L'importance de la mortalité et la fréquence des gros enfants chez les diabétiques et les prédiabétiques. Sem Hôp 31:652–5.

Morishima M, Ando M, Takao A. 1991. Visceroatrial heterotaxy syndrome in the NOD mouse with particular reference to the atrial sinus. Teratology 44:91–100.

Morison SE. 1971. The European Discovery of America: the northern voyages. AD 500–1600. Oxford University, New York.

Morris MA, Grandis AS, Litton JC. 1985. Glycosylated hemoglobin concentration in early gestation associated with neonatal outcome. Am J Obstet Gynecol 153:651–4.

Morris NM, Udry JR, Chase CL. 1975. Shifting age-parity distribution of births and the decrease in infant mortality. Am J Public Health 65:359–62.

Mosenthal HO, Barry E. 1950. Criteria for and interpretation of normal glucose tolerance tests. Ann Intern Med 33:1175–94.

Moss JM, Connor EJ. 1965. Pregnancy complicated by diabetes: report of 102 pregnancies including eleven treated with oral hypoglycemic drugs. Med Ann DC 34:253–60.

Moss JM, Mulholland HB. 1951. Diabetes and pregnancy: with special reference to the prediabetic state. Ann Intern Med 34:678–91.

Moyer JH, Womack CR. 1950. Glucose tolerance. I. A comparison of 4 types of diagnostic tests in 103 control subjects and 26 patients with diabetes. Am J Med Sci 219:161–73.

Mufarrij IK, Kilejian VO. 1963. Anencephaly. Obstet Gynecol 22:657–61.

Müller F, O'Rahilly R. 1989. Mediobasal prosencephalic defects, including holoprosencephaly and cyclopia, in relation to the development of the human forebrain. Am J Anat 185:391–414.

Murphy DP. 1929. Outcome of 625 pregnancies in women subjected to pelvic radium or roentgen irradiation. Am J Obstet Gynecol 18:179–87.

Murphy DP. 1933. Excretion of ovary stimulating hormone in urine during pregnancy: its relation to urinary output. Surg Gynecol Obstet 56:914–7.

Murphy DP. 1939. Congenital Malformations: a study of parental characteristics with special reference to the reproductive process. University of Pennsylvania, Philadelphia.

Murphy EA. 1966. A scientific viewpoint on normalcy. Perspect Biol Med 9:333–48.

Murphy J, Peters J, Morris P, et al. 1984. Conservative management of pregnancy in diabetic women. Br Med J 288:1203–5.

Murphy NJ, Bulkow LR, Schraer CD, et al. 1993. Prevalence of diabetes mellitus in pregnancy among Yup'ik Eskimos, 1987–1988. Diab Care 16 Suppl 1:315–7.

Muylder XD. 1984. Perinatal complications of gestational diabetes: the influence of the timing of the diagnosis. Eur J Obstet Gynecol Reprod Biol 18:35–42.

Mylvaganam R, Stowers JM, Steel JM, et al. 1983. Insulin immunogenicity in pregnancy: maternal and fetal studies. Diabetologia 24:19–25.

Myrianthopoulos NC. 1985. Malformations in Children From One to Seven Years: a report from the Collaborative Perinatal Project. Liss, New York.

Myrianthopoulos NC, Chung CS. 1974. Congenital malformations in singletons: epidemiological analysis. Birth Defects 10(11):1–58.

Naeye RL. 1965. Infants of diabetic mothers: a quantitative morphologic study. Pediatrics 35:980–8.

Naeye RL. 1979. The outcome of diabetic pregnancies: a prospective study. Ciba Found Symp 63:227–41.

Naeye RL. 1990. Maternal bidy weight and pregnancy outcome. Am J Clin Nutr 52:273–9.

Naggan L, MacMahon B. 1967. Ethnic differences in the prevalence of anencephaly and spina bifida in Boston, Massachusetts. N Engl J Med 277:1119–23.

Nakhooda AF, Like AA, Chappel CI, et al. 1976. The spontaneously diabetic Wistar rat: metabolic and morphologic studies. Diabetes 26:100–12.

Nathanson JN. 1950. The excessively large fetus as an obstetric problem. Am J Obstet Gynecol 60:54–63.

National Center for Health Statistics. 1992. Annual summary of births, marriages, divorces, and deaths: United States, 1991. Mon Vital Stat Rep 40 (13):1–28.

National Center for Health Statistics. 1998. Births, marriages, divorces, and deaths for October 1997. Mon Vital Stat Rep 46 (10):1–20.

National Diabetes Data Group. 1979. Classification and diagnosis of diabetes mellitus and other categories of glucose intolerance. Diabetes 28:1039–57.

Nau H. 1987. Species differences in pharmacokinetics, drug metabolism, and teratogenesis. In: Nau H, Scott WJ, eds. Pharmacokinetics in Teratogenesis. Vol. 1. CRC, Boca Raton, pp. 81–106.

Navarrete VN, Torres IH, Rivera IR, et al. 1967. Maternal carbohydrate disorder and congenital malformations. Diabetes 16:127–9.

Naylor AF. 1974. Sequential aspects of spontaneous abortion: maternal age, parity, and pregnancy compensation artifact. Soc Biol 21:195–204.

Naylor CD. 1989. Diagnosing gestational diabetes mellitus: is the gold standard valid? Diab Care 12:565–72.

Naylor CD, Sermer M, Chen E, et al. 1997. Selective screening for gestational diabetes mellitus. N Engl J Med 337:1591–6.

Neave C. 1967. Congental Malformations in Offspring of Diabetics. Doctor of Public Health Thesis, Harvard University, Boston.

Neave C. 1984. Congenital malformations in offspring of diabetics. Perspect Paediatr Pathol 8:213–22.

Neel JV. 1958. A study of major congenital defects in Japanese infants. Am J Hum Genet 10:398–445.

Neel JV. 1970. The genetics of diabetes mellitus. In: Camerini-Dávalos RA, Cole HS, eds. Early Diabetes. Academic Press, New York, pp. 3–10.

Neilson DR, Bolton RN, Prins RP, et al. 1991. Glucose challenge testing in pregnancy. Am J Obstet Gynecol 164:1673–9.

Nelson HB, Gillespie L, White P. 1953. Pregnancy complicated by diabetes mellitus. Obstet Gynecol 1:219–25.

Nelson RL. 1986. Diabetes and pregnancy: control can make a difference. Mayo Clin Proc 61:825–9.

Neufeld ND. 1987. Infants of diabetic mothers: prenatal care and outcomes for the infant. Mt. Sinai J Med 54:266–71.

Nevinny H, Schretter G. 1930. Zuckerkrankheit und Schwangerschaft. Arch Gynäk 140:397–427.

Newman TB. 1985. Etiology of ventricular septal defects: an epidemiologic approach. Pediatrics 76:741–9.

Newsholme A. 1910. Report by the Medical Officer on Child Mortality. Supplement to the 30th Annual Report. Local Government Board, London.

Nicolini U, Kustermann A, Gargiulo M, et al. 1986. Esiti perinatali nelle gravide diabetiche:1963–75 e 1978–83. Ann Ost Gin 107:243–50.

Nielsen GL, Hostrup P. 1990. Malformations in 238 diabetic pregnancies: no correlation between HbA_{1c} and malformations. Diabetologia 33:A138.

Nielsen GL, Nielsen PH. 1993. Outcome of 328 pregnancies in 205 women with insulin-dependent diabetes mellitus in the county of Northern Jutland from 1976 to 1990. Eur J Obstet Gynecol Reprod Biol 50:33–8.

Nielsen GL, Nielsen PH. 1994. Results of 312 pregnancies among White class B-F mothers in Northern Jutland from 1976 to 1992. Dan Med Bull 41:115–8.

Nishimura H, Takano K, Tanimura, T, et al. 1968. Normal and abnormal development of human embryos: first report of the analysis of 1,213 intact embryos. Teratology 1:281–90.

Niswander KR, Gordon M. 1972. The Women and their Pregnancies. Saunders, Philadelphia.

Nordlander E, Hanson U, Persson B. 1989. Factors influencing neonatal morbidity in gestational diabetic pregnancy. Br J Obstet Gynecol 96:671–8.

Northern Regional Survey Steering Group. 1992. Fetal abnormality: an audit of its recognition and management. Arch Dis Child 67:770–4.

Nothmann M, Hermstein A. 1932. Diabetes und Gravidität. I. Mitteilung. Arch Gynäk 150:287–301.

Nowack E. 1965. Die sensible Phase bei der Thalidomid-Embryopathie. Humangenetik 1:516–36.

O'Rahilly R, Müller F. 1989. Interpretation of some median anomalies as illustrated by cyclopia and symmelia. Teratology 40:409–22.

O'Shaughnessy R, Russ J, Zuspan FP. 1979. Glycosylated hemoglobins and diabetes mellitus in pregnancy. Am J Obstet Gynecol 135:783–90.

O'Sullivan JB. 1961. Gestational diabetes: unsuspected, asymptomatic diabetes in pregnancy. N Engl J Med 264:1082–5.

O'Sullivan JB. 1975. Insulin treatment for gestational diabetes. In: Camerini-Dávalos RA, Coles HS, eds. Early Diabetes. Academic Press, New York, pp. 447–53.

O'Sullivan JB. 1979. Gestational diabetes: factors influencing the rates of subsequent diabetes. In: Sutherland HW, Stowers JM, eds. Carbohydrate Metabolism in Pregnancy and the Newborn 1978. Springer, Berlin, pp. 425–34.

O'Sullivan JB. 1980. Establishing criteria for gestational diabetes. Diab Care 3:437–9.

O'Sullivan JB, Gellis SS, Dandrow RV, et al. 1966. The potential diabetic and treatment in pregnancy. Obstet Gynecol 27:683–9.

O'Sullivan JB, Mahan CM. 1964. Criteria for the oral glucose tolerance test in pregnancy. Diabetes 13:278–85.

O'Sullivan JB, Mahan CM. 1966. Glucose tolerance test: variability in pregnant and nonpregnant women. Am J Clin Nutr 19:345–51.

O'Sullivan JB, Mahan CM, Charles D, et al. 1973a. Screening criteria for high-risk gestational diabetic patients. Am J Obstet Gynecol 116:895–900.

O'Sullivan JB, Mahan CM, Charles D, et al. 1974. Medical treatment of the gestational diabetic. Obstet Gynecol 43:817–21.

Oakley GP, Erickson JD, James LM, et al. 1994. Prevention of folic acid-preventable spina bifida and anencephaly. In: Bock G, Marsh J, eds. Neural Tube Defects. Wiley, Chichester, pp. 212–31.

Oakley W. 1953. Prognosis in diabetic pregnancy. Br Med J 1:1413–5.

Oakley W. 1965. The treatment of pregnancy in diabetes mellitus. In: Leibel BS, Wrenshall GA, eds. On the Nature and Treatment of Diabetes Mellitus. Excerpta Medica, Amsterdam, pp. 673–8.

Oats JN, Beischer NA. 1986. Gestational diabetes. Aust NZ J Obstet Gynecol 26:2–10.

Ober C, Simpson JL. 1986. Diabetes mellitus: preventing anomalies through maternal metabolic intervention. Clin Obstet Gynecol 29:558–68.

Olofsson P, Liedholm H, Sartor G, et al. 1984. Diabetes and pregnancy: a 21-year Swedish material. Acta Obstet Gynecol Scand Suppl 122:3–62.

Olsen CL, Hughes JP, Youngblood LG, et al. 1997. Epidemiology of holoprosencephaly and phenotypic characteristics of affected children: New York State, 1984–1989. Am J Med Genet 73:217–26.

Ooshima Y, Shiota K. 1991. Congenital malformations in genetically diabetic mice, yellow KK. Teratology 44:13B.

Opitz JM. 1994. Associations and syndromes: terminology in clinical genetics and birth defects epidemiology. Am J Med Genet 49:14–20.

Opperman W, Gugliucci C, O'Sullivan MJ, et al. 1975. Gestational diabetes and macrosomia. In: Camerini-Dávalos RA, Cole HS, eds. Early Diabetes. Academic Press, New York, pp. 455–69.

Orchard TJ, Dorman JS, LaPorte RE, et al. 1986. Host and environmental interactions in diabetes mellitus. J Chron Dis 39:979–1000.

Ornoy A, Ratzo, N, Greenbaum C, et al. 1994. The development of children born to diabetic mothers at the age of 6–10 years. Teratology 50:25A.

Osler W. 1885. The Gulstonian Lectures, on malignant endocarditis. Br Med J 1:467–70.

Österlund K, Rantakallio P. 1964. Perinatal mortality in diabetic pregnancies. Ann Paediatr Fenn 10:84–91.

Otani H, Tanaka O, Tatekawi R, et al. 1991. Diabetic environment and genetic disposition as causes of congenital malformations in NOD mouse embryos. Diabetes 40:1245–50.

Ounsted M, Moar VA, Cockburn J, et al. 1984. Factors associated with the intellectual ability of children born to women with high risk pregnancies. Br Med J 228:1038–41.

Padmanabhan R, Al-Zuhair AG. 1988. Congenital malformations and intrauterine growth retardation in streptozotocin induced diabetes during gestation in the rat. Reprod Toxic 1:117–25.

Palacin M, Lasunción MA, Martin A, et al. 1985. Decreased uterine blood flow in the diabetic pregnant rat does not modify the augmented glucose transfer to the fetus. Biol Neonat 48:197–203.

Palmer LJ, Barnes RH. 1945. Pregnancy in the diabetic. West J Surg Obstet Gynecol 53:195–202.

Palumbo L. 1954. Diabetes mellitus complicated by pregnancy. N Carol Med J 15:120–3.

Pampfer S, Hertogh RD, Vanderheyden I, et al. 1990. Decreased inner cell mass proportion in blastocysts from diabetic rats. Diabetes 39:471–6.

Pang D. 1993 Sacral agenesis and caudal spinal cord malformations. Neurosurgery 32:755–78.

Pang D, Hoffman HJ. 1980. Sacral agenesis with progressive neurological deficit. Neurosurgery 7:118–26.

Pardou A, Dodion J, Loeb H. 1977. Mortality and morbidity in newborns of insulin dependent diabetic mothers. Acta Paediatr Belg 30:165–70.

Parisot MJ. 1911. Les troubles de la fonction génitale chez les diabétiques: leur pathogénie. Bull Mem Soc Med Hôp Paris 35:95–110.

Park SC, Mathews RA, Zuberbuhler JR, et al. 1977. Down syndrome with congenital heart malformation. Am J Dis Child 131:29–37.

Parsons E, Randall LM, Wilder RM. 1926. Pregnancy and diabetes. Med Clin North Am 10:679–88.

Passarge E. 1965. Congenital malformations and maternal diabetes. Lancet 1:324–5.

Passarge E, Lenz W. 1966. Syndrome of caudal regression in infants of diabetic mothers: observations of further cases. Pediatrics 37:672–5.

Pastor X, Domenech P, Jorba JM, et al. 1988. Somatometric study in the infant of gestational diabetic mother. In: Weiss PA, Coustan DR, eds. Gestational Diabetes. Springer, New York, pp. 171–5.

Paterson SJ. 1944. Iniencephalus. J. Obstet Gynecol Br Emp 51:330–3.

Paton DM. 1948. Pregnancy in the prediabetic patient. Am J Obstet Gynecol 56:558–60.

Patrick SL, Moy CS, LaPorte RE. 1989. The world of insulin-dependent diabetes mellitus: what international epidemiological studies reveal about the etiology and natural history of IDDM. Diab Metab Rev 5:571–8.

Patterson JW, Lazarow A, Levey S. 1949. Alloxan and dialuric acid: their stabilities and ultraviolet absorption spectra. J Biol Chem 177:187–96.

Patterson M, Burnstein N. 1949. Diabetes and pregnancy: a clinical analysis. Arch Intern Med 83:390–401.

Pauli RM, Reiser CA. 1994. Wisconsin stillbirth service program. II. Analysis of diagnoses and diagnostic categories in the first 1,000 referrals. Am J Med Genet 50:135–53.

Paxton J, ed. 1987. The Statesman's Year-Book. St. Martin's Press, New York.

Peacock I, Hunter JC, Walford S, et al. 1979. Self-monitoring of blood glucose in diabetic pregnancy. Br Med J 2:1333–6.

Pease JC, Smallpiece V, Lennon GC. 1951. Diabetes and pregnancy. Br Med J 1:1296–8.

Peck RW, Price DE, Lang GD, et al. 1991. Birthweight of babies born to mothers with type 1 diabetes: is it related to blood glucose control in the first trimester? Diab Med 8:258–62.

Peckham CH. 1931. Diabetes mellitus and pregnancy. Bull Johns Hopkins Hosp 49:184–201.

Pedersen J. 1952. Course of diabetes during pregnancy. Acta Endocrinol 9:342–64.

Pedersen J. 1954a. Fetal mortality in diabetic pregnancies. Diabetes 3:199–204.

Pedersen J. 1954b. Weight and length at birth of infants of diabetic mothers. Acta Endocrinol 16:330–42.

Pedersen J. 1975. Goals and end-points in management of diabetic pregnancy. In: Camerini-Dávalos RA, Cole HS, eds. Early Diabetes. Academic Press, New York, pp. 381–91.

Pedersen J. 1977. The Pregnant Diabetic and Her Newborn: problems and management. Munksgaard, Copenhagen.

Pedersen J. 1979. Congenital malformations in newborns of diabetic mothers. In: Sutherland HW, Stowers JM, eds. Carbohydrate Metabolism and the Newborn 1978. Springer, Berlin, pp. 264–76.

Pedersen J, Brandstrup E. 1956. Foetal mortality in pregnant diabetics: strict control of diabetes with conservative obstetric management. Lancet 1:607–10.

Pedersen J, Mølsted-Pedersen L. 1965. Prognosis of the outcome of pregnancies in diabetics: a new classification. Acta Endocrinol 50:70–8.

Pedersen J, Mølsted-Pedersen L. 1978. Congenital malformations: the possible role of diabetes care outside pregnancy. Ciba Found Symp 63:265–71.

Pedersen J, Mølsted-Pedersen LA, Andersen B. 1974. Assessors of fetal perinatal mortality in diabetic pregnancy: analysis of 1,332 pregnancies in the Copenhagen series, 1946–1972. Diabetes 23:302–5.

Pedersen J, Osler M. 1958. Development of ossification centres in infants of diabetic mothers. Acta Endocrinol 29:467–72.

Pedersen J, Schondel A. 1949. Follow-up examination of children of diabetic mothers. Acta Paediatr Suppl 77:203–4.

Pedersen JF, Mølsted-Pedersen L. 1979. Early growth retardation in diabetic pregnancy. Br Med J 1:18–9.

Pedersen JF, Mølsted-Pedersen L. 1981. Early fetal growth delay detected by ultrasound marks increased risk of congenital malformation in diabetic pregnancy. Br Med J 283:269–71.

Pedersen JF, Mølsted-Pedersen L. 1985. The possibility of an early growth delay in White's Class A diabetic pregnancy. Diabetes 34 Suppl 2:47–9.

Pedersen JF, Mølsted-Pedersen L, Mortensen HB. 1984. Fetal growth delay and maternal hemoglobin A_{1c} in early diabetic pregnancy. Obstet Gynecol 64:351–2.

Pedowitz P, Shlevin EL. 1952. The pregnant diabetic. Bull NY Acad Med 28:440–53.

Pedowitz P, Shlevin EL. 1955. The pregnant diabetic patient. Am J Obstet Gynecol 69:395–404.

Pedowitz P, Shlevin EL. 1964. Review of management of pregnancy complicated by diabetes and altered carbohydrate metabolism. Obstet Gynecol 23:716–29.

Peel J, Oakley W. 1949. The management of pregnancy in diabetics. In: Transactions of the XIIth British Congress of Obstetrics and Gynecology. Austral, London, pp. 161–84.

Pehrson SL. 1974. A study of the relationship between some prediabetic stigmas, glucose tolerance in late pregnancy and the birthweight of the children. Acta Obstet Gynecol Scand Suppl 33:1–152.

Peller S. 1923. Die Säulingssterblichkeit nach dem Kriege. I. Wein Klin Wochenschr 36:799–801.

Peller S. 1948. Mortality, past and future. Popul Stud 1:411–56.

Pengelly CDR. 1961. Pregnancy in the diabetic. Practitioner 186:96–101.

Penrose LS. 1957. The genetics of anencephaly. J Ment Def Res 1:4–15.

Perrot LJ, Williamson S, Jimenez JF. 1987. The caudal regression syndrome in infants of diabetic mothers. Ann Clin Lab Med 17:211–20.

Perry J, Bonnett CA, Hoffer MM. 1970. Vertebral pelvic fusions in the rehabilitation of patients with sacral agenesis. J Bone Joint Surg 52A:288–94.

Persson B, Gentz J. 1984. Follow-up of children of insulin-dependent and gestational diabetic mothers. Acta Paediatr Scand 73:349–58.

Persson B, Hanson U. 1993. Insulin dependent diabetes in pregnancy: impact of maternal blood glucose control on the offspring. J Paediatr Child Health 29:20–3.

Persson B, Gentz J, Möller E. 1984. Follow-up of children of insulin dependent (type I) and gestational diabetic mothers: growth pattern, glucose tolerance, insulin response, and HLA types. Acta Paediatr Scand 73:778–84.

Persson B, Gentz J, Stangenberg M. 1979. Neonatal problems. In: Sutherland HW, Stowers JM, eds. Carbohydrate Metabolism in Pregnancy and the Newborn 1978. Springer, Berlin, pp. 376–91.

Persson B, Hanson U. 1993. Insulin dependent diabetes in pregnancy: impact of maternal blood glucose control on the offspring. J Paediatr Child Health 29:20–3.

Petersen MB. 1989. Status at 4–5 years in 90 children of insulin-dependent diabetic mothers. In: Sutherland HW, Stowers JM, Pearson DW, eds. Carbohydrate Metabolism in Pregnancy and the Newborn. IV. Springer, New York, pp. 353–61.

Petersen MB, Pedersen SA, Greisen G, et al. 1988. Early growth delay in diabetic pregnancy: relation to psychomotor development at age 4. Br Med J 296:598–600.

Pettitt DJ, Bennett PH, Knowler WC, et al. 1985. Gestational diabetes mellitus and impaired glucose tolerance during pregnancy: long-term effects on obesity and glucose tolerance in the offspring. Diabetes 34 Suppl 2:119–22.

Pettitt DJ, Knowler WC, Baird HR, et al. 1980. Gestational diabetes: infant and maternal complications of pregnancy in relation to third-trimester glucose tolerance in the Pima Indians. Diab Care 3:458–64.

Philipson EH, Kalhan SC, Rosen MG, et al. 1985. Gestational diabetes mellitus: is further improvement necessary? Diabetes 34 Suppl 2:55–60.

Phillipou G. 1991. Relationship between normal oral glucose tolerance test in women at risk for gestational diabetes and large for gestational age infants. Diab Care 14:1092–5.

Phillips WA, Cooperman DR, Lindquist TC, et al. 1982. Orthopedic management of lumbosacral agenesis: long-term follow-up. J Bone Joint Surg 64A:1282–94.

Pijlman BM, de Koning WB, Wladimiroff JW, et al. 1989. Detection of fetal structural malformations by ultrasound in insulin-dependent pregnant women. Ultrasound Med Biol 15:541–43.

Pinget M, Krummel Y, Gandar R. et al. 1979. Incidence de la maladie diabétique sur l'age de survenue des premières règles. Nouv Presse Med 8:3664.

Pinsky L. 1985. Informative morphogenetic variants: minor congenital anomalies revisited. In: Kalter H, ed. Issues and Reviews in Teratology. Vol. 3. Plenum Press, New York, pp. 135–70.

Piper JM, Langer O. 1993. Does maternal diabetes delay fetal pulmonary maturity? Am J Obstet Gynecol 168:783–6.

Pirart J. 1955. The so-called prediabetic syndrome of pregnancy. Acta Endocr 20:192–208.

Pitt DB, Findlay II, Cole WG, et al. 1982. Case report: femoral hypoplasia-unusual facies syndrome. Aust Paediatr 18:63–6.

Plauchu M, Pousset G, Chapu H, et al. 1970. Diabète et grossesse. J Med Lyon 51:169–72.

Poland BJ, Miller JR, Harris M, et al. 1981. Spontaneous abortion: a study of 1961 women and their conceptuses. Acta Obstet Gynecol Scand Suppl 102:5–32.

Polednak AP. 1986. Birth defects in blacks and whites in relation to prenatal development: a review and hypothesis. Hum Biol 58:317–36.

Polednak AP, Janerich DT. 1985. Maternal factors in congenital limb-reduction defects. Teratology 32:41–50.

Pomeranze J, Stone ML, King EJ. 1959. The obstetric importance of obesity and "benign" glycosuria in prediagnosis diabetes. Obstet Gynecol 13:181–4.

Porter IH, Hook EB, eds. 1980. Human Embryonic and Fetal Death. Academic Press, New York.

Post RH, White P. 1958. Tentative explanation of the high incidence of diabetes. Diabetes 7:27–32.

Potter EL, Adair FL. 1943. Clinical-pathological study of the infant and fetal mortality for a ten-year period at the Chicago Lying-in Hospital. Am J Obstet Gynecol 45:1054–65.

Powell-Griner E. 1986. Perinatal mortality in the United States: 1950–81. Mon Vital Stat Rep Suppl 34 (12):1–16.

Powell-Griner E. 1989. Perinatal mortality in the United States: 1981–85. Mon Vital Stat Rep Suppl 37(10):1–12.

Powell-Griner E, Woolbright A. 1990. Trends in infant deaths from congenital anomalies: results from England and Wales, Scotland, Sweden, and the United States. Int J Epidemiol 19:391–8.

Pradat P. 1992a. A case-control study of major congenital heart defects in Sweden: 1981–1986. Eur J Epidemiol 8:789–96.

Pradat P. 1992b. Epidemiology of major heart defects in Sweden, 1981–1986. J Epidemiol Comm Health 46:211–5.

Pyke DA. 1962. Prediabetes. In: Pyke DA, ed. Disorders of Carbohydrate Metabolism. Lippincott, Philadelphia, pp. 95–112.

Rahbar S. 1968. An abnormal hemoglobin in red cells of diabetics. Clin Chim Acta 22:296–8.

Rahbar S, Blumenfeld O, Ranney HM. 1969. Studies of an unusual hemoglobin in patients with diabetes mellitus. Biochem Biophys Res Comm 36:838–43.

Rakieten N, Rakieten ML, Hadkarni MV. 1963. Studies on the diabetogenic action of streptozotocin (HSC-37917). Canc Chemother Rep 29:91–8.

Ramos-Arroyo MA, Rodriguez-Pinilla E, Cordero JF. 1992. Maternal diabetes: the risk for specific birth defects. Eur J Epidemiol 8:503–8.

Randall LM. 1947. Pregnancy associated with diabetes. Am J Obstet Gynecol 54:618–25.

Rasmussen SA, Moore CA, Khoury MJ, et al. 1996. Descriptive epidemiology of holoprosencephaly and arhinenecephaly in Metropolitan Atlanta, 1968–1992. Am J Med Genet 66:320–33.

Record RG. 1961. Anencephalus in Scotland. Br J Prev Soc Med 15:93–105.

Reddi AS, Opperman W, Velasco CA, et al. 1975. Early genetic diabetes in the KK mouse. In: Camerini-Dávalos RA, Cole HS, eds. Early Diabetes. Academic Press, New York, pp. 413–25.

Reece EA, Hobbins JC. 1986. Diabetic embryopathy: pathogenesis, prenatal diagnosis and prevention. Obstet Gynecol Surv 41:325–35.

Reece EA, Winn HN, Smikle C, et al. 1990. Sonographic assessment of growth of the fetal head in diabetic pregnancies compared with normal gestations. Am J Perinatol 7:18–22.

Regemorter NV, Dodion J, Druart C, et al. 1984. Congenital malformations in 10,000 consecutive births in a university hospital: need for genetic counseling and prenatal diagnosis. J Paediatr 104:386–90.

Reid M, Hadden D, Harley JM, et al. 1984. Fetal malformations in diabetics with high haemoglobin A_{1c} in early pregnancy. Br Med J 298:1001.

Reis RA, DeCosta EJ, Allweiss MD. 1950. The management of the pregnant diabetic woman and her newborn infant. Am J Obstet Gynecol 60:1023–39.

Reis RA, DeCosta EJ, Allweiss MD. 1952. Diabetes and Pregnancy. Thomas, Springfield, Illinois.

Reis RA, DeCosta EJ, Gerbie AB. 1958. Pregnancy in the diabetic woman. Am J Obstet Gynecol 76:1148–50.

Reis RR. 1956. Discussion. In: White et al. 1956, pp. 68–9.

Rerup CC. 1970. Drugs producing diabetes through damage of the insulin secreting cells. Pharmacol Rev 22:485–518.

Reveno WS. 1923. Insulin in diabetic coma, complicating pregnancy. JAMA 81:2101–2.

Richards MR, Merritt KK, Samuels MH, et al. 1955. Congenital malformations of the cardiovascular system in a series of 6,053 infants. Pediatrics 15:12–32.

Rike PM, Fawcett RM. 1948. Diabetes in pregnancy. Am J Obstet Gynecol 56:484–93.

Ring PA. 1961. Congenital abnormalities of the femur. Arch Dis Child 36:410–7.

Rizzo G, Arduini D, Romanini C. 1991. Cardiac function in fetuses of type I diabetic mothers. Am J Obstet Gynecol 164:837–43.

Rizzo TA, Dooley SL, Metzger BE, et al. 1995. Prenatal and perinatal influences on long-term psychomotor development in offspring of diabetic mothers. Am J Obstet Gynecol 173:1753–8.

Rizzo TA, Ogata ES, Dooley SL, et al. 1994. Perinatal complications and cognitive development in 2- to 5-year-old children of diabetic mothers. Am J Obstet Gynecol 171:706–12.

Roach E, DeMyer W, Conneally PM, et al. 1975. Holoprosencephaly: birth data, genetic and demographic analyses of 30 families. Birth Defects 11(3):294–313.

Robert MF, Neff RK, Hubbell JP, et al. 1976. Association between maternal diabetes and the respiratory-distress syndrome in the newborn. N Engl J Med 294:357–60.

Roberts RN, Moohan JM, Foo RL, et al. 1993. Fetal outcome in mothers with impaired glucose tolerance in pregnancy. Diab Med 10:438–43.

Roccella EJ, Bowler AE, Horan M. 1987. Epidemiologic considerations in defining hypertension. Med Clin North Am 71:785–801.

Rogers SC, Weatherall JA 1976. Anencephalus, Spina Bifida, and Congenital Hydrocephalus: England and Wales 1964–1972. Office of Population, Censuses and Surveys, HMSO, London.

Rolland C. 1954. Diabetes in pregnancy. Edinb Med J 61:257–72.

Roman E, Stevenson AC. 1983. Spontaneous abortion. In: Barron SL, Thomson AM, eds. Obstetrical Epidemiology. Academic Press, London, pp. 61–87.

Ronsheim J. 1933. Diabetes and pregnancy. Am J Obstet Gynecol 25:710–4.

Rose BI, Graff S, Spencer R, et al. 1988. Major congenital anomalies in infants and glycosylated hemoglobin levels in insulin-requiring diabetic mothers. J Perinatol 8:309–11.

Rosenberg M. 1924. Glycosurie, Diabetes und Acidose bei Schwangeren. Klin Woch 3:1561–5.

Rosendahl K, Markestad T, Lie RT. 1992. Congenital dislocation of the hip: a prospective study comparing ultrasound and clinical examination. Acta Paediatr 81:177–81.

Rosenn B, Combs CA, Khoury J, et al. 1994. Glycemic thresholds for spontaneous abortion and congenital malformations in insulin-dependent diabetes mellitus. Obstet Gynecol 84:515–20.

Rosenn B, Miodovnik M, Combs CA, et al. 1991. Pre-conception management of insulin-dependent diabetes: improvement of pregnancy outcome. Obstet Gynecol 77:846–9.

Rosenthal M, McMahan CA, Stern MP, et al. 1985. Evidence of bimodality of two hour plasma glucose concentrations in Mexican Americans: results from the San Antonio heart study. J Chron Dis 38:5–16.

Ross OA, Spector S. 1952. Production of congenital abnormalities in mice by alloxan. Am J Dis Child 84:647–8.

Roth MP, Dott B, Alembik Y, et al. 1987. Malformations congénitales dans une série de 66,068 naissances consécutives. Arch Fr Pediatr 44:173–6.

Roversi DG, Gargiulo M, Nicolini U, et al. 1977. Diabéte de la mère et risque peri-natal: reduction du risque perinatal lors de grossesses chez les diabétiques, par la recherche d'un strict équilibre métabolique de la maladie maternelle, 479 cas (1963–1975). Rev Med Suisse Roman 97:401–12.

Roversi GD, Canussio V, Gargiulo M. 1975. Insulin in gestational diabetes. In: Camerini-Dávalos RA, Coles HS, eds. Early Diabetes. Academic Press, New York, pp. 469–75.

Rowe BR, Rowbotham CJ, Barnett AH. 1987. Pre-conception counselling, birth weight, and congenital abnormalities in established and gestational diabetic pregnancy. Diab Res 6:33–5.

Rowe RD, Freedom RM, Mehrizi A, et al. 1981. The Neonate with Congenital Heart Disease. Saunders, Philadelphia.

Rowland TW, Hubbell JP, Nadas AS. 1973. Congenital heart disease in infants of diabetic mothers. J Pediatr 83:s815–20.

Rubenstein MA, Bucy JG. 1975. Caudal regression syndrome: the urologic implications. J Urol 114:934–7.

Rubin A. 1958. Studies in human reproduction. II. The influence of diabetes mellitus in men upon reproduction. Am J Obstet Gynecol 76:25–9.

Rubin A, Murphy DP. 1958. Studies in human reproduction. III. The frequency of congenital malformations in the offspring of nondiabetic and diabetic individuals. J Pediatr 53:579–85.

Ruoff W. 1903. Glycosuria gravidarum. Am Med 5:663–65.

Rushforth NB, Bennett PH, Steinberg AG, et al. 1971. Diabetes in the Pima Indians: evidence of bimodality in glucose tolerance distributions. Diabetes 20:756–65.

Rushton DI. 1985. The nature and causes of spontaneous abortions with normal karyotypes. In: Kalter H, ed. Issues and Reviews in Teratology. Vol. 3. Plenum Press, New York, pp. 21–63.

Russell DS. 1949. Observations on the Pathology of Hydrocephalus. MRC Special Report Series No. 265. HMSO, London.

Russell HE, Aitken GT. 1963. Congenital absence of the sacrum and lumbar vertebrae with prosthetic management. J Bone Joint Surg 45A:501–8.

Sachon C, Grimaldi A, Bosquet F, et al. 1994. Grossesse diabétique: bilan et perspective à partir de l'étude de 212 grossesses diabétiques suivies entre 1985 et 1992. Ann Med Intern 145:391–7

Sadler LS, Robinson LK, Msall ME. 1995. Diabetic embryopathy: possible pathogenesis. Am J Med Genet 55:363–66.

Sadovnik AD, Baird PA. 1985. Congenital malformations associated with anencephaly in liveborn and stillborn infants. Teratology 32:355–62.

Saint-Hilaire IG. 1832–37. Histoire Générale et Particulière des Anomalies de l'Organisation chez l'Homme et les Animaux: ouvrage comprenant des recherches sur les caractères, la classification, l'influence physiologique et pathologique, les rapports généraux, les lois et les causes des monstruosités, des variétés et vices de conformation, ou traité de tératolgie. Baillière, Paris.

Saintonge J, Côté R. 1984. Fetal brain development in diabetic guinea pigs. Pediatr Res 18:650–3.

Saintonge J, Côté R. 1983. intrauterine growth retardation and diabetic pregnancy: two types of fetal malnutrition. Am J Obstet Gynecol 146:194–8.

Salans LB, Graham BJ, eds. 1982. Proceedings of a task force on animals appropriate for studying diabetes mellitus and its complications. Diabetes 31 Suppl 1:1–102.

Salvioli GP, Dallacasa P, Bottiglioni F, et al. 1976. Prognosi dei figli nati da madri affete da diabete mellito. Min Pediatr 28:212–6.

Salzberger M, Liban E. 1975. Diabetes and antenatal fetal death. In: Shafrir E, ed. Contemporary Topics in the Study of Diabetes and Metabolic Endocrinology. Academic Press, New York, pp. 97–102.

Sanctis CD. 1969. Il neonato di madre diabetica: orientamenti clinico-terapeutici. Min Pediatr 21:2139–44.

Sarnat HB, Case ME, Graviss R. 1976. Sacral agenesis: neurologic and neuropathologic features. Neurology 26:1124–9.

Saugstad LF. 1981. Weight of all births and infant mortality. J Epidemiol Comm Health 35:185–91.

Saunders N, Paterson C. 1991. Can we abandon Naegele's rule? Lancet 337:600–601.

Saxén L. 1983. Twenty years of study of the etiology of congenital malformations in Finland. In: Kalter H, ed. Issues and Reviews in Teratology. Vol. 1. Plenum Press, New York, pp. 73–110.

Saxén L, Klemetti A, Härö AS. 1974. A matched-pair register for studies of selected congenital defects. Am J Epidemiol 100:297–306.

Schaefer UM, Songster G, Xiang A, et al. 1997. Congenital malformations in offspring of women with hyperglycemia first detected during pregnancy. Am J Obstet Gynecol 117:1165–71.

Schmid J, Kunz J, Sutter R. 1984. Diabetes und Schwangerschaft. Gynecol Rund 24:197–209.

Schmidt MI, Matos MC, Branchstein L, et al. 1994. Variation in glucose tolerance with ambient temperature. Lancet 344:1054–5.

Schwalbe E. 1906. Die Morphologie der Missbildungen des Menschen und der Tiere. Gustav Fischer, Jena.

Schwaninger D. 1973. Katamnestische Untersuchungen von Kindern diabetischer Mütter. Schweiz Med Woch 103:1130–4.

Schwartz JG, Phillips WT, Blumhardt MR, et al. 1994. Use of a more physiologic oral glucose solution during screening for gestational diabetes mellitus. Am J Obstet Gynecol 171:685–90.

Schwartz M, Schneeweiss J, Bock E. 1960. Über perinatale Sterblichkeit von Kindern diabetischer Mütter. Schweiz Med Wochenschr 90:751–4.

Schwartz ML, Brenner WE. 1982. The need for adequate and consistent diagnostic classifications for diabetes mellitus diagnosed during pregnancy. Am J Obstet Gynecol 143:119–24.

Schwartz W, Poulsen HK, Andersen PE. 1982. Sirenomelia: the caudal regression syndrome. Mon Kinderheilk 130:565–6.

Second International Workshop-Conference on Gestational Diabetes Mellitus. 1985. Summary and recommendations. Diabetes 34 Suppl 2:123–6.

Sehgal NN. 1976. Pregnancy in diabetic women: a review of five years' experience at the Sacramento Medical Center. W Va Med J 72:81–7.

Seligman SA. 1963. Hazards facing the neonate. Proc R Soc Med 56:1019–21.

Sells CJ, Robinson NM, Brown Z, et al. 1994. Long-term developmental follow-up of infants of diabetic mothers. J Pediatr 125:S9–17.

Selman JJ. 1932. The results of glucose tolerance tests in pregnant women. Ohio State Med J 28:184–8.

Sentrakul P, Potter EL. 1966. Pathologic diagnosis on 2,681 abortions at the Chicago Lying-in Hospital, 1957–1965. Am J Public Health 56:2083–92.

Sepe SJ, Connell FA, Geiss LS, et al. 1985. Gestational diabetes: incidence, maternal characteristics, and perinatal outcome. Diabetes 34 Suppl 2:13–6.

Shanberg AM, Rosenberg MT. 1989. Partial transposition of the penis and scrotum with anterior urethral diverticulum in a child born with the caudal regression syndrome. J Urol 142:1060–2.

Shands AR, Bundens WD. 1966. Congenital malformations of the spine: an analysis of the roentgenograms of 700 children. Bull Hosp Joint Dis 17:110–33.

Shapiro S, Schlesinger ER, Nesbitt EL Jr 1965. Infant and Perinatal Mortality in the United States. U.S. Government Printing Office, Washington, DC.

Shepard TH, Fantel AG, Fitzsimmons J. 1989. Congenital defects among spontaneous abortuses: twenty years of monitoring. Teratology 39:325–32.

Shepard TH, Fantel AG, Mirkes PE. 1988. Collection and scientific use of human embryonic and fetal material: 25 years of experience. In: Kalter H, ed. Issues and Reviews in Teratology. Vol. 4. Plenum Press, New York, pp. 129–62.

Sheridan-Pereira M, Drury MI, Baumgart R, et al. 1983. Haemoglobin A_1 in diabetic pregnancy: an evaluation. Ir J Med Sci 152:261–7.

Sheumack DR. 1949. Diabetes mellitus and pregnancy. Med J Aust 2:553–8.

Shields LE, Gan EA, Morphy HF, et al. 1993. The prognostic value of hemoglobin A_{1c} in predicting fetal heart disease in diabetic pregnancies. Obstet Gynecol 81:954–7.

Shiota K. 1993. Teratothanasia: prenatal loss of abnormal conceptuses and the prevalence of various malformations during human gestation. Birth Defects 29:189–99.

Shir MM. 1939. Diabetes in pregnancy with observations in 28 cases. Am J Obstet Gynecol 37:1032–5.

Sicree RA, Hoet JJ, Zimmet P, et al. 1986. The association of non-insulin-dependent diabetes with parity and still-birth occurrence amongst five Pacific populations. Diab Res Clin Pract 2:113–22.

Siddiqi T, Rosenn B, Mimouni F, et al. 1991. Hypertension during pregnancy in insulin-dependent diabetic women. Obstet Gynecol 77:514–9.

Sievers G. 1969. Discussion. In: Swinyard CA, ed. Limb Development and Deformity: problems of evaluation and rehabilitation. Thomas, Springfield, pp. 232–48.

Silverman BL, Rozzo T, Green OC, et al. 1991. Long-term prospective evaluation of offspring of diabetic mothers. Diabetes 40 Suppl 2:121–5.

Simpson JL. 1978. Genetics of diabetes mellitus (DM) and anomalies in offspring of diabetic mothers. Semin Perinatol 2:383–94.

Simpson JL, Elias S, Martin AO, et al. 1983. Diabetes in pregnancy, Northwestern University Series (1977–1981). I. Prospective study of anomalies in offspring of mothers with diabetes mellitus. Am J Obstet Gynecol 146:263–70.

Simpson JL, Mills JL, Moren A, et al. 1989. Drug ingestion during pregnancy: infrequent exposure in a contemporary United States sample. Am J Perinatol 6:244–51.

Sindram IS. 1951. De sectio Caesarea bij diabetes mellitus. Ned Tijd Geneesk 95:2686–94.

Singer DB. 1984. The placenta in pregnancies complicated by diabetes mellitus. Perspect Paediatr Pathol 8:199–212.

Sisson WR. 1940. The neonatal problem in infants of diabetic mothers. JAMA 115:2040–4.

Skipper E. 1933. Diabetes mellitus and pregnancy: a clinical and analytical study (with special observations upon thirty-three cases). Q J Med 2:353–80.

Skyler JS. 1989. Diabetes and pregnancy: consensus and controversy. In: Sutherland HW, Stowers JM, Pearson DW, eds. Carbohydrate Metabolism in Pregnancy and the Newborn. IV. Springer, New York, pp. 363–72.

Skyler JS, O'Sullivan MJ, Robertson EG, et al. 1989. Blood glucose control during pregnancy. Diab Care 3:69–76.

Slot JB, Sande PL, Terpstra J. 1967. Diabetes mellitus and pregnancy. Folia Med Neerl 10:77–84.

Small M, Cassidy L, Leiper JM, et al. 1986. Outcome of pregnancy in insulin-dependent (type 1) diabetic women between 1971 and 1984. Q J Med 61:1159–69.

Smith DW. 1971. Minor malformations: their relevance and significance. In: Hook EB, Janerich DT, Porter IH, eds. Monitoring, Birth Defects and Environment: the problem of surveillance. Academic Press, New York, pp. 169–75.

Smith GV, Smith OW. 1935. Further quantitative determinations of prolan and estrin in pregnancy, with especial reference to late toxemia and eclampsia. Surg Gynecol Obstet 61:27–35.

Smith NC. 1989. Epidemiology of spontaneous abortion in insulin-dependent diabetic women. In: Sutherland HW, Stowers JM, Pearson DW, eds. Carbohydrate Metabolism and the Newborn–IV. Springer–Verlag, New York, pp. 75–81.

Smith R. 1994. Promoting research into peer review. Br Med J 309:143–4.

Smith RS, Comstock CH, Lorenz RP, et al. 1997. Maternal diabetes mellitus: which views are essential for fetal echocardiography? Obstet Gynecol 90:575–9.

Smithells RW, Newman CG 1992. Recognition of thalidomide defects. J Med Genet 29:716–23.

Smorenberg-School ME, Heringa GM. 1983. Diabetes mellitus en zwangerschap; behandelung en resultaten in de periode 1969–1982. Ned Tijdschr Geneeskd 127:1999–2003.

Smorenberg-Schoorl ME, Klomp J, Sluyter AH, et al. 1970. De behandeling van de diabetische zwangere. Ned Tijdschr Verlosled 70:341–8.

Snell LM, Little BB, Knoll KA, et al. 1992. Reliability of birth certificate reporting of congenital anomalies. Am J Perinatol 9:219–22.

Soares JA, Dornhorstt A, Beard RW. 1997. The case for screening for gestational diabetes. Br Med J 315:737–8.

Soler NG, Soler SM, Malins JM. 1978. Neonatal morbidity among infants of diabetic mothers. Diab Care 1:340–50.

Soler NG, Walsh CH, Malins JM. 1976. Congenital malformations in infants of diabetic mothers. Q J Med 45:303–33.

Soni AL, Kishan J, Mir NA, et al. 1989. Cyclopic malformation in infants of diabetic mothers. Ind J Pediatr 56:141–4.

Spellacy WN, Miller S, Winegar A, et al. 1985. Macrosomia—maternal characteristics and infant complications. Obstet Gynecol 66:158–61.

Spiegelman M, Marks HH. 1946. Age and sex variations in the prevalence and onset of diabetes mellitus. Am J Public Health 36:26–33.

Spiers PS. 1982. Does growth retardation predispose the fetus to congenital malformation? Lancet 1:312–3.

Spooner EW, Hook, EB, Farina MA, et al. 1988. Evaluation of a temporal increase in ventricular septal defects: estimated prevalence and severity in northeastern New York, 1970–1983. Teratology 37:21–8.

Stallone LA, Ziel HK. 1974. Management of gestational diabetes. Am J Obstet Gynecol 119:1091–4.

Stanley FJ, Priscott PK, Johnston R, et al. 1985. Congenital malformations in infants of mothers with diabetes and epilepsy in Western Australia, 1980–1982. Med J Aust 143:440–3.

Steel JM. 1988. Preconception, conception, and contraception. In: Reece EA, Coustan DR, eds. Diabetes Mellitus in Pregnancy: principles and practice. Churchill Livingstone, New York, pp. 601–20.

Steel JM, Johnstone FD 1992. Pre-pregnancy clinics for diabetic women. Lancet 340:918–9.

Steel JM, Johnstone FD, Duncan LJ 1980. Abnormal infants of diabetic mothers. Lancet 1:771.

Steel JM, Johnstone FD, Smith AF, et al. 1984a. The pre-pregnancy clinic approach. In: Sutherland HW, Stowers JM, eds. Carbohydrate Metabolism in Pregnancy and the Newborn. Livingstone, Edinburgh, pp. 75–86.

Steel JM, Johnstone SD, Corrie JE 1984b. Early assessment of gestation in diabetics. Lancet 2:975–6.

Steel JM. Johnstone FD, Smith AF. 1989. Prepregnancy preparation. In: Sutherland HW, Stowers JM, Pearson DWM, eds. Carbohydrate Metabolism in Pregnancy and the Newborn-IV. Springer-Verlag, New York, pp. 120–39.

Steel JM, Johnstone FD, Hepburn DA, et al. 1990. Can prepregnancy care of diabetic women reduce the risk of abnormal babies? Br Med J 301:1070–4.

Steel JM, Livingstone FD, Smith AF, et al. 1982. Five years' experience of a "prepregnancy" clinic for insulin-dependent diabetics. Br Med J 285:353–6.

Steel JM, Wu PS, Johnstone FD, et al. 1995. Does early growth delay occur in diabetic pregnancy? Br J Obstet Gynecol 102:224–7.

Steer C, Campbell S, Davies M, et al. 1989. Spontaneous abortion rates after natural and assisted conception. Br Med J 299:1317–8.

Stehbens JA, Baker GL, Kitchell M. 1977. Outcome at ages 1, 3, and 5 years of children born to diabetic women. Am J Obstet Gynecol 127:408–14.

Steindel E, Mohnike A. 1971. Über Häufigkeit und Verlauf der schwangerschaften bei Diabetikerinnen und Frauen mit Schwangerschaftsglukosurien in Berlin im Zeitraum von 1963 bis 1970. Deut Gesundheit 26:2075–9.

Stengel A. 1904. Diabetes as a complication of pregnancy. U Penn Med Bull 17:296–9.

Stephens JW, Page OC, Hare RL. 1963. Diabetes and pregnancy: a report of experiences in 119 pregnancies over a period of ten years. Diabetes 12:213–9.

Stern L, Ramos A, Light I. 1965. Congenital malformations and diabetes. Lancet 1:1393–4.

Stern MP. 1988. Type II diabetes mellitus: interface between clinical and epidemiological investigation. Diab Care 11:119–26.

Stern MP, Rosenthal M, Haffner SM. 1985. A new concept of impaired glucose tolerance: relation to cardiovascular risk. Arteriosclerosis 5:311–4.

Stevenson AC, Warnock HA. 1959. Observations on the results of pregnancies in women resident in Belfast. I. Data relating to all pregnancies ending in 1957. Ann Human Genet 23:382–94.

Stevenson AC, Johnston HA, Stewart MI, et al. 1966. Congenital malformations: a report of a study of series of consecutive births in 24 centres. Bull WHO 34 Suppl:1–127.

Stevenson AE 1956. Pregnancy complicated by diabetes mellitus: a review of 119 cases. Br Med J 2:1514–8.

Stevenson DK, Hopper AO, Cohen RS, et al. 1982. Macrosomia: causes and consequences. J Pediatr 100:515–20.

Stevenson RE, Jones KL, Phelan MC, et al. 1986. Vascular steal: the pathogenetic mechanism producing sirenomelia and associated defects of the viscera and soft tissues. Pediatrics 78:451–7.

Stocker JT, Heifetz SA. 1987. Sirenomelia: a morphological study of 33 cases and review of the literature. Perspect Pediatr Pathol 10:7–50.

Stoll C, Alembik Y, Dott B, et al. 1992. An epidemiologic study of environmental and genetic factors in congenital hydrocephalus. Eur J Epidemiol 8:797–803.

Stoll C, Alembik Y, Roth MP, et al. 1989. Risk factors in congenital heart disease. Eur J Epidemiol 5:382–91

Stone DH. 1992. RE "Completeness of the discharge diagnoses as a measure of birth defects in the hospital record." Am J Epidemiol 136:498–9.

Strong RM. 1925. The order, time and rate of ossification of the albino rat (*Mus Norvegicus Albinus*) skeleton. Am J Anat 36:313–51.

Stroup NE, Edmonds L, O'Brien TR. 1990. Renal agenesis and dysgenesis: are they increasing? Teratology 42:383–96.

Stubbs SM. 1987. Personal communication.

Stubbs SM, Doddridge MC, John PN, et al. 1987. Haemoglobin A_1 and congenital malformation. Diab Med 4:156–9.

Styrud J, Thunberg L, Nybacka O, et al. 1995. Correlations between maternal metabolism and deranged development in the offspring of normal and diabetic rats. Pediatr Res 37:343–53.

Sutherland HW, Fisher PM. 1982. Fetal loss and maternal glucose intolerance: a retrospective study. Päd Päd 17:279–86.

Sutherland HW, Pedersen JF, Mølsted-Pedersen L. 1981. Treatment of diabetic pregnancy with special reference to fetal growth. In: Van Assche FA, Robertson WB, eds. Fetal Growth Retardation. Livingstone, Edinburgh, pp. 197–207.

Sutherland HW, Pritchard CW. 1986. Increased incidence of spontaneous abortion in pregnancies complicated by maternal diabetes mellitus. Am J Obstet Gynecol 155:135–8.

Sutherland I. 1949. Stillbirths: their epidemiology and social significance. Oxford University, London.

Svanteson G. 1953. Diabetes mellitus och graviditet. Nord Med 49:533–6.

Szabó M, Tóth T, Tóth Z, et al. 1986. Fetal malformation and serum alpha-fetoprotein concentration of diabetic mothers. Zentralbl Gynecol 108:1228–36.

Taeusch HW, Ballard TR, Avery ME 1991. Schaffer and Avery's Diseases of the Newborn. Saunders, Philadelphia.

Taffel S. 1978. Congenital Anomalies and Birth Injuries Among Live Births: United States, 1973–74. National Center for Health Statistics, Hyattsville, Maryland.

Takano K, Nishimura H. 1967. Congenital malformations induced by alloxan diabetes in mice and rats. Anat Rec 158:303–12.

Takano K, Tanimura T, Nishimura H. 1965. The susceptibility of the offspring of alloxan-diabetic mice to a teratogen. J Embryol Exp Morphol 14:63–73.

Takeuchi A, Benirschke K. 1961. Renal venous thrombosis of the newborn and its relation to maternal diabetes: report of 16 cases. Biol Neonat 3:237–56.

Tanigawa K, Kawaguchi M, Tanaka O, et al. 1991. Skeletal malformations in rat offspring: long-term effect of maternal insulin-induced hypoglycemia during organogenesis. Diabetes 40:1115–21.

Tatekawi R, Otani H, Tanaka O, et al. 1989a. Chromosome analysis in preimplantation stage embryos of non-obese diabetic (NOD) mice. Cong Anom 29:7–13.

Tatewaki R, Otani J, Tanaka O, et al. 1989b. A morphological study on the reproductive organs as a possible cause of developmental abnormalities in diabetic NOD mice. Histol Histopathol 4:343–58.

Tatewaki R, Hashimoto R, Tanigawa K, et al. 1995. Relationship between associations of NOR and chromosomal anomalies in the abnormal embryos of nonobese diabetic and STZ-diabetic mouse. Biol Neonat 67:132–9.

Taylor FW. 1899. Diabetes mellitus and pregnancy. Bost Med Surg J 140:205–7.

Tchobroutsky C. 1991. Blood glucose levels in diabetic and non-diabetic subjects. Diabetologia 34:67–73.

Tchobroutsky C, Breart GL, Rambaud DC, et al. 1985. Correlation between fetal defects and early growth delay observed by ultrasound. Lancet 1:706.

Tchobroutsky C, Vray MM, Altman J-J 1991. Risk/benefit ratio of changing late obstetrical strategies in the management of insulin-dependent diabetic pregnancies: a comparison between 1971–1977 and 1978–1985 periods in 389 pregnancies. Diab Metab 17:287–94.

Tegnander E, Eik-Nes SH, Johansen OJ, et al. 1995. Prenatal examination of heart defects at the routine fetal examination at 18 weeks in a non-selected population. Ultrasound Obstet Gynecol 5:372–80.

Teramo K, Kuusisto AN, Raivio KU. 1979. Perinatal outcome of insulin-dependent diabetic pregnancies. Ann Clin Res 11:146–55.

Teramoto S, Hatakenaka N, Shirasu Y. 1991. Effects of the A^y gene on susceptibility to hydrocortisone fetotoxicity and teratogenicity in mice. Teratology 44:101–6.

Tevaarwerk GJ, Harding PG, Milne KJ, et al. 1981. Pregnancy in diabetic women: outcome with a program aimed at normoglycemia before meals. Can Med Ass J 125:435–42.

Thalhammer O, Lachmann D, Scheibenreiter S. 1968. "Caudale Regression" beim Kind einer 18 jährigen Frau mit Prädiabetes. Z Kinderchir 102:346–55.

Theile U, Rückel E, Hust U. 1985. Kinder diabetischer Eltern—zur Frage von Entwicklungsstörungen während der Schwangerschaft mit besonderer Berücksichtigung des sogenannten Riesenkindes. Z Geburtsh Perinat 189:79–83.

Thomson AM, Barron SL. 1983. Perinatal mortality. In: Barron SL, Thomson AM, eds. Obstetrical Epidemiology. Academic Press, London, pp. 347–98.

Thosteson GC. 1953. Diabetes and pregnancy. Harper Hosp Bull 11:245–7.

Tiisala R, Michelsson K, Wist A. 1967. Observations on the perinatal period of infants of diabetic mothers. Ann Paediatr Fenn 13:9–16.

Tingle CD. 1926. A contribution to the study of the causation of foetal death. Arch Dis Child 1:255–78.

Titus RS. 1937. Diabetes in pregnancy from the obstetric point of view. Am J Obstet Gynecol 33:386–92.

Tochino Y. 1987. The NOD mouse as a model of type 1 diabetes. Crit Rev Immunol 8:49–81.

Tolstoi E. 1949. Treatment of diabetes mellitus: the controversy of the past decade. Clin J Med 30:1–7.

Tolstoi E, Given WP, Douglas RG. 1953. Management of the pregnant diabetic. JAMA 153:998–1002.

Toumilehto J, Korhonen HJ, Kartovaara L, et al. 1991. Prevalence of diabetes-mellitus and impaired glucose tolerance in the middle-aged population of three areas in Finland. Int J Epidemiol 20:1010–17.

Traub AI, Harley JM, Cooper TK, et al. 1987. Is centralized hospital care necessary for all insulin-dependent pregnant diabetics? Br J Obstet Gynecol 94:957–72.

Traub AI, Harley JM, Montgomery DA, et al. 1983. Pregnancy and diabetes—the improving prognosis. Ulster Med J 52:118–24.

Tunçer M, Tunçer M. 1981. Congenital malformations and diabetes mellitus. Turk J Pediatr 23:157–69.

U.S. Bureau of the Census. 1961. Historical Statistics of the United States: colonial times to 1957. U.S. Department of Commerce, Washington, DC.

Ueda K, Nishida Y, Oshima K, et al. 1979. Congenital rubella syndrome: correlation of gestational age at the time of maternal rubella with type of defect. J Pediatr 94:763–5.

Ullrich E. 1979. Gewusst und/oder nachgeschlagen: kaudale Hypoplasie. Med Akt 5:45.

Uriu-Hare JY, Stern JS, Keen CL. 1989. Influence of maternal dietary Zn on expression of diabetes-induced teratogenicity in rats. Diabetes 38:1282–90.

Uriu-Hare JY, Stern JS, Reaven GM, et al. 1985. The effects of maternal diabetes on trace element status and fetal development in the rat. Diabetes 34:1031–40.

Vadheim CM. 1983. Pregnancy with Diabetes: Washington State, 1978–1980. Ph.D. Thesis, University of Washington, Seattle, Washington.

Vadheim CM. 1989. Genetics of diabetes mellitus. In : Draznin B, Melmed S, Leroith D, eds. Molecular and Cellular Biology of Diabetes Mellitus. Vol. 1. Insulin secretion. Liss, New York, pp. 139–48.

Vaes G, Meyer R de. 1957. Étude histochimique du glycogène utérin chez la lapine: ses variations au cours du diabète alloxanique et sous l'action de la cortisone. Ann Endocrinol 18:828–40

Vallance-Owen J, Braithwaite F, Wilson JS, et al. 1967. Cleft lip and palate deformities and insulin antagonism. Lancet 2:912–4.

Van Allen DC, Petersen MC, Lin-Dyken, DC, et al. 1995. Delays in diagnosis in children with sacral anomalies. Am J Med Genet 55:251–2.

Van Allen MI, Brown, ZA, Plovie B, et al. 1994. Deformations in infants of diabetic and control pregnancies. Am J Med Genet 53:210–15.

Van Allen MI, Myhre S. 1991. New multiple congenital anomalies syndrome in a stillborn infant of consanguinous parents and a prediabetic pregnancy. Am J Med Genet 38:523–8.

van der Wal KG, Mulder JW. 1993. Median cleft lip without holoprosencephaly: case report. Int J Oral Maxillofac Surg 22:39–41.

Vasilenko P, Mead JP, Slaughter T, et al. 1989. Detrimental effects of maternal diabetes on growth and development of offspring in the rat. Diabetes 33:91A.

Veille J-C, Sivakoff M, Hanson R, et al. 1992. Interventricular septal thickness in fetuses of diabetic mothers. Obstet Gynecol 79:51–4.

Ventura SJ, Martin JA, Taffel SM, et al. 1992. Advance report of final natality statistics, 1992. Mon Vital Stat Rep 43(5) Suppl:1–88.

Vercheval M, Hertogh R de, Pampfer S, et al. 1990. Experimental diabetes impairs rat embryo development during the preimplantation period. Diabetologia 33:187–91.

Verrotti A, Chiarelli F, Capani F, et al. 1993. Prediabetes: genetic, immunological and metabolic aspects. Panminerva Med 35:179–85.

Viberti G. 1995. A glycemic threshhold for diabetic complications? N Engl J Med 332:1292–3.

Victor A. 1974. Normal blood sugar variation during pregnancy. Act Obstet Gynecol Scand 53:37–40.

Villumsen AL. 1970. Environmental Factors in Congenital Malformations: a prospective study of 9,006 human pregnancies. F.A.D.L.s, Copenhagen.

Villumsen AL, Zachau-Christiansen B. 1963. Incidence of malformations in the newborn in a prospective child health study. Bull Soc R Belg Gynecol Obstet 33:95–105.

Visser GH, Bedekam DJ, Mulder EJ, et al. 1985. Delayed emergence of fetal behaviour in type-1 diabetic women. Early Human Dev 12:167–72.

von Noorden C. 1910. Die Zuckerkrankheit und ihre Behandlung. Hirschwald. Berlin.

Wald NJ, Cuckle H, Boreham J, et al. 1979. Maternal serum alpha-fetoprotein and diabetes mellitus. Br J Obstet Gynecol 86:101–5.

Walden RH, Logosso RD, Brennan L. 1971. Pierre Robin syndrome in association with combined congenital lengthening and shortening of the long bones: case report. Plast Reconstr Surg 48:80–2.

Walker A. 1928. Diabetes mellitus and pregnancy. J Obstet Gynecol Br Emp 35:271–81.

Wang J, Palmer RM, Chung CS. 1988. The role of major gene in clubfoot. Am J Hum Genet 42:772–6.

Warburton D, Fraser FC. 1964. Spontaneous abortion risks in man: data from reproductive histories collected in a medical genetics unit. Am J Hum Genet 16:1–25.

Ward RJ, Readhead SM. 1970. The effect of alloxan-induced diabetes on the foetal toxicity of thalidomide, carbutamide and myleran in rats. In: The Problems of Species Difference and Statistics in Toxicology. Proceedings of the European Society for the Study of Drug Toxicity. Vol. 11. Exerpta Medica Foundation, Amsterdam, pp. 151–66,

Wareham NJ, O'Rahilly S. 1998. The changing classification and diagnosis of diabetes. Br Med J 317:359–60.

Warkany J. 1971. Congenital Malformations: notes and comments. YearBook Medical, Chicago.

Warkany J. 1977. History of teratology. In: Wilson JG, Fraser FC, eds. Handbook of Teratology. Vol. 1. Plenum Press, New York, pp. 3–45.

Warkany J. 1978. Terathanasia. Teratology 17:187–92.

Warkany J, Kalter H. 1961. Congenital malformations. N Engl J Med 265:993–1001, 1046–52.

Warkany J, Nelson RC. 1941. Skeletal abnormalities in the offspring of rats reared on deficient diets. Anat Rec 79:83–100.

Warren S, LeCompte PM. 1952. The Pathology of Diabetes Mellitus. Lea & Febiger, Philadelphia.

Warrner RA, Cornblath M. 1969. Infants of gestational diabetic mothers. Am J Dis Child 117:678–83.

Watanabe G, Ingalls TH. 1963. Congenital malformations in the offspring of alloxan-diabetic mice. Diabetes 12:66–72.

Watson C. 1968. A follow-up study of children born to diabetic mothers, with particular reference to frequency of congenital abnormalities. Arch Dis Child 43:746–7.

Watson C. 1970. Prognosis for infants born to diabetic mothers, with particular reference to the prevalence of congenital abnormalitites. Int J Gynecol Obstet 8:212–3.

Watson CM. 1973. Late Prognosis for Children Born to Diabetic Mothers. M.D. Thesis, University of London.

Weber DJ. 1992. The Spanish Frontier in North America. Yale University, New Haven, Connecticut.

Weicker H. 1963. Klinik und Epidemiologie der Thalidomid-Embryopathie. Bull Soc Roy Belg Gynecol Obstet 33:21–7.

Weicker H. 1969. Epidemiological and etiological considerations in the increase of limb malformations in Germany. In: Swinyard CA, ed. Limb Development and Deformity: problems of evaluation and rehabilitation. Thomas, Springfield, Illinois, pp. 225–32.

Weiner CP. 1988. Effect of varying degrees of "normal" glucose metabolism on maternal and perinatal outcome. Am J Obstet Gynecol 159:862–70.

Weiss PA, Hofmann HM, Winter RR, et al. 1986. Diagnosis and treatment of gestational diabetes according to amniotic fluid insulin levels. Arch Gynecol 239:81–92.

Weitz R, Laron Z. 1976. Height and weight of children born to mothers with diabetes mellitus. Isr J Med Sci 12:195–8.

Welch. P, Aterman K. 1984. The syndrome of caudal dysplasia: a review, including etiologic considerations and evidence of heterogeneity. Pediatr Pathol 2:313–27.

Wentzel P, Jansson L, Eriksson UJ. 1995. Diabetes in pregnancy: uterine blood flow and embryonic development in the rat. Pediatr Res 38:598–606.

West KM. 1971. Epidemiology of diabetes. In: Fajans SS, Sussman KE, eds. Diabetes Mellitus: diagnosis and treatment. American Diabetes Association, New York, pp. 121–6.

West KM. 1975. Substantial differences in the diagnostic criteria used by diabetes experts. Diabetes 24:641–4.

West KM. 1978. Epidemiology of Diabetes and its Macrovascular Complications. American Diabetes Association, New York.

West KM, Wulff JA, Reigel DG, et al. 1964. Oral carbohydrate tolerance tests. Arch Intern Med 113:641–8.

Wheller JJ, Reiss R, Allen HD. 1990. Clinical experience with fetal echocardiography. Am J Dis Child 144:49–53.

White P. 1935. Pregnancy complicating diabetes. Surg Gynecol Obstet 61:324–32.

White P. 1946. Pregnancy complicating diabetes. In: Joslin EP, Root HF, White P, et al., eds. The Treatment of Diabetes Mellitus. Lea & Febiger, Philadelphia, pp. 769–84.

White P. 1949. Pregnancy complicating diabetes. Am J Med 7:609–16.

White P. 1950. Diabetes in pregnancy. Trans Int Cong Obstet Gynecol 4:382–7.

White P. 1952. Pregnancy complicating diabetes. In: Joslin EP, Root HF, White P, et al., eds. The Treatment of Diabetes Mellitus. Lea & Febiger, Philadelphia, pp. 676–98.

White P. 1965. Pregnancy and diabetes, medical aspects. Med Clin North Am 49:1015–24.

White P. 1971. Pregnancy and diabetes. In: Marble A, White P, Bradley RF, et al., eds. Joslin's Diabetes Mellitus. Lea & Febiger, Philadelphia, pp. 581–98.

White P. 1974. Diabetes in pregnancy. Clin Perinatol 1:331–47.

White P. 1978. Classification of obstetric diabetes. Am J Obstet Gynecol 130:228–30.

White P, Gillespie L, Sexton L. 1956. Use of female sex hormone therapy in pregnant diabetic patients. Am J Obstet Gynecol 71:57–69.

White P, and Hunt H. 1943. Pregnancy complicating diabetes. J Clin Endocrinol Metab 3:500–11.

White P, Koshy P, Duckers J. 1953. The management of pregnancy complicating diabetes and of diabetic mothers. Med Clin North Am 39:1481–96.

White P, Titus RS, Joslin EP, et al. 1939. Prediction and prevention of late pregnancy accidents in diabetes. Am J Med Sci 198:482–92.

Whiteford ML, Tolmie JL. 1996. Holoprosencephaly in the west of Scotland. J Med Genet 33:578–84.

Whitehouse FW, Lowrie WL, Hodgkinson CP. 1956. Diabetes and pregnancy. J Mich State Med Soc 55:1211–7.

Whitely JM, Adams TW. 1952. Diabetes and pregnancy. West J Surg 60:98–107.

Whitely JM, Adams TW, Parrott MH. 1953. Diabetes and pregnancy. West J Surg 61:439–47.

Whittaker PG, Aspillaga MO, Lind T. 1983. Accurate assessment of early gestational age in normal and diabetic women by serum human placental lactogen concentration. Lancet 2:304–5.

Whittle MJ, Anderson D, Lowensohn RI, et al. 1979. Estriol in pregnancy. VI. Experience with unconjugated plasma estriol assays and antepartum fetal heart rate testing in diabetic pregnancies. Am J Obstet Gynecol 135:764–72.

Wiener HJ. 1924. Diabetes mellitus in pregnancy. Am J Obstet Gynecol 7:710–18.

Wilcox AJ, Russell IT. 1983. Birthweight and perinatal mortality. II. On weight-specific mortality. Int J Epidemiol 12:319–25.

Wilcox AJ, Weinberg CR, O'Connor JF, et al. 1988. Incidence of early loss of pregnancy. N Engl J Med 319:189–94.

Wilder RM, Parsons E. 1928. Treatment of diabetes during pregnancy. Col Med 25:372–82.

Wilkerson HL. 1959. Pregnancy and the prediabetic state. Ann NY Acad Sci 82:219–28.

Wilkerson HL, O'Sullivan JB. 1963. A study of glucose tolerance and screening criteria in 752 unselected pregnancies. Diabetes 12:313–8.

Wilkerson HL, Remein QR. 1957. Studies of abnormal carbohydrate metabolism in pregnancy: the significance of impaired glucose tolerance. Diabetes 6:324–9.

Willhoite MB, Bennert HW, Palomaki GE, et al. 1993. The impact of preconception counseling on pregnancy outcomes: the experience of the Maine Diabetes in Pregnancy Program. Diab Care 16:450–5.

Williams EC, Wills L. 1929. Studies in blood and urinary chemistry during pregnancy: blood sugar curves. Q J Med 22:493–505.

Williams JJ. 1930. Obstetrics. Appleton, New York.

Williams JW. 1909. The clinical significance of glycosuria in pregnant women. Am J Med Sci 137:1–26.

Williger VM. 1965. Fetal outcome in the diabetic pregnancy. Am J Obstet Gynecol 94:57–60.

Wilson GN, Howe M, Stover JM. 1985 Delayed development sequences in rodent diabetic embryopathy. Pediatr Res 19:1337–40.

Wilson JG. 1960. Factors involved in causing congenital malformations. Bull NY Acad Med 36:145–57.

Wilson JG. 1973. Environment and Birth Defects. Academic Press, New York.

Wilson JS, Vallance-Owen J. 1966. Congenital deformities and insulin antagonism. Lancet 2:940–1.

Wolfe RR, Way GL. 1977. Cardiomyopathies in infants of diabetic mothers. Johns Hopkins Med J 140:177–80.

Wolff E. 1948. La Science des Monstres. Gallimard, Paris.

Woolf B. 1947. Studies on infant mortality. Br J Soc Med 2:73–125.

World Health Organization. 1977. Recommended definitions, terminology and format for statistical tables related to the perinatal period and use of a new certificate for cause of perinatal deaths. Acta Obstet Gynecol Scand 56:247–53.

World Health Organization. 1985. Diabetes mellitus: Report of a WHO Study Group. Tech Rep Ser 727. WHO, Geneva.

World Health Organization Multinational Project for Childhood Diabetes Group. 1991. Familial insulin-dependent diabetes mellitus (IDDM) epidemiology: standardization of data from the DIAMOND Project. Bull WHO 69:767–77.

Worm M. 1955. Menstruation und Fertilität bei Diabetes mellitus. Zentralbl Gynecol 77:886–93.

Worm M. 1960. Behandlung, Geburtsleitung und Ergebnisse bei 300 Entbindungen diabetischer Frauen. In: Prenatal Care. Noordhoff, Groningen, pp. 140–5.

Wrenshall GA, Hetenyi G, Feasby WR. 1962. The Story of Insulin: forty years of success against diabetes. Indiana University, Bloomington.

Wright AD. 1984. Diabetes in pregnancy. In: Natrass M, Santiago JV, eds. Recent Advances in Diabetes. Chuchill Livingstone, Edinburgh, pp. 239–54.

Wright AD, Nicholson HO, Pollock A, et al. 1983. Spontaneous abortion and diabetes mellitus. Postgrad Med J 59:295–8.

Yamashita Y, Kawano Y, Kuriya N, et al. 1996. Intellectual development of offspring of diabetic mothers. Acta Paediatr 85:1192–6.

Yankauer A. 1990. What infant mortality tells us. Am J Public Health 80:653–4.

Yen IH, Khoury MJ, Erickson JD, et al. 1992. The changing epidemiology of neural tube defects: United States, 1968–1989. Am J Dis Child 146:857–61.

Ylinen K, Aula P, Stenmann UH, et al. 1984. Risk of minor and major fetal malformations in diabetics with high haemoglobin A_{1c} values in early pregnancy. Br Med J 289:345–6.

Ylinen K, Hekali R, Teramo K. 1981a. Haemoglobin A_{1c} during pregnancy of insulin-dependent diabetics and healthy controls. J Obstet Gynecol 1:223–8.

Ylinen K, Raivio K, Teramo K. 1981b. Haemoglobin A_{1c} predicts the perinatal outcome in insulin-dependent diabetic pregnancies. Br J Obstet Gynecol 88:961–7.

Yssing M. 1975. Long-term prognosis of children born to mothers diabetic when pregnant. In: Camerini-Dávalos RA, Cole HS, eds. Early Diabetes. Academic Press, New York, pp. 575–86.

Yudkin JS, Alberti KG, McLarty DG, et al. 1990. Impaired glucose tolerance. Br Med J 301:397–401.

Zachau-Christiansen B, Villumsen AL, Sinkbaek SA. 1962. Antihistaminpraeparater og graviditet. Ugeskr Laeger 124:1843–4.

Zanardo V, Pesenti P, Mittiga SM, et al. 1983. Embriofetopatia nei nati di madri con diabete gravidico e di madri con diabete insulino-dependente. Paediatr Med Chir 5:185–8.

Zarowitz H, Moltz A. 1966. Management of diabetes in pregnancy. Obstet Gynecol 27:820–6.

Zilliacus H. 1950. Pregnancy and diabetes mellitus. Acta Endocrinol 4:63–78.

Zusman I, Ornoy A. 1986. The effect of maternal diabetes and high sucrose diets on the intrauterine development of rat fetuses. Diab Res 3:153–9.

INDEX